Clinical Aspects
of
Perinatal Medicine

Clinical Aspects
of
Perinatal Medicine

Volume I

EDITOR

Manohar Rathi, M.D.

Chairman, Department of Pediatrics

Director, Perinatal Medicine

Christ Hospital

Oak Lawn, Illinois;

Associate Professor of Pediatrics

Rush Medical College

Chicago, Illinois

MACMILLAN PUBLISHING COMPANY
New York
Collier Macmillan Canada, Inc.
Toronto
Collier Macmillan Publishers
London

Macmillan Publishing Company
866 Third Avenue, New York, New York 10022

Collier Macmillan Canada, Inc.
Collier Macmillan Publishers • London

Library of Congress Cataloging in Publication Data
Main entry under title:

Clinical aspects of perinatal medicine.

Includes bibliographies and index.
1. Pregnancy, Complications of. 2. Infants (Newborn)
—Diseases. I. Rathi, Manohar.
RG571.C55 1985 618.3′2 83–72519
ISBN 0–02–398660–3 (v. 1)

Printing: 1 2 3 4 5 6 7 8   Year: 5 6 7 8 9 0 1 2 3

Preface

In recent decades, as substantial progress has been made in controlling maternal morbidity and mortality, attention has shifted increasingly to the management of problems affecting the fetus and the newborn infant. The rapid advances occurring today in perinatal patient care make periodic updates, such as this volume provides, a virtual necessity for clinicians who wish to keep current. A distinguished group of specialists in various aspects of perinatal medicine has contributed the chapters that follow. The breadth of their experience and points of view will make this book a valuable reference for all physicians and allied health personnel involved in the care of the high-risk mother and infant.

M.R.

Acknowledgments

I am grateful to the contributors for their cooperation in preparing the manuscripts, to my associates for their help and support, and to the publishers for their continued interest in this work. Above all, I am thankful to my secretaries, Ms. Mary Rago and Ms. MaryAnn Cichowski, for their hard work in making this publication possible.

Manohar Rathi, M.D.

Contributors

Girdhar D. Ahuja, M.D.   Medical Director, Division of Neonatology, St. Francis Hospital Center, Beech Grove, Indiana

Alice F. Andrews, M.D.   Assistant Professor of Pediatrics, University of Michigan Medical School, Ann Arbor, Michigan; Attending Neonatologist, Wayne County General Hospital, Westland, Michigan

Jacob V. Aranda, M.D., Ph.D.   Associate Professor of Pediatrics and of Pharmacology and Therapeutics, Queen Elizabeth II Research Scientist for Diseases in Children; Director, Developmental and Perinatal Pharmacology Unit, The Montreal Children's Hospital and The McGill University Faculty of Medicine, Montreal, Quebec

Robert H. Bartlett, M.D.   Professor of Surgery, University of Michigan Medical School; Head, Section of General Surgery, University of Michigan Hospitals, Ann Arbor, Michigan

Stephen J. Boros, M.D.   Associate Professor of Pediatrics, University of Minnesota Medical School, Minneapolis, Minnesota; Director of Neonatology, Children's Hospital, St. Paul, Minnesota

Nancy J. Brent, R.N., M.S., J.D.   Private Law Practice, Chicago, Illinois; Professor of Nursing, St. Xavier College, Graduate Program, Chicago, Illinois

Cheryl L. Ehrhart, R.N., M.S.   Maternal Child Clinical Specialist, Nursing Education Department, University of Chicago Medical Center, Chicago, Illinois

Judith Gibbs, M.D.   Developmental Pharmacology and Perinatal Research Unit, McGill University-Montreal Children's Hospital, Montreal, Quebec

Glen R. Graves, M.D.   Division of Newborn Medicine, Department of Pediatrics, The University of Mississippi Medical Center, Jackson, Mississippi

Carl Hunt, M.D.   Professor and Vice Chairman, Department of Pediatrics, Northwestern University Medical School; Head, Division of Neonatology, Children's Memorial Hospital, Chicago, Illinois

Charles J. Ingardia, M.D. Director, Maternal-Fetal Medicine and Obstetrics, Hartford Hospital, Hartford, Connecticut; Assistant Professor of Obstetrics and Gynecology, University of Connecticut School of Medicine, Farmington, Connecticut

James H. Jose, M.D. Director, Pediatric Intensive Care Unit, Scottish Rite Children's Hospital, Atlanta, Georgia

Vasundhara Kakodkar, M.D. Attending Neonatologist, Christ Hospital, Oak Lawn, Illinois

Michael D. Klein, M.D. Associate Professor of Surgery, Wayne State University School of Medicine; Associate Chief of General Pediatric Surgery, Children's Hospital of Michigan, Detroit, Michigan

Russell K. Laros, Jr., M.D. Professor of Obstetrics and Gynecology and Vice Chairman, Department of Obstetrics and Gynecology and Reproductive Sciences, University of California School of Medicine, San Francisco, California

Gail A. Liberg, M.P.A., O.T.R.L. Pediatric Occupational Therapist, Christ Hospital, Oak Lawn, Illinois

Edward A. Liechty, M.D. Assistant Professor of Pediatrics, West Virginia University School of Medicine; Attending Neonatologist, West Virginia University Medical Center, Morgantown, West Virginia

Paul R. Meier, M.D. Assistant Professor of Obstetrics and Gynecology, Division of Maternal Fetal Medicine, University of Colorado School of Medicine, Denver, Colorado

Carlos Mendez-Bauer, M.D. Chairman, Perinatal Medicine, Cook County Hospital; Professor of Obstetrics and Gynecology, Chicago Medical School, Chicago, Illinois

John Patrick O'Grady, M.D. Chief, Maternal-Fetal Medicine, and Associate Professor, Department of Reproductive Biology, Case Western Reserve University, University Hospitals of Cleveland, Cleveland, Ohio

Daksha M. Patel, M.D. Medical Director of Newborn Nurseries, Department of Pediatrics, Schumpert Medical Center, Shreveport, Louisiana

Graham E. Quinn, M.D. Associate Surgeon, Division of Pediatric Ophthalmology, Children's Hospital of Philadelphia, Philadelphia, Pennsylvania

Manohar L. Rathi, M.D. Chairman, Department of Pediatrics, and Director, Perinatal Medicine, Christ Hospital, Oak Lawn, Illinois; Associate Professor, Rush Medical College, Chicago, Illinois

Philip G. Rhodes, M.D. Professor of Pediatrics, and Director, Newborn Medicine, University of Mississippi Medical Center, Jackson, Mississippi

Joyce Roberts, C.N.M., Ph.D., F.A.A.N. Professor and Director, Graduate Nurse-Midwifery Program, University of Colorado Health Sciences Center, Denver, Colorado

Ann C. Schoup, M.Div. Chaplain, Neonatal Intensive Care, and Director, Department of Pastoral Care, Christ Hospital, Oak Lawn, Illinois

Richard L. Schreiner, M.D. Professor of Pediatrics, Indiana University School of Medicine; Director of Neonatal Perinatal Medicine, Riley Children's Hospital, Indianapolis, Indiana

Dona J. Snyder, R.N., Ph.D. Associate Professor of Nursing, Maternal-Child Health Division, Marcella Niehoff School of Nursing, Loyola University of Chicago, Chicago, Illinois

Michael J. Tidd, M.D. Medical Director, Research and Development, Norwich Eaton Pharmaceuticals Inc., Norwich, New York

Kent Ueland, M.D. Professor of Gynecology and Obstetrics, and Chief, Section of Maternal-Fetal Medicine, Stanford University Medical Center, Stanford, California

Contents

1 Control of Uterine Activity: A Clinical Approach   *1*
John Patrick O'Grady, M.D.

2 Initiation of Parturition with Drugs   *28*
Kent Ueland, M.D.

3 Management of Preterm Labor   *36*
Charles J. Ingardia, M.D.

4 Which Position in Labor?   *48*
Joyce Roberts, R.N., C.N.M., Ph.D., and Carlos Mendez-Bauer, M.D.

5 Cesarean Section: Enough is Enough   *67*
Paul R. Meier, M.D.

6 Autoimmune Thrombocytopenia and Pregnancy   *74*
Russell K. Laros, Jr., M.D.

7 Thromboembolic Disease in Obstetrics and Gynecology   *83*
Russell K. Laros, Jr., M.D.

8 Pregnancy-Induced Hypertension: New Perspectives on
an Old Disorder   *90*
John Patrick O'Grady, M.D.

9 Management of Dangerous Cardiovascular Lesions During
Pregnancy   *110*
Kent Ueland, M.D.

10 Management of Perinatal Infections   *131*
Charles J. Ingardia, M.D.

11 Psychosocial Effects of Long-Term Antepartal
Hospitalization   *149*
Dona J. Snyder, R.N., Ph.D.

12 Spiritual and Emotional Issues When Pregnancy Fails   *164*
Ann C. Schoup, M. Div.

13 Selected Legal Aspects of Perinatal Care   *171*
Nancy J. Brent, R.N., M.S., J.D.

14 Neonatology Practice: A New Challenge   *182*
    Girdhar L. Ahuja, M.D.

15 Arterial Oxygen Monitoring: Using the Searle Umbilical
    Artery Catheter-Tip Electrode in Neonates   *193*
    Manohar L. Rathi, M.D., Vasundhara Kakodkar, M.D., and Michael J.
    Tidd, M.D.

16 New Concepts in the Treatment of Acute Respiratory
    Failure   *209*
    Carl Hunt, M.D.

17 Respiratory Distress in the Infant of the Diabetic Mother   *215*
    Philip G. Rhodes, M.D., and Daksha M. Patel, M.D.

18 Neonatal High-Frequency Ventilation: A Review   *221*
    Stephen J. Boros, M.D.

19 Extracorporeal Membrane Oxygenation for Newborn
    Respiratory Failure   *232*
    Michael D. Klein, M.D., Alice French Andrews, M.D., and Robert H.
    Bartlett, M.D.

20 Perinatal Aspiration Syndromes   *249*
    James H. Jose, M.D., and Richard L. Schreiner, M.D.

21 Bronchopulmonary Dysplasia   *264*
    Philip G. Rhodes, M.D., Glen R. Graves, M.D., and Daksha M. Patel,
    M.D.

22 Congenital Abdominal Wall Defects   *269*
    Michael D. Klein, M.D.

23 Neonatal Polycythemia/Hyperviscosity   *283*
    Edward A. Liechty, M.D., and Richard L. Schreiner, M.D.

24 Retinopathy of Prematurity   *302*
    Graham E. Quinn, M.D.

25 Congenital Eye Infections   *314*
    Graham E. Quinn, M.D.

26 Stimulation Programs in the Neonatal Intensive Care
    Nursery   *334*
    Gail A. Liberg, M.P.A., D.T.R., Cheryl L. Ehrhart, R.N., M.S., and
    Manohar L. Rathi, M.D.

27 Drugs and Breast Feeding   *355*
    Jacob V. Aranda, M.D., Ph.D., and Judith Gibbs, M.D.

    Index   *369*

1

Control of Uterine Activity: A Clinical Aproach

John Patrick O'Grady, M.D.

Shall we say that nature blind check'd her hand and chang'd her
mind, just when she had exactly wrought a finished pattern without
fault.
Charles Lamb

Introduction and Overview

Premature birth is a principal cause of perinatal morbidity and mortality. In the United States, premature labor occurs in 5 to 8 percent of all pregnancies, but accounts for 80 percent of perinatal mortality [1]. Epidemiologic studies indicate that premature labor is more frequent under certain conditions and is related to distinct obstetrical complications [2]. For example, the Obstetrical Statistical Cooperative study collected data between 1970 and 1976 on 240,474 deliveries. This study identified a group of high risk factors associated with a threefold or greater increase in premature delivery (Table 1–1).

In addition, poor nutrition, limited access to prenatal care, poor hygiene, which influences the bacterial and viral flora of the reproductive tract, and a higher incidence of pregnancies in younger and older age groups predispose to early delivery [3,4]. Other factors felt to be important in the early onset of labor include smoking during pregnancy, substance abuse, residence at high altitude, and cyanotic heart disease.

The development of effective agents to stop or delay labor has been enthusiastically heralded by clinicians as an opportunity to reduce perinatal mortality and morbidity. However, perinatal statistics can be markedly improved without resort to tocolytic agents [5]. Further, the drugs in most common use, the beta-sympathomimetics, carry clear and important ma-

1

Table 1–1

Premature Delivery Associated with High Risk Factors

Placental abnormalities, abruption placentae, placenta previa
Eclampsia, preeclampsia
Multiple gestation
Nephritis
Hyperemesis, liver disease
Anemia (Hgb < 8 g)
Mullerian anomaly
Prior history of premature delivery (two or more)

Obstetrical Statistical Cooperative Data, modified from Johnson, J.W.C., Dubin, N.H. Prevention of preterm labor. *Clin. Obstet. Gynecol.* 23:51–73, 1980.

ternal risks [6]. Finally, many patients are not found to be candidates for tocolysis with any agent at the time of admission to a hospital [7]. These facts emphasize that prevention of preterm labor is an important obstetric issue that requires both further study and application of population screening protocols to determine how prematurity can best be prevented. However, the clinician must still evaluate and treat patients with uterine activity who are remote from term. In this chapter I discuss the clinical diagnosis, evaluation, and management of premature labor and critically evaluate the benefits and hazards of treatment with currently available tocolytic agents.

Onset of Parturition

Despite significant advances in our understanding of labor physiology, we are as yet unable to clearly define the mechanisms that trigger labor [8,9]. Uterine motility in pregnant women is known to be influenced by many factors, including myometrial stretch, the ratio of estrogens to progesterone [10], changes in uterine blood flow [11], prostaglandin synthesis [12,13], and oxytocin release [14]. Although there is evidence that endocrine changes initiated by the fetus may be responsible for triggering the onset of labor at an appropriate time near term [9,15], it is also clear that a variety of nonspecific stimuli (e.g., uterine bleeding, chorioamnionitis, premature rupture of the membranes) may intervene at an earlier and inappropriate time to initiate uterine activity.

The synchronization of the irregular but recurrent uterine activity of late pregnancy into the rhythmic and coordinate action of labor depends upon the production of gap junctions between myometrial cells [16]. *In vitro,* increasing the estrogen/progesterone ratio favors the formation of gap junctions. Prostaglandins stimulate and indomethacin inhibits this

Figure 1–1

Current concept of actin-myosin interaction, mediated by the availability of myosin light-chain kinase. *(From Huszar, G. Current concepts of myometrial control in tocolytic agents. In Merrill–National Laboratories (ed.), Tocolytic Agents. New York: Biomedical Information Corp., 1980, pp. 1–14.)*

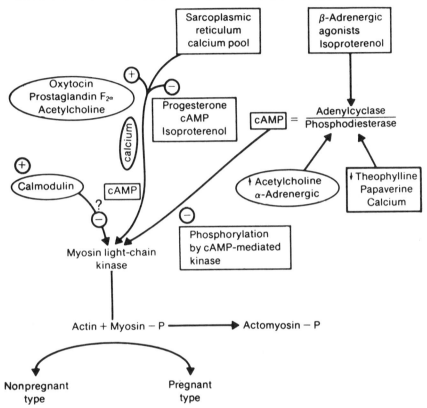

process. Thus, formation of myometrial gap junctions, and the accompanying increase in coordinate uterine activity, is controlled by pregnancy sex steroids through a prostaglandin-dependent mechanism [16]. This formation neatly ties together biophysical ultrastructural events (gap junction formation) with the endocrine changes of advanced gestation (change in estrogen/progesterone ratio) as coordinate labor ensues.

Biochemically, smooth muscle contraction results from actin-myosin interaction, which is dependent upon calcium ion availability [16,17]. Actin-myosin interaction is controlled by reversible enzymatic phosphorylation of a muscle protein, myosin light chain (MLC). The enzyme responsible for this phosphorylation is MLC kinase. Activity of MLC kinase is calcium dependent. Actin-myosin interaction is inhibited by another enzyme, MLC phosphatase, which dephosphorylates the myosin molecule,

3

thus preventing contraction. Finally, calcium ion and calmodulin, a calcium-dependent regulatory protein, must be present for MLC kinase activity. MLC kinase activation is further complexed by cyclic adenosine monophosphate–dependent protein kinase inhibition. The various pharmacologic agents and hormones known to alter uterine excitability act ultimately to alter the availability of either MLC kinase or calcium, the major cofactor. These complex events are best understood in graphic presentation (Fig. 1–1).

Patient Identification and Prophylaxis

The management of patients with premature labor begins with prevention [3]. Avoidance of early-onset labor is more important than any drug therapy in reducing the overall incidence of prematurity [2,5,18–20]. As Boylan and O'Driscoll [5] point out, improvements in perinatal loss related to preterm labor can be strongly influenced by demographic and socioeconomic changes in the sample population. Creasy and coworkers [3,19,21] have shown how a program for early detection of patients at risk for preterm labor, involving patient and professional education and more judicious use of tocolytic agents, can lead to fewer preterm deliveries. Such approaches deserve additional clinical study and more extensive application.

Prospective management consists of early prenatal care, improved nutrition, prophylaxis of urinary tract and reproductive tract infections, identification of women with a past history of premature labor, and careful attention to the progression of the current pregnancy.

Patients who have experienced an episode of painless dilatation of the cervix in the second trimester may have an incompetent cervical os. In some cases, ultrasonic examination during pregnancy may reveal early dilatation of the lower uterine segment. Serial cervical examinations in suspected cases may reveal early cervical effacement or dilatation, or both. In the interval between pregnancies, diagnosis can be made by pelvic examination, calibration of the cervical canal with Hegar dilators, or hysterosalpingography. A hysterosalpingogram in the late puerperium to detect a possible uterine anomaly is indicated in every patient who has delivered prematurely. In properly selected patients, these conditions are amenable to surgical correction by cervical cerclage or metroplasty.

Clinical Diagnosis and Patient Selection

Clinical selection of patients for pharmacologic inhibition of premature labor is fraught with uncertainties. Labor is characterized by regular uterine contractions at intervals of less than 10 minutes accompanied by progressive cervical dilatation or effacement. Once labor has advanced with cervical dilatation greater than 4 cm, especially in the face of membrane rupture, it is difficult to inhibit. Therefore, it is imperative to identify early signs of impending labor. Yet many patients admitted with the presumptive diagnosis of premature labor have uterine irritability only and respond to bed rest with or without sedation [22]. The problem of uterine activity without cervical change is common and confuses the interpretation of many clinical studies of the efficacy of various agents in labor. prevention.

This clinical setting is not uncommon and many "easy-stops" were so because the patient was never in true labor. Appropriate management is complicated in patients remote from term who have regular uterine activity. Even without cervical change, if the contractions are perceived as uncomfortable by the patient, the clinician all too often has difficulty in avoiding the use of tocolytics. To wait for definitive dilatation and effacement is the correct, scientific approach, given the high percentage of "placebo responders," but it risks cervical progression and may compromise membrane integrity. To treat without necessity results in inappropriate anxiety, expense, and inflated statistical "success."

At the time of hospital admission, patients with premature uterine activity require careful evaluation in the attempt to identify treatable factors. Physical examination, with maternal vital signs, urinalysis, pelvic examination with cervical culture, and a complete blood cell count should be performed. Continuous external Doppler electronic fetal monitoring or careful abdominal palpation and fetal heart tone auscultation should be initiated by a trained observer (Table 1–2).

If uterine activity is persistent or is unresponsive to oral or intravenous hydration, or if cervical change is documented, and the use of tocolytic agents is contemplated, a more extensive evaluation is necessary. Blood should be drawn for measuring baseline levels of electrolytes, hematocrit-hemoglobin, white cell and differential counts, and serum glucose. Real-time ultrasound is used to document fetal and placental position and provide measurements for dating estimation. Finally, amniocentesis should

Table 1–2
Premature Labor: Patient Evaluation

Initial	Secondary
History	Complete blood cell count, electrolytes
Physical examination (including cervical assessment)	Blood glucose
	Real time ultrasound exam
Urinalysis	Amniocentesis
External electronic	Amniotic fluid maturity profile
Fetal monitoring	
Observation	

5

Table 1–3
Clinical Factors in Treatment
of Premature Labor

Vaginal bleeding
Integrity of the membranes
Fetal gestational age
Placental locale
Fetal position
Fetal well-being
Cervical dilatation

be considered. Immediate clinical considerations in a patient with premature uterine activity are outlined in Table 1–3.

As shown in Table 1–4, some factors contraindicate tocolytic treatment, modified by the features of each individual case. Obviously, in the face of a hemodynamically unstable patient either from blood loss or from septicemia, the use of powerful pharmacologic agents, such as beta-sympathomimetics, that promote tachycardia or hypotension are to be avoided [6]. Similarly, aggressive use of parenteral tocolytic drugs in patients beyond 34 weeks of gestation is rarely indicated, as the risks of such treatment generally outweigh the potential benefits.

Uterine activity in the face of vaginal bleeding accompanied by mild to moderate uterine irritability, but with normal coagulation studies, constitutes a difficult clinical dilemma. The presumptive diagnosis in the majority of cases is marginal sinus rupture or mild abruptio placentae. In some instances on more careful evaluation, a low-lying placenta or a placenta previa is identified. Unusually, the patient may progress to clinical abruptio. It is unclear how best to proceed in these instances. In general, tocolysis is contraindicated in the face of uterine bleeding or abruptio. However, all clinicians have managed similar cases where tocolytic agents

Table 1–4
Contraindications to Tocolysis

Absolute	Relative
Known myocardial dysfunction	Diabetes mellitus
Cardiac rhythm disturbance	Twin (multiple) gestation
Amnionitis or septicemia	Hemorrhage
Nonviable fetus	Low-lying placentation
Abruptio placentae	Membrane rupture
Eclampsia	Advanced labor
Hyperthyroidism	Hypertension
Fetal anomaly	

were used with apparent safety and possibly beneficial effect. Our experience has been that in the majority of instances of mild bleeding and uterine irritability, uterine activity abates spontaneously. Thus, tocolytic treatment constitutes any unnecessary risk and may simply mask the progression of a more serious clinical condition. However, the prohibition against treatment is not absolute; the decision to use tocolytics hinges on the unique circumstances of each case. Before administering a tocolytic, however, the clinician must be certain that coagulopathy is absent, blood loss is not hemodynamically significant, and the fetus is in stable condition.

Before an agent is administered, a period of observation is appropriate. Twenty to 50 percent of cases with premature uterine activity respond to bed rest or infusion of intravenous fluid [1,13,22]. Such responses may be due to beneficial effects of recumbency in cervical tension or to changes in uterine blood flow. Whether patients responding to hydration and positioning would have ceased their uterine activity spontanously regardless of positioning is problematic.

Valenzuela et al. [22] studied the use of bed rest, intravenous hydration (500 ml of 5% dextrose–0.45% NaCl), and parenteral morphine sulfate (8 mg intramuscularly) in 184 consecutive singleton pregnancies in women admitted for suspected premature labor. Fifty-five percent of patients so treated with intact membranes, cervical dilatation of less than 4 cm, and no chorioamnionitis stopped contracting. However, when the patients who were responsive to hydration or sedation were followed to term, they proved to have a 2.6 times increased likelihood of preterm delivery or tocolytic drug use, or both, than the general hospital obstetric population. This experience suggests that preterm uterine activity that is marked enough to cause patients to seek hospital evaluation is not as benign as is commonly supposed. In this study, the parenteral morphine used in conjunction with simple hydration likely contributed little to the observed effect, since similar results occur without the use of narcotic sedation.

Bed rest and fluid infusion may not be a placebo. Bed rest has been studied carefully for its effect in twin gestation [23–26]. Not all studies agree on the benefits of resting; however, substantial evidence indicates that fetal outcome is better in rested gravidas as a result of increased birth weight [23,24] and prolonged gestation [26].

Resting in left lateral recumbency increases uterine blood flow, promotes fetal growth, prolongs gestation, and, when accompanied by hydration, inhibits uterine activity in a substantial percentage of patients. However, the work of Valenzuela et al. [22] indicates that patients whose "false labor" responds to such measures need continued close clinical observation once discharged, and that these patients should not be assumed to be normal. In sum, resting and hydration deserve a trial in suspected premature labor if clinical circumstances are not pressing.

7

Clinical Use of Tocolytic Agents

Ritodrine (Yutopar) is the only pharmacologic agent approved for use as a tocolytic in the United States [6,7]. A number of additional agents (terbutaline, magnesium sulfate, isoxsuprine, indomethacin) remain in clinical use as drugs approved by the Food and Drug Administration but without specific approval for the indication of tocolysis. Other agents, including hexoprenaline, are undergoing clinical trials.

Ritodrine is neither tolerated nor appropriate in all clinical instances. For example, patients intolerant to the side effects of ritodrine may tolerate an effective dose of terbutaline. In insulin-requiring diabetics or in hypertensive patients, beta-sympathomimetics are relatively contraindicated, and other agents such as magnesium sulfate are more appropriate.

The use of an approved drug for an unapproved indication is the clinical practice of medicine. It is prudent to discuss with the patient and document in the record the reasons for the use of any potent agent, especially under these circumstances. The choice of a tocolytic agent should be governed by considerations of greatest efficacy and the lowest possible fetal and maternal risk, with clear goals in mind. Considerations of nursing assistance, staff familiarity with particular agents, the patient's medical condition, and the availability of pediatric and anesthetic assistance are all germane to this choice. Experience at the Oregon Health Sciences University has led us to develop familiarity with several drugs (magnesium sulfate, terbutaline, ritodrine). The clinical circumstances and peculiarities of each case are used to decide when therapy is necessary and which agent is best. In our experience, complete reliance on a single tocolytic agent is both inappropriate and unrealistic.

Progestational Agents

The importance of progesterone and the ratio of progesterone to estrogen in human parturition is unsettled [8,10,13,15]. Progesterone appears to block the ability of the myometrium to conduct the action potentials required for rhythmic uterine contractions [9]. This is likely modulated through intracellular gap junctions [16]. In a number of species, but not humans, demonstrable decline of progesterone occurs immediately before the onset of labor [27–29]. Csapo has been the greatest proponent for an effect of progesterone on uterine activity. He proposes a scheme for the onset of labor involving progesterone withdrawal, thereby releasing the uterus from inhibition. The increased uterine excitation resulting from the decline in progesterone is promoted by the now uninhibited effects of prostaglandins, estradiol, and oxytocin leading toward the coordinate uterine activity of labor [28].

8

The exact mechanism of the myometrial "progesterone" block and its importance in the onset of labor in primates requires additional study. In clinical use, progestational agents have had a limited role in inhibition of premature labor, except as prophylactic agents. There is evidence that 17-hydroxyprogesterone caproate (Delalutin) inhibits premature labor in patients with a prior history of premature labor or spontaneous abortion [30,31]. Additionally, selected progestational agents may be effective for treating active, premature labor [1,32]. In a small $(N = 24)$, nonrandomized series, Kauppila et al. [32] utilized intravenous cortisol with simultaneous intramuscular 17-hydroxyprogesterone caproate in patients with premature labor occurring at 27 to 36 weeks; they found that this therapy was as effective as intravenous ritodrine. Such preliminary work is interesting but needs confirmation by well-designed prospective, randomized studies.

The clinical role for progestational agents in premature labor is unclear [33]. The prophylactic therapy suggested by Johnson et al. [30,31] has not achieved popularity, due largely to concerns of the use of progestational agents in early pregnancy. However, progestational treatment deserves consideration after the first trimester in patients with histories of premature delivery, documented fetal viability and normality, and the absence of Müllerian abnormalities. Whether combinations of parenteral progestational agents will prove useful to control active labor remains unestablished.

Ethyl Alcohol

Ethanol is one of the oldest and most familiar agents to obstetricians. Pharmacologically, ethyl alcohol inhibits the myometrium directly. Alcohol also interferes with the release of oxytocin and antidiuretic hormone [13]. The efficacy of ethanol has been both supported [34] and challenged [13]. In sum, there appears reasonable evidence of its ability to arrest premature labor [15,34]. As a tocolytic, ethanol (9.5%) is administered intravenously in a loading dose of 7.5 ml/kg of body weight over 2 hours. This is followed with 1.5 mg/kg per hour as a maintenance dose for an additional 6 to 10 hours. Thereafter, ethanol is administered orally or other agents are given [13,34]. Patients often experience nausea and restlessness during treatment, and it is advantageous to administer an antiemetic at the outset. The level of patient intoxication varies. Constant and close supervision is mandatory. Vomiting, aspiration, dehydration, lactic acidosis, and hypoglycemia (in diabetic patients) are potential complications [3].

Adverse fetal effects have been observed with ethanol but are uncommon. Ethyl alcohol crosses the placenta, exposing the fetus to levels approaching or equal to maternal concentration, and fetal depression is possible; especially in premature infants [35]. Acute ethyl alcohol exposure may also adversely affect fetal umbilical circulation, predisposing to hypoxia and acidosis [36].

Although there is evidence of the efficacy of ethanol in premature labor, there is little current indication for its clinical use [13,33]. The maternal side effects of intoxication and somnolence can be at best unpleasant and occasionally dangerous. Patient compliance and comprehension are adversely affected at times when they are most critical. Finally, more effective agents are available [37–39]. However, studies combining alcohol with other agents suggest that combined therapies have promise in selected cases. Ethanol will continue in the obstetric armamentarium, but only as a second-line tocolytic agent.

Magnesium Sulfate

Magnesium sulfate ($MgSO_4$) is a drug long in use in obstetrics in the United States for preeclampsia. Magnesium sulfate is not an antihypertensive agent, and it is administered principally to preeclamptic patients as an anticonvulsant. Interest in magnesium as a potential tocolytic grew from observations that tetanic uterine contractions would respond to rapid magnesium infusions, and that patients treated with magnesium for preeclampsia often required augmentation with pitocin to achieve delivery [40]. Magnesium has its effect on the myometrium through blocking calcium availability to MLC kinase [41]. Of interest, maternal serum levels of magnesium have been reported to be low-normal in patients with preterm labor [42]. The implications of this observation on the mechanism of uterine activity remain at best unclear.

For use as a tocolytic agent, magnesium is given intravenously in a fashion similar to its use for preeclampsia. After a 4- to 6-g intravenous loading dose administered over 15 to 20 minutes, a maintenance infusion of 2 g/h is initiated [38]. Hourly checks of urinary output and maternal deep tender reflexes are mandatory, since magnesium is renally excreted [41]. Thereafter, levels of 4.5 to 6.5 mg/dl are maintained by adjustment of the infusion rate.

None of the reviews of $MgSO_4$ use in the United States mention use of an oral form once a course of parenteral treatment has been completed. In the majority of instances once labor control has been achieved for 12 to 24 hours, either oral beta-mimetics have been instituted or all therapy has been discontinued [42]. There is a report of the use of oral therapy for continued tocolysis with maintenance of a therapeutic magnesium level [33]. However, because magnesium salts are poorly and incompletely absorbed from the gastrointestinal tract (leading to their principal oral use as cathartic agents), it is unlikely that oral magnesium therapy will prove to be either successful or well tolerated [43] (Table 1–5).

Table 1-5
Magnesium Sulfate Tocolysis[a]

Administer loading dose of 4–6 g of $MgSO_4$ over a 15 to 20-minute period

Maintain 2 to 3 g/hour by infusion pump

Titrate to maintain a Mg^{++} concentration of 4.5 to 6.5 mg/dl or to uterine response (or both)

Checks hourly vital signs, deep tendon reflexes, and urinary output

Attempt to taper and terminate infusion after 12 to 24 hours

Thereafter, convert to oral beta-mimetic agent if appropriate, or else no therapy

SOURCES: Steer, C.M., Petrie, R.H. A comparison of magnesium sulfate and alcohol for the prevention of premature labor. *Am. J. Obstet. Gynecol.* 128:1–4, 1977. Elliot, J.P. Magnesium sulfate as a tocolytic agent. *Am. J. Obstet. Gynecol.* 147:277–284, 1983.

Maternal complications from treatment are rare, but potentially serious and are due principally to failure of adequate magnesium excretion in patients with reduced renal function. In Elliott's review [42], the incidence of side effects was 7 percent, but in only 2 percent of 355 patients did side effects necessitate discontinuation of the drug. Pulmonary edema has been reported with the use of magnesium as a tocolytic, but the incidence is low (1 percent) [42,44].

Magnesium sulfate does not have large, prospective, controlled studies supporting its efficacy as a tocolytic agent. Clinical studies by Elliott et al. [42], Steer and Petrie [38], and Spisso et al. [45] provide data indicating that, as a tocolytic, magnesium is successful in delaying delivery by 24 or more hours in 60 to 85 percent of treated patients. The randomized study of Miller et al. [46] compared $MgSO_4$ with terbutaline in a total of 29 patients. No difference was noted in the ability of either agent to delay delivery, although untoward side effects were more common in the terbutaline-treated patients.

As a tocolytic agent, magnesium has definite advantages. Nurses and physicians are well accustomed to its administration and complications. Also, magnesium is especially useful in diabetic or hypertensive patients for whom other agents are contraindicated. Finally, there is reasonable evidence of efficacy for $MgSO_4$, and maternal side effects severe enough to curtail therapy are uncommon.

However, magnesium sulfate also has distinct disadvantages. There is no acceptable oral form. In addition, magnesium crosses the placenta and may affect the fetus. Although the clinical importance of transplacental transfer is debated, in some cases it clearly is a factor in neonatal depression [41]. Overdosage can lead to maternal apnea or paralysis or, rarely to pulmonary edema.

In sum, magnesium sulfate is the clear agent of choice in limited circumstances and is reasonably effective and safe [41,42,46]. Magnesium may be the safest tocolytic agent available, considering wide clinical experience with the drug and the limited potential for maternal and fetal complications.

Beta-Sympathomimetics

Ahlquist [47] and Lands et al. [48] have identified and characterized alpha and beta receptors in the action of sympathomimetic amines on smooth muscle. Beta$_1$ receptors occur principally in heart, bowel, and adipose tissue, whereas beta$_2$ receptors are located in the uterus, vascular smooth muscle, and bronchioles. An ideal beta-sympathomimetic drug would avoid beta$_1$ stimulation while acting selectively on beta$_2$ receptors. Such specificity is not possible with current agents, and all available drugs lose specificity when administered in progressively higher doses [13,49].

Beta-sympathomimetics reduce the availability of intracellular calcium ions and inhibit the phosphorylation of myosin light chains. By failure to activate the enzyme MLC kinase, MLC phosphorylation is blocked, the interaction of actin-myosin is inhibited, and uterine smooth muscle thus relaxes [7,16,50,51] (see Figure 1–1).

Administration of beta-mimetic compounds produces major metabolic effects that can result in serious derangements of blood chemistry [6,7,52,53–55]. Beta-sympathomimetics stimulate cyclic adenosine monophosphate-mediated pathways leading to gluconeogenesis. Insulin concentration rises by direct action on beta-adrenegic receptors in the pancreas. The net result is a prompt rise in serum glucose ketonemia, lipemia, and hyperlacticacidemia. Hyperglycemia in normal patients and the rapid development of ketoacidosis in insulin-requiring diabetics has been observed with administration of beta-sympathomimetics [6,55,56].

When beta-sympathomimetics are administered intravenously, serum potassium rapidly falls because of shifts from the extracellular to the intracellular space. This is partially due to cell membrane hyperpolarization with intracellular sodium and hydrogen ions exchanged for extracellular potassium [55]. Total body potassium does not decline during beta-sympathomimetic treatment. Potassium simply shifts into another compartment. Serum potassium levels return to normal after several hours without specific therapy. However, we have encountered clinical difficulties with anesthesiologists unwilling to provide general anesthetics to patients who are tocolysis failures, but have depressed serum potassium concentrations. Concern is also raised about hypokalemia in the occasional patient with symptomatic arrhythmia evoked or unmasked by beta-mimetics. We have favored administration of D5W in lactated Ringers (Hartmann's solution), including 20 meq of potassium as our basic infusion solution, when beta-sympathomimetics are administered. In our experience, this maintains near-normal serum potassium. We have not encountered complications with this treatment and continue to favor its use, although others argue that such therapy is unnecessary [55].

The measured hemoglobin and hematocrit decline during beta-sympathomimetic administration. This is due partially to hydration and partially to intravascular recruitment of extravascular fluid and inhibition of renal sodium excretion [6]. This can be a trap for the unwary, as patients may evidence low hemoglobin levels. Transfusion should be avoided, as it is often unnecessary, contributes to vascular overload, and carries the usual risks of reaction, antibody formation, and hepatitis.

Beta-sympathomimetics have been associated with serious complications including cardiac arrhythmias [6], acidosis [57], cerebral vasospasm (in patients with a migraine history) [6], hypotension (especially in the face of maternal hemorrhage), angina [58], and maternal death [6,59,60]. However, among the maternal complications of beta-mimetics, the one that has received the most attention, yet remains illusive in etiology, is pulmonary edema [6,49,60–72]. This potentially serious problem has been reported for all of the major beta-sympathomimetics, including isoxsuprine [69], fenoterol [69], ritodrine [60,62,66,63,70], and terbutaline [64,65,67,68,73]. The cause of this complication, involving some 5% of treated patients, is not established, but some clinical correlations are clear [64]. Pulmonary edema is unusual with periods of beta-sympathomimetic administration less than 12 hours [69]. Patients with pulmonary edema are frequently found to be substantially overhydrated, have prolonged tachycardia secondary to drug effects, and may have complications of amnionitis [6,64,72].

The reported association between pulmonary edema and corticosteroid administration is likely serendipitous. Most patients who develop pulmonary edema were aggressively treated for the purpose of preventing delivery to achieve a corticosteroid effect. Clinicians may thus preselect patients for heroic tocolysis with a particular goal in mind. In this setting, practitioners are more willing to continue tocolysis in the face of increasing maternal symptoms.

Large doses of another beta-mimetic agent, epinephrine, are known to produce pulmonary edema in both human and animal models [69]. Although in dogs this effect may be due to ventricular failure [74], evidence for this mechanism in humans is lacking [6]. The findings of normal pulmonary artery wedge pressure with increased cardiac output [68] by intracardiac catheterization and echocardiographic evidence of enhanced ventricular performance in patients with both ritodrine [49] and terbutaline [61] indicates that pulmonary edema does develop without frank ventricular dysfunction.

The recent studies of Hauth et al. [71,72] in pregnant baboons with parenteral ritodrine infusion deserve careful review. Six control and six treatment animals at various gestational ages were restrained, anesthetized, multiply catheterized, and then studied during fluid or ritodrine (or both) infusion over 23 hours. Neither pulmonary edema nor increases in extravascular lung water were observed despite prolonged ritodrine administration and heroic fluid challenge. Hyperdynamic cardiac function and progressive fluid retention were observed similar to that previously noted in humans. The authors observed that the pulmonary capillary wedge pressure increase was maximal during this same time interval as the nadir of the colloid oncotic pressure.

The authors suggested that if this process continued, increasing volumes of fluid would transudate into the maternal lung and eventually overcome the compensatory mechanisms (largely lymphatic) for fluid removal, thus eventually leading to pulmonary edema. They also postulated that the acute myocardia ischemia suggested by the symptoms of some patients with beta-mimetic pulmonary edema might precipitate acute cardiac dysfunction and pulmonary congestion in some cases.

The onset and rapid recovery of patients with beta-mimetic-related pulmonary edema is not consistent with membrane injury as seen in the adult respiratory distress syndrome. The arguments of Hankins and Hauth would be more compelling if they had managed to produce pulmonary edema or even increases in lung water in their experimental animals, which they did not. A rising pulmonary capillary wedge pressure in the presence of a myocardial hyperdynamic state in the face of rapid fluid infusion or vascular expansion may not indicate ventricular failure or myocardial fatigue as these authors suggest. This latter point needs emphasis as treatment for beta-mimetic pulmonary edema should not be directed at enhancing myocardial contractility, but instead at reducing heart rate and cardiac output demands by judicious use of diuretics and termination of beta-mimetic drug therapy. Unfortunately, in this study an anesthetized animal preparation was used, and no evidence of frank ventricular failure was observed as evidenced by the progressive increases in cardiac index and the absence of pulmonary edema. The wedge pressure observations are interesting, but the manner of measurement, number of observations, and standard deviations are not reported, making interpretation difficult. The hypothesis that they forward is interesting, but only incompletely substantiated by the data reported.

The principal treatment for pulmonary edema is avoidance. Pulmonary edema occurs most often in a subclass of patients with prolonged (>12 hours) drug administration accompanied by moderate to generous fluid infusion with a corresponding decline in central hematocrit and, not infrequently, with drug-induced hypokalemia. Therefore, parenteral beta-mimetic administration beyond 12 hours must be closely monitored with careful attention to patient symptomatology. Persisting symptomatic tachycardia, restlessness, complaints of dyspnea, and clinical findings of bronchial breath sounds and end inspiratory crepitations are all signs that the patient is being pressed too vigorously, and the infusion should be stopped or tapered.

If pulmonary edema occurs, the correct treatment is symptomatic. The infusion is stopped. The parturient should be set upright, and oxygen should be administered. Small doses of furosemide (10 to 20 mg) may be given, but are often not required. Digitalis, corticosteroids, dopamine, and a number of other potentially dangerous agents have been administered to these patients [69]. Such polypharmacy is unnecessary and maybe dangerous.

We have made a practice of restricting intravenous fluids to 2 L per 24 hours and have been reluctant to treat patients parenterally with beta–mimetics for more than 12 hours. These changes and increased attention to patient symptomology have meant a virtual disappearance of pulmonary edema as a complication of beta-mimetic-related pulmonary edema. On our service, one case has occurred in the last two years, and that patient was transferred after heroic tocolysis in another institution.

The serious cardiovascular problems encountered with beta-mimetics are due to their use in patients with unrecognized cardiovascular disease or because of heroic attempts to control premature uterine activity. Both terbutaline [61] and ritodrine [49] lose beta selectivity at higher dose ranges and exhibit potent ionotropic and chronotropic effects. As both rate and contractility are important determinants of myocardial oxygen demand, beta-mimetics should be used sparingly, if at all, in patients with structural or ischemic heart disease.

Serious problems with hyperglycemia can also complicate beta-mimetic therapy [6,61]. These drugs should be used with great care, if at all, in insulin-requiring diabetics. Care should also be exercised in apparently normal patients, as vigorous beta-mimetic treatment may evoke rapid onset hyperglycemia in women with no prior evidence for glucose intolerance. Coadministration of corticosteroids can exacerbate this effect. All patients receiving these drugs need a baseline blood glucose before initiating the infusion and one or more repeat determinations after several hours of therapy.

Although there is strong clinical belief in the efficacy of tocolytic agents to control premature uterine activity, the older supporting literature is mixed. Newer evidence for the efficacy of beta-mimetics is more reassuring [75–79]. Ingemarrson [79] states that data from Sweden on preterm delivery indicate that beta-mimetics are responsible for a significant decrease in preterm deliveries occurring before week 32. Further, there is now good evidence for fetal safety of beta-mimetics [7,80,81]. The long-term effects of beta-sympathomimetics have been reviewed by Karlsson [80], who observed no significant adverse long-term effects in infants. Necropsies of infants who were treated with beta-mimetics who subsequently succumbed to various causes, principally complications of extreme prematurity, were reviewed. Myocardial necrosis, a lesion produced in animal on models by isoproterenol, a related sympathomimetic, was absent. No specific structural abnormalities could be attributed to the drug therapy.

The first beta-mimetic agent in general use was isoxsuprine [13,15]. Standard isoxsuprine treatment commences with an intravenous infusion of 0.25 mg/minute increasing to 0.75 to 1.0 mg/minute sequentially according to maternal tolerance and uterine effect [15,29,82]. After control of uterine activity the infusion rate is tapered. Thereafter, 10 to 15 mg is given intramuscularly for 6 to 10 additional doses. Oral doses of 10 to 20 mg every 6 hours follow. The oral dose is titrated to a mild maternal tachycardia, overall tolerance, and control of perceived uterine contractions.

Although found to be an effective agent, isoxsuprine commonly results in maternal hypotension and tachycardia, which seriously limit its usefulness [29,82,83]. In contrast to newer beta-mimetics, isoxsuprine has been associated with potentially serious neonatal complications apparently closely related to hypotension. Depression is most marked in infants of less than 33 weeks of gestation delivered when a high drug concentration is present [83]. Thus, premature infants delivered due to drug failure with a drug-free interval of 2 hours or less are at high risk for hypoglycemia, hypocalcemia, ileus, and hypotension. The difficulties inherent in assuring a drug-free interval before delivery and the greater efficacy of newer agents severely limits the desirability of isoxsuprine as a tocolytic agent.

The beta-mimetics in most common use are ritodrine [84] and terbutaline [85,86]. Other agents, including fenoterol, hexoprenaline, and salbutamol, have been studied for tocolytic effect [33]. Hexoprenaline may prove to have less cardiovascular effect than the other agents and thus may be more desirable for obstetrical emergencies [7]. However, a healthy skepticism is appropriate, as similar claims were initially made for each currently available agent.

The efficacy of ritodrine in inhibiting premature labor is supported by controlled, double-blind studies conducted in both Europe [77] and the United States [76]. In the American study, involving 313 singleton pregnancies (although flawed in experimental design), there were statistically significant reductions in neonatal death and respiratory distress syndrome in the ritodrine-treated group. The treated patients were more likely to reach greater than 36 weeks and delivered neonates exceeding 2,500 g in birth weight. Finally, ritodrine treatment prolonged gestation by 32.6 days (mean) in treated pregnant women versus 21.3 days (mean) for gravidas in the control group ($P < 0.001$).

Terbutaline has also been proved effective in inhibiting premature labor in a placebo-controlled, double-blind study [86]. Comparison studies with other agents and additional, uncontrolled studies have also provided evidence for the clinical efficacy of terbutaline [87,88].

Clinical Use of Beta-Mimetics

Techniques for the use of tocolytic agents vary dependent upon the experience in different institutions and beliefs about which agent, route of administration, or schedule is best. At the Oregon Health Sciences University Hospital, the situation is no less arbitrary, albeit consistent. (Table 1–6). We use three parenteral tocolytic agents, magnesium sulfate, terbutaline, and ritodrine, but in different clinical settings. Oral preparations of both terbutaline and ritodrine are also employed. Ethyl alcohol, diazoxide, prostaglandin inhibitors, calcium-blocking agents, and progestational compounds are not used at this institution as tocolytics.

Patients less than 34 weeks of gestation admitted with obvious uterine activity, with or without intact membranes are given 250 μg of terbutaline subcutaneously to arrest labor and permit initial evaluation [85]. Active maternal bleeding, fetal distress, hypertension, arrhythmia, or a history of cardiac disease precludes immediate use of this or any other beta-mimetic agent. In five years of utilizing subcutaneous terbutaline in this manner, on more than 400 gravidas, we have observed no significant maternal or fetal complications. Ultrasound, amniocentesis, and appropriate laboratory studies can then proceed. The terbutaline dose may be repeated in 1 to 4 hours, if contractions persist. We also use a similar dose schedule in transfer patients where maintenance of an infusion pump or intravenous line used during ambulance and air transport is difficult. Both intramuscular (5 to 10 mg) and small intravenous doses of ritodrine (4 to 6 mg) presumably have the same effect and may be equally safe [89,90]. However, we have been pleased with our results with terbutaline, and our nursing personnel are comfortable with this form of administration. On occasion, similar doses of subcutaneous terbutaline are used for uterine relaxation to permit obstetrical maneuvers, especially late third trimester external cephalic version. Intravenous terbutaline at a dose of 2.5 to 10.0 μg/minute for 10 to 15 minutes has also been used at other centers for such obstetrical manipulations [91,92].

In patients for whom long-term tocolysis is appropriate, intravenous ritodrine is administered by infusion pump (150 to 300 μg/minute). Graded increases in dose are used until either intolerance or control of uterine activity occurs. We follow a procedure similar to that outlined by Lipshitz [7], where the maternal pulse is used as a clinical marker of drug effect (Table 1–7). Doses in excess of 300 μg/minute will occasionally be administered if the maternal pulse is less than 120 to 140 beats per minute and the parturient is otherwise tolerating the infused dose. Close clinical observation is maintained during the infusion. After a uterine controlling dose is reached, that rate of administration is generally maintained for six hours, and then progressive tapering to a lower dose is attempted. Any infusion lasting greater than 12 hours requires careful reevaluation. If the

Table 1-6

Clinical Use of Tocolytic Agents[a]

Agent	Dose/Route/Frequency	Comments
Beta-sympathomimetics:		
Terbutaline	250 μg subcutaneously, 1–4 h,[b] 2.5–10 mg, perorally, 2–4 h	Useful for obstetrical procedures and to arrest labor for evaluation, alternative oral therapy
Ritodrine	150–350 mμg, intravenously by pump,[c] 10–20 mg, perorally, 4–6 h	Increase dose 50 mμg/min every 15 min with titration to maternal pulse or effect, rarely should be used parenterally beyond 12 hours
MgSO$_4$	Load: 4–6 g intravenously, 15–20 min[d] Maintenance: 1–3 g, intravenously, 1 h	Close attention to output, reflexes; maintain serum levels, 4.5–6.5 mg/dl, by varying the infusion rate

[a] As practiced at Oregon Health Sciences University in patients unresponsive to lateral recumbancy bed rest and hydration. See text for details.

[b] SOURCE: Stubblefield, P.G., Heyl. P.S. Treatment of premature labor with subcutaneous terbutaline. *Obstet. Gynecol.* 59:457–462. 1982.

[c] SOURCES: Lipshitz, J. Beta-adrenergic agonists. *Semin. Perinatol.* 5:252–265. 1981. Niebyl, J.R.. Johnson, J.W.C. Inhibition of preterm labor. *Clin Obstet. Gynecol.* 23:115–126. 1980. Barden, T.P. Ritodrine hydrochloride: an FDA-approved tocolytic agent for use in the United States. I. Pharmacology, clinical history, administration, side effects and safety. *Obstet. Gynecol.* 56:1–6, 1980.

[d] SOURCES: Petrie, R.H. Tocolysis using magnesium sulfate. *Semin. Perinatol.* 5:266–273. 1981. Elliott. J.P. Magnesium sulfate as a tocolytic agent. *Am. J. Obstet. Gynecol.* 147:277–284, 1983.

Table 1–7
Administration of Betamimetic Agents

Intake and output every hour
Vital signs every 30 minutes
Electrolytes initially then every 8 hours
Restriction of intravenous fluids to 2ϑ/24 hours
Plasma glucose initially then finger stick blood glucose every 1–4 hours
Stepped dose increases by intravenous infusion pump with a maximum of 12
    hours of parenteral administration before reevaluation.

controlling dose is accompanied by persisting maternal tachycardia or patient symptomology (or both), conversion to magnesium sulfate is entertained, or else oral therapy is instituted.

Some patients may be candidates for tocolysis, but have relative contraindications to the use of beta-mimetic agents. In hypertensives, insulin-requiring diabetics, and patients intolerant to parenteral beta-mimetics, we administer magnesium sulfate as the drug of first choice. If control is adequate, patients are reassessed at 12 to 24 hours for continuation or conversion to an oral agent. We no longer administer intravenous terbutaline.

Prostaglandin Inhibitors

There is increasing evidence that prostaglandins play a significant role in parturition, although the control mechanisms are incompletely understood [12,93,94]. Release of prostaglandins from uterine sites (decidua, myometrium, amnion) initiates human parturition. Prostaglandins are also apparently involved in the major structural changes that occurs in the cervix just before the onset of labor. Various prostaglandin preparations have proven efficacy in the preparation of an unfavorable cervix for induction [95,96] or the initiation of labor [12,97]. These observations have led to trials of prostaglandin-inhibiting agents to block premature labor [13,93,98,99].

Initial studies using indomethacin (50 mg initially and then 25 mg/4 hours for 24 hours) in a prospective randomized and double-blinded trial indicate significant efficacy and neonatal safety [99]. Brief courses of such agents (less than 24 hours) and careful restriction to pregnancies less than 34 weeks of gestation are important to avoid adverse side effects [93,99]. The eventual role for prostaglandin inhibitors in tocolysis has not been established, nor has their long-term safety been sufficiently documented. They may be useful for intense, brief treatment or selected cases where other agents are contraindicated or ineffective. The interested reader is referred to the recent reviews of Neibyl [93] and Novy and Liggins [12].

Other Agents

Consideration of calcium channel blocking agents for hypertension and tocolysis is a natural step considering the central role of calcium in the physiology of smooth muscle contraction. Calcium channel blockers function by reducing the availability of free cytoplasmic calcium [100–102]. These agents have found clinical application in nonpregnant patients in the treatment of angina, cardiac arrhythmias, and hypertension [103].

Nicardipine, a potent calcium antagonist, is effective in halting labor in rabbits and is not antagonized by prostaglandins [104]. In human volunteers, another calcium blocker, nifedipine, has been shown to be effective in inhibiting menstrual contractions [102] as well as uterine activity induced by exogenous prostaglandin for midtrimester abortion [105]. There is limited experience with nifedipine in premature labor [93,106]. The efficacy of these drugs and the apparent absence of major cardiovascular changes accompanying the use of these drugs make them particularly attractive as potential tocolytics. Clinical investigation of these agents in obstetrics is commencing, and initial reports are promising.

Evaluation of Tocolysis

Tocolysis involves consideration of benefit versus risk. The maternal complications of treatment, although uncommon, can rarely be serious and even fatal. Certain subclasses of patients are not good candidates for treatment with the commonly used and potent agents, the beta-mimetics. Women with hypertension, known cardiac arrhythmia, or cardiovascular dysfunction are at high risk for complication. Patients with multiple gestation, diabetes mellitus, hemorrhage, or ruptured membranes are also in a high risk category for complications and should be treated with tocolytic agents only after the most careful consideration [6,64].

Although the principal role of tocolytic agents is in arresting premature labor, other uses are under investigation. There may be a role for beta–mimetics or other tocolytics in producing uterine relaxation to permit *in utero* resuscitation [107–109]. In limited studies, improvement in fetal scalp pH and electronic monitoring tracings have been shown in cases of fetal compromise. Further well-planned studies are necessary, but it appears that the uterorelaxing effect of beta-mimetics will have a role in the treatment of fetal distress.

Tocolytics also have a role in obstetrical manipulations, including uterine relaxation for cerclage placement as well as in external cephalic version or in complicated twin delivery [79,91,92,110,111].

Finally, there is limited evidence to indicate that beta-mimetic therapy reduces the incidence of neonatal respiratory distress syndrome [7,112,113]. Both animal data and data from human tocolytic trials suggest surfactant release and reduced incidence of respiratory distress. The mechanism is not clear, but may be related to the cyclic adenosine monophosphate release known to accompany parenteral beta-mimetics administration or to more prompt reabsorption of pulmonary fluid.

Conclusions

A number of pharmacologic agents have proved to be potent inhibitors of uterine activity. Ritodrine, terbutaline, and magnesium sulfate are by far the most popular tocolytics. Although clearly efficacious, these drugs also have a potential for serious maternal injury, including death [6,114]. The current problem for the clinician is to make appropriate choices in the use of these potent agents to improve fetal chances without excessive or unnecessary maternal risks.

It is important to note that many, if not most, patients at risk for premature labor are not candidates for tocolysis by the time they arrive at the hospital [19], and many patients evaluated for possible tocolysis will be excluded from treatment for sound obstetrical reasons [115]. Without better preventative measures, tocolysis is unlikely to impact importantly on the overall incidence of prematurity [5,20,19,115], but may clearly be of benefit in individual cases.

References

1. Cohen, W.R., Friedman, E.A. Etiology and management of premature labor. *Curr. Prob. Obstet. Gynecol.* 1:3–42, 1978.
2. Johnson, J.W.C., Dubin, N.H. Prevention of preterm labor. *Clin. Obstet. Gynecol.* 23:51–73, 1980.
3. Creasy, R.K., Gummer, B.A., Liggins, G.C. System for predicting spontaneous preterm birth. *Obstet. Gynecol.* 55:692–696, 1980.
4. Kaltreider, D.F., Kohl, S. Epidemiology of preterm delivery. *Clin. Obstet. Gynecol.* 23:17–31, 1980.
5. Boylan, P., O'Driscoll, K. Improvement in perinatal mortality rate attributed to spontaneous preterm labor without use of tocolytic agents. *Am. J. Obstet. Gynecol.* 145:781–783, 1983.
6. Benedetti, T.J. Maternal complications of parenteral B-sympathomimetic therapy for premature labor. *Am. J. Obstet. Gynecol.* 145:1–6, 1983.
7. Lipshitz, J. Beta-adrenergic agonists. *Semin. Perinatol.* 5:252–265, 1981.
8. Challis, J.R.G., Mitchell, B.F. Hormonal control of preterm and term parturition. *Semin. Perinatol.* 5:192–202, 1981.
9. Thornburn, G.D. Past and present concepts on the initiation of parturition. In MacDonald, P.C., Porter, J. (eds.), *Initiation of Parturition: Prevention of Prematurity. Report of the 4th Ross Conference on Obstetric Research.* Columbus, Ohio: Ross Laboratories, 1983, p. 2–11.

21

10. Csapo, A. Progesterone "block." *Am. J. Anat.* 98:273–291, 1956.
11. Neibyl, J.R., Blake, D.A., Johnson, J.W.C., King, T.M. Pharmacologic inhibition of preterm labor. *Obstet. Gynecol Surv.* 33:507–515, 1978.
12. Novy, M.J., Liggins, G.C. Role of prostaglandins, prostacyclin and thromboxanes in the physiologic control of the uterus and in parturition. *Semin. Perinatol.* 4:45–66, 1980.
13. Neibyl, J.R., Johnson, J.W.C. Inhibition of preterm labor. *Clin. Obstet. Gynecol.* 23:115–126, 1980.
14. Sellers, S. M., Hodgson, H.T., Mountfield, L.A., et al. Is oxytocin involved in parturition? *Br. J. Obstet. Gynaecol.* 88:725–729, 1981.
15. Fuller, W.E. Management of premature labor. *Clinic. Obstet. Gynecol.* 21:533–545, 1978.
16. Huszar, G. Biology and biochemistry of myometrial contractility and cervical maturiation. *Semin. Perinatol.* 5:216–235, 1981.
17. Carsten, M.E., Miller, J.D. Regulation of myometrial contractions. In MacDonald, P.C., Porter, J. (eds.), *Initiation of Parturition: Prevention of Prematurity. Report of the 4th Ross Conference on Obstetric Research.* Columbus, Ohio: Ross Laboratories, 1983, pp. 166–171.
18. Editorial: Drug treatment of premature labor. *Br. Med. J.* 283:395, 1981.
19. Creasy, R.K. Implications of treatment of preterm labor. In MacDonald, P.C., Porter, J. (eds.), *Initiation of Parturition: Prevention of Prematurity. Report of the 4th Ross Conference on Obstetric Research.* Columbus, Ohio: Ross Laboratories, 1983, pp. 173–181.
20. Zlatnik, F. The applicability of labor inhibition to the problem of prematurity. *Am. J. Obstet. Gynecol.* 113:704–706, 1972.
21. Herron, M.A., Katz, M., Creasy, R.K. Evaluation of a preterm birth prevention program: preliminary report. *Obstet. Gynecol.* 59:452–456, 1982.
22. Valenzuela, G., Cline, S., Hayaski, R.H. Followup of hydration and sedation in the pretherapy of premature labor. *Am. J. Obstet. Gynecol.* 147:396–398, 1983.
23. Jeffrey, R.L., Bowes, W.A., Jr., Delaney, J.J. Role of bed rest in twin gestation. *Obstet. Gynecol.* 43:822–826, 1974.
24. Misenhimer, H.R., Kaltkeider, D.F. Effects of decreased prenatal activity in patients with twin pregnancy. *Obstet. Gynecol.* 51:692–694, 1978.
25. Weekes, A.R.L., Menzies, D.N., DeBoer, C.H. The relative efficacy of bed rest, cervical suture, and no treatment in the management of twin pregnancy. *Br. J. Obstet. Gynaecol.* 84:161–164, 1977.
26. Persson, P.H., Grennest, L., Geunser, G., Kullanden, S. On improved outcome of twin pregnancies. *Acta. Obstet. Gynecol. Scand.* 58:3–7, 1979.
27. Guilliams, S., Held, B. Contemporary management and conduct of preterm labor and delivery: a review. *Obstet. Gynecol. Surv.* 34:248–255, 1979.
28. Csapo, A.I. The "seesaw" theory of parturition. *Ciba Found. Symp.* 47:159, 1977.
29. Csapo, A.I., Herczog, J. Arrest of premature labor by isoxsuprine. *Am. J. Obstet. Gynecol.* 129:482–491, 1977.
30. Johnson, J.W.C., Austin, K.L., Jones, G.S. Efficacy of 17α-hydroxyprogesterone caproate in the prevention of premature labor. *N. Engl. J. Med.* 293:675–680, 1975.

22

31. Johnson, J.W.C., Lee, P.A., Zachary, A.S., Calhoun, S. High risk prematurity—progestin treatment and steroid studies. *Obstet. Gynecol.* 54:412–418, 1979.
32. Kauppila, A., Hartikainen-Sorri, A.L., Janne, O., et al. Suppression of threatened premature labor by administration of cortisol and 17α-hydroxyprogesterone caproate: comparison with ritodrine. *Am. J. Obstet. Gynecol.* 138:404–408, 1980.
33. Carson, G.D. Tocolytic therapy. *Curr. Probl. Obstet. Gynecol.* 6:48–49, 1983.
34. Fuchs, A.R., Fuchs, F. Ethanol for prevention of preterm birth. *Semin. Perinatol.* 5:236–250, 1981.
35. Zervoudakis, I.A., Krauss, A., Fuchs, F., Wilson, K.H. Infants of mothers treated with ethanol for premature labor. *Am. J. Obstet. Gynecol.* 137:713–717, 1980.
36. Joffe, J.M. Letter: alcohol and pregnancy. *Science* 22:1244–1246, 1983.
37. Lauersen, N.H., Merkatz, I.R., Tejani, N., et al. Inhibition of premature labor: a multi-center comparison of ritodrine and ethanol. *Am. J. Obstet. Gynecol.* 127:837–845, 1977.
38. Steer, C.M., Petrie, R.H. A comparison of magnesium sulfate and alcohol for the prevention of premature labor. *Am. J. Obstet. Gynecol.* 128:1–4, 1977.
39. Spearing, G. Alcohol, indomethacin, and salbutamol. *Obstet. Gynecol.* 53:171–174, 1979.
40. Petrie, R.H. Stopping premature labor with magnesium sulfate. *Contemp. Ob/Gyn.* 11:187–192, 1978.
41. Petrie, R.H. Tocolysis using magnesium sulfate. *Semin. Perinatol.* 5:266–273, 1981.
42. Elliott, J.P. Magnesium sulfate as a tocolytic agent. *Am. J. Obstet. Gynecol.* 147:277–284, 1983.
43. Goodman, L.S., Gilman, A. (eds.) The pharmacological basis of therapeutics, 5th ed. New York: MacMillan Publishing Co., Inc., p. 880.
44. Elliot, J.P., O'Keefe, D.F., Greenberg, P., Freeman, R.K. Pulmonary edema associated with magnesium sulfate and beta-methasone administration. *Am. J. Obstet. Gynecol.* 134:717–719, 1979.
45. Spisso, K.R., Harbert, G.M., Thiagarajah, S. The use of magnesium sulfate as the primary tocolytic agent to prevent premature delivery. *Am. J. Obstet. Gynecol.* 142:840–845, 1982.
46. Miller, J.M., Jr., Keane, M.W.D., Horger, E.O. A comparison of magnesium sulfate and terbutaline for the arrest of premature labor: a preliminary report. *J. Reprod. Med.* 27:348–351, 1982.
47. Ahlquist, R.P. A study of adrenotropic receptors. *Am. J. Physiol.* 153:586–600, 1948.
48. Lands, A.M., Arnold, A., Mcauliff, J., et al. Differentiation of receptor systems activated by sympathomimetic amines. *Nature* 214:597–598, 1967.
49. Hosenpud, J.D., Morton, M.J., O'Grady, J.P. Cardiac stimulation during ritodrine hydrochloride tocolytic therapy. *Obstet. Gynecol.* 62:52–58, 1983.
50. Huszar, G. Current concepts of myometrial control in tocolytic agents. In Merrill-National Laboratories (ed.), *Tocolytic Agents.* New York: Biomedical Information Corp., 1980, pp. 1–14.

51. Scheid, C.R., Honeyman, T.W., Fay, F.S. Mechanism of b-adrenergic relaxation of smooth muscle. *Nature* 277:32–36, 1979.
52. Cotton, D.B., Strassnen, H.T., Lipson, L.G., Goldstein, D.A. The effects of terbutaline on acid base, serum electrolytes, and glucose homeostasis during the management of premature labor. *Am. J. Obstet. Gynecol.* 141:617–623, 1981.
53. Kirkpatrick, C., Quenon, M., Desir, D. Blood amions and electrolytes during ritodrine infusion in preterm labor. *Am. J. Obstet. Gynecol.* 138:523–526, 1980.
54. Spellacy, W.N., Cruz, A.C., Buhi, W.C., Birk, S.A. The acute effects of ritodrine infusion on maternal metabolism measurements of levels of glucose, insulin, glucagon, triglycerides, cholesterol, placental lactogen, and chorionic gonadotropin. *Am. J. Obstet. Gynecol.* 131:736–742, 1978.
55. Gross, T.L. How tocolytics affect mother, fetus and neonate. *Contemp. Ob/Gyn,* 19:1–6, 1982.
56. VanLierde, M., Buysschaert, M., deHertogh, R., et al., Administration intraveineuse de ritodrine chez la diabetique insulino-dependante enceinte. *J. Gyn. Obstet. Biol. Repr.* 11:869–875, 1982.
57. Desir, D., VanCoevorden, A., Kirkpatrick, C., Caufriez, A. Ritodrine-induced acidosis in pregnancy. *Br. Med. J.* 2:1194, 1978.
58. Tye, K.H., Desser, K.B., Benchimol, A. Angina pectoris associated with use of terbutaline for premature labor. *JAMA* 244:692–693, 1980.
59. Domenichini, Y., Thoulon, J.M. The cardiovascular complications of the use of beta-mimetic drugs in obstetrics. *J. Gynecol. Obstet. Biol. Reprod.* 11:861–867, 1982.
60. Milliez, J., Sureau, C. A case report of maternal death associated with beta–mimetics and beta–methasone administration in premature labor. *Eur. J. Obstet. Gynecol. Reprod. Biol.* 11:95–100, 1980.
61. Wagner, J.M., Morton, M.J., Johnson, K., et al. Terbutaline and maternal cardiac function. *JAMA* 246:2697–2701, 1981.
62. Philipsen, T., Eriksen, P.S., Lynggard, F. Pulmonary edema following ritodrine-saline infusion in premature labor. *Obstet. Gynecol.* 58:304–308, 1981.
63. Elliott, H.R., Abdulla, U. Pulmonary edema associated with ritodrine infusion and beta–methasone administration in premature labor. *Br. Med. J.* 2:799–800, 1978.
64. Katz, M., Robertson, P.A., Creasy, R.K. Cardiovascular complications associated with terbutaline treatment for premature labor. *Am. J. Obstet. Gynecol.* 139:605–608, 1981.
65. Jacobs, M.M., Knight, A.B., Arias, F. Maternal pulmonary edema resulting from beta-mimetic and glucocorticoid therapy. *Obstet. Gynecol.* 56:56–69, 1980.
66. Tinga, D.J., Aarnoudse, J.G. Letter: post-partum pulmonary edema associated with preventative therapy for premature labor. *Lancet* 1:1026–1027, 1979.
67. Brodey, P.A., Fisch, A.E., Huffaker, J. Acute pulmonary edema resulting from treatment for premature labor. *Radiology* 140:631–633, 1981.
68. Benedetti, T.J., Hargrove, J., Rosene, K.A. Maternal pulmonary edema during premature labor inhibition. *Obstet. Gynecol.* 59(Suppl.):333–375, 1982.

69. Guernsey, B.G., Villarreal, Y., Snyder, M.D., Gabert, H.A. Pulmonary edema associated with the use of beta–mimetic agents in preterm labor. *Am. J. Hosp. Pharm.* 38:1942–1948, 1981.

70. Abramovici, H., Lewin, A., Lissak, A., Palant, A. Maternal pulmonary edema occurring after therapy with ritodrine for premature uterine contractions. *Acta Obstet. Gynecol. Scand.* 59:555, 1980.

71. Hauth, J.C., Hamkins, G.D., Kuehl, T.J., Pierson, W.P. Ritodrine hydrochloride infusion in pregnant baboons. I. Biophysical effects. *Am. J. Obstet. Gynecol.* 146:916–924, 1983.

72. Hankins, G.D., Hauth, J.C., Kuehl, T.J., et al. Ritodrine hydrochloride infusion in pregnant baboons. II. Sodium and water compartments alternations. *Am. J. Obstet. Gynecol.* 147:254–259, 1983.

73. Stubblefield, P.G. Pulmonary edema occurring after therapy with dexamethasone and terbutaline for premature labor: a case report. *Am. J. Obstet. Gynecol.* 132:341–342, 1978.

74. Ersoz, N., Finestone, S.C. Adrenaline-induced pulmonary edema and its treatment: a report of two cases. *Br. J. Anaesth.* 43:709–712, 1971.

75. Schilthnis, M.S., Aarnoudse, J.G. Fetal death associated with severe ritodrine induced ketoacidosis. *Lancet* 1:1145, 1980.

76. Merkatz, I.R., Peter, J.B., Barden, T.P. Ritodrine hydrochloride: a beta–mimetic agent for use in preterm labor. *Obstet. Gynecol.* 56:7–12, 1980.

77. Wesselius-de Casparis, A., Thiery, M., YoLeSian, A., et al. Results of double-blind, multi-centre study with ritodrine in premature labor. *Br. Med. J.* 3:144–147, 1971.

78. Creasy, R.K., Golbus, M.S., Laros, R.K., et al. Oral ritodrine maintenance in the treatment of preterm labor. *Am. J. Obstet. Gynecol.* 137:212–219, 1980.

79. Ingemarrson, I. Use of β–receptor agonists in obstetrics. *Acta Obstet. Gynecol. Scand.* Suppl. 108:29–34, 1982.

80. Karlsson, K. β-receptor agonists in pregnancy: long term effects in preterm children. *Acta Obstet. Gynecol. Scand.* 108(Suppl.):71–72, 1982.

81. Huisjes, H.J., Touwen, B.C.L. Neonatal outcome after treatment with ritodrine: a controlled study. *Am. J. Obstet. Gynecol.* 147:250–253, 1983.

82. Schenken, R.S., Hayashi, R.H., Valenzuela, G.V., Castillo, M.S. Treatment of premature labor with beta–sympathomimetics: results with isoxuprine. *Am. J. Obstet. Gynecol.* 137:773–780, 1980.

83. Brazy, J.E., Little, V., Grimm, J., Pupkin, M. Risk/benefit considerations for the use of isoxsuprine in the treatment of premature labor. *Obstet. Gynecol.* 58:297–302, 1981.

84. Barden, T.P. Ritodrine hydrochloride: an FDA-approved tocolytic agent for use in the United States. I. Pharmacology, clinical history, administration, side effects and safety. *Obstet. Gynecol.* 56:1–6, 1980.

85. Stubblefield, P.G., Heyl, P.S. Treatment of premature labor with subcutaneous terbutaline. *Obstet. Gynecol.* 59:457–462, 1982.

86. Ingemarsson, I. Effect of terbutaline on premature labor. *Am. J. Obstet. Gynecol.* 125:520–524, 1976.

87. Brown, S.M., Tejani, N.A. Terbutaline sulfate in the prevention of recurrence of premature labor. *Obstet. Gynecol.* 57:22–25, 1981.

88. Wallace, R.L., Caldwell, D.L., Ansbacher, R., Otterson, W.N. Inhibition of premature labor by terbutaline. *Obstet. Gynecol.* 51:387–392, 1978.

89. Spellacy, W.N., Cruz, A.C., Birk, S.A., Buhi, W.C. Treatment of premature labor with ritodrine: a randomized controlled study. *Obstet. Gynecol.* 54:220–223, 1979.

90. Schreyer, P.J., Caspi, E., Snir, E., et al. Metabolic effects of intramuscular and oral administration of ritodrine in pregnancy. *Obstet. Gynecol.* 57:730–733, 1981.

91. Fall, O., Nilsson, B.A. External cephalic version in breech presentation under tocolysis. *Obstet. Gynecol.* 53:712–715, 1979.

92. VanDorsten, J.P. Safe and effective external cephalic version with tocolysis. *Contemp. Ob/Gyn.* 19:44–59, 1982.

93. Neibyl, J.R. Prostaglandin synthetase inhibitors. *Semin. Perinatol.* 5:274–286, 1981.

94. Turnbull, A.C. Human parturition: historic development and overview. In MacDonald, P.C., Porter, J. (eds.), *Initiation of Parturition: Prevention of Prematurity. Report of the 4th Ross Conference on Obstetric Research.* Columbus, Ohio: Ross Laboratories, 1983, pp. 87–94.

95. Prins, R.P., Bolton, R.N., Mark, C., et al. Cervical ripening with intravaginal prostaglandin E2 gel. *Obstet. Gynecol.* 61:459–462, 1983.

96. Tromans, P.M., Beazley, J.M., Shenonda, P.I. Comparative study of estradial and prostaglandin E2 vaginal gel for ripening the unfavorable cervix before induction of labor. *Br. Med. J.* 282:679–681, 1981.

97. Wingerup, L., Ulmsten, U. Single application of prostaglandin E2 in a viscous gel for induction of labor at term in patients with favorable cervix. *Acta Obstet. Gynecol. Scand.* 60:17–19, 1981.

98. Coceani, F., Olley, P.M. (eds.). On the use of blockers of prostaglandin synthesis in the control of labor. In *Advances in Prostaglandin and Thromboxane Research,* vol. 4, New York: Raven Press, 1978, pp. 301–305.

99. Neibyl, J.R., Blake, D.A., White, R.D., et al. The inhibition of premature labor with indomethacin. *Am. J. Obstet. Gynecol.* 136:1014–1019, 1980.

100. McAllister, R.G. Clinical pharmacokinetics of calcium channel antagonists. *J. Cardiovasc. Pharmacol.* 4(Suppl.):340–345, 1982.

101. Krebs, R., Graefe, K.H., Ziegler, R. Effects of calcium entry antagonists in hypertension. *Clin. Exp. Hypertens.* A4:271–284, 1982.

102. Forman, A., Andersson, K.E., Ulmsten, U. Inhibition of myometrial activity by calcium antagonists. *Semin. Perinatol.* 5:288–294, 1981.

103. Nifedipine for angina pectoris. *The Medical Letter.*, 24:39–41, 1982.

104. Csapo, A.I., Puri, C.P., Tarro, S., Henzl, M.R. Deactivation of the uterus during normal and premature labor by the calcium antagonist Nicardipine. *Am. J. Obstet. Gynecol.* 142:483–491, 1982.

105. Andersson, K.E., Ingemarsson, I., Ulmsten, U., Wingerup, L. Inhibition of prostaglandin-induced uterine activity by nifedipine. *Br. J. Obstet. Gynaecol.* 86:175–179, 1979.

106. Ulmsten, U., Andersson, K.E., Wingerup, L. Treatment of premature labor with the calcium antagonist nifedipine. *Arch. Gynecol.* 229:1–5, 1980.

107. Esteban-Altirriba, J. Treatment of fetal distress. In Merrill-National Laboratories (ed.), *Tocolytic Agents.* New York: Bio-medical Information Corp., 1980, pp. 69–75.

108. Lipshitz, J. Use of a β2-sympathomimetic drug as a temporizing measure in the treatment of acute fetal distress. *Am. J. Obstet. Gynecol.* 129:31–36, 1977.

109. Arias, F. Intrauterine resuscitation with terbutaline: a method for the management of acute intrapartum fetal distress. *Am. J. Obstet. Gynecol.* 131:39–43, 1978.

110. Lipshitz, J. Beta-mimetics for tocolysis or obstetrical procedures. In Merrill-National Laboratories (ed.), *Tocolytic Agents*. New York: Biomedical Information Corp., 1980, pp. 77–82.

111. Chervenak, F.A., Johnson, R.E., Berkowitz, R.L., Hobbins, J.C. Intrapartum external version of the second twin. *Obstet. Gynecol.* 62:160–165, 1983.

112. Bergman, B., Hedner, T. Antepartum administration of terbutaline and the incidence of hyaline membrane disease in preterm infants. *Acta Obstet. Gynecol. Scand.* 57:217–221, 1978.

113. Esteban-Altirriba, J. Fetal lung maturation. In Merrill-National Laboratories (ed.), *Tocolytic Agents*. New York: Biomedical Information Corp., 1980, pp. 41–49.

114. Neibyl, J.R. Drugs for inhibition of premature labor. *Clin. Pharmacol.* 6:53–63, 1979.

115. Tejani, N.A., Verma, U.L. Effect of tocolysis on incidence of low birth weight. *Obstet. Gynecol.* 61:556–558, 1983.

2

Initiation of Parturition with Drugs

Kent Ueland, M.D.

The Initiation of Spontaneous Labor

In some animals the factors responsible for triggering labor have been delineated. In humans, however, the initiating factor has not been defined, and two prominant schools of thought prevail: the oxytocin theory—production of oxytocin by the fetus with transfer to the mother—and the prostaglandin (PGE_2, $PGF_{2\alpha}$) theory—stimulation of prostaglandin production in the decidua ($PGF_{2\alpha}$) and the cervix (PGE_2) by as yet an unidentified substance or event. Recent work by Fuchs et al. [1] suggests that both mechanisms may be involved. The fetus produces oxytocin, which is transferred to the mother, inducing contractions by stimulating the release of prostaglandins. The factor in the entire scheme that has not been answered to date is what turns on the fetal oxytocin production.

The sex steroids are most likely not involved in the initiation of human parturition. Investigations so far have not been able to demonstrate the estrogen surge that precedes parturition in, for example, sheep and rabbits. This may be attributable to the fact that blood sampling has not been carried out frequently enough.

An increased knowledge and understanding about parturition and uterine muscle physiology has allowed the obstetrician to manipulate the pregnant uterus more effectively. One can now both start and stop labor almost at will. However, there remains one obstacle in induction of labor that needs to be overcome, i.e., the unfavorable or unripe cervix. The success rate of induced labor is directly related to the Bishop score at the onset [2]. Recent evidence, however, indicates that one may now prime the cervix without inducing myometrial contraction by the direct intra-cervical application of small amounts of PGE_2 gel [3]. This allows for the successful induction of labor with oxytocin 8 to 12 hours later.

Induction of Labor with Oxytocin

In 1980 the Food and Drug Administration recommended against the use of oxytocin for elective induction of labor and required that the package insert contain the following important notice:

> Pitocin is not indicated for the elective induction of labor because available data and information are inadequate to define the benefits-to-risks consideration in the use of the drug product. Elective induction of labor is defined as the initiation of labor in an individual with a term pregnancy who is free of medical indications for the initiation of labor.

This overreaction on the part of this government body was likely prompted by such factors as iatrogenic prematurity resulting from elective induction of labor and possibly failed elective induction resulting in cesarean section.

In my mind this has significantly hampered the practice of normal obstetrics, particularly by the conscientious practitioner who induced labor electively at term only when fetal maturity was assured and the Bishop score was favorable.

In 1968 Friedman et al. [4] carried out a study evaluating the success rate of elective induction of labor at term and relating it to the preinduction Bishop score. Table 2–1 summarizes their results. When the Bishop score

Table 2–1

Induction Failures—Bishop Score
(408 Multiparas)

Bishop Score	% Failure
1–4	19.5
5–8	4.8
9–13	0.0

SOURCE: modified from Friedman, E.A., Niswarder, K. R., Bayonet-Rivera, N.P., Sachtleben, M.R. Relation of prelabor evaluation to inducibility and the course of labor. *Obstet. Gynecol.* 28:495–501, 1966.

29

Table 2–2
Induction of Labor—Common Indications

Maternal Indications	Fetal Indications
Hypertension	Diabetes
Premature rupture of membranes	Rh sensitization
Intrauterine fetal death	Intrauterine growth retardation
Deteriorating maternal illness	Prolonged pregnancy
Hydramnios, fetal anomaly	Anomalies
incompatible with life	

was 9 or greater, all patients were induced successfully. When the Bishop score was less than 5, the failure rate was 19.5%.

Oxytocin is approved for induction of labor in patients with a medical indication for the initiation of labor. The most common medical and obstetrical indications are listed in Table 2–2.

Oxytocin for induction of labor should only be used intravenously in a dilute solution. Some form of a controlled infusion device is required. A two-bottle piggy-back system should be utilized where the oxytocin-containing solution is infused into the tubing of an existing main-line intravenous catheter. The recommended starting dose is 0.5 to 2 mU/minute. The rate should not be increased more frequently than every 15 to 30 minutes, and the increment should be 1 to 2 mU/minute until the desired normal labor pattern is achieved. Electronic fetal heart rate monitoring is imperative, and direct electrocardiographic monitoring is preferred, as is the direct measurement of intrauterine pressure with a catheter. The frequency of contractions normally range between two and five per 10 minutes. The tonus between contractions should be maintained at levels below 12 to 15 mmHg. The intensity of normal contractions range between 30 and 50 mmHg in the early first stage of labor to between 50 and 75 mmHg late in the first stage and in the second stage of labor. These values must be considered as general guidelines, since the individual variation is great.

Some of the contraindications to oxytocin stimulation are listed in Table 2–3. With proper use and continuous fetal and maternal surveillance, the risks to both mother and fetus are small. Nonetheless, uterine hypertonus is occasionally encountered and can result in fetal compromise. Discontinuing the infusion, giving O_2 by mask, and making sure the mother is positioned on her side are invariably the only therapeutic measures required to correct it. Hypertonus occurs most commonly at the onset of the infusion. If the uterus appears irritable before initiating the infusion or if the patient is having irregular contractions, begin the infusion at the lowest dose, 0.5 mU/minute. Once the infusion has been established hypertonus is rarely encountered, but may occassionally occur when the

Table 2–3
Contraindications to Uterine Stimulation

Absolute	Relative
Fetal distress	Overdistended uterus
Central placenta previa	Grand multiparity
Unfavorable fetal position	Breech presentation
Proven cephalo-pelvic disproportion	Previous low transverse cesarean section
Scar in myometrium	Prematurity

rate of the infusion is increased. Uterine hypertonus is invariably the reason why the oxytocin infusion needs to be stopped or decreased. Hyperstimulation in the form of contractions that are too intense is exceedingly rare. When the infusion is restarted after an episode of hyperstimulation, begin at the lowest rate of 0.5 mU/minute. It should be remembered that hypertonus occurs in up to 2 percent of normal spontaneous unstimulated labors.

Induction of Labor with Prostaglandins

The prostaglandins, particularly PGE_2, have been used to induce labor by various routes of administration. They have been given intravenously, orally, oromucosally, extraamniotically, intravaginally, and intracervically. The route of administration determines the frequency and severity of the systemic side effects. Local applications, i.e., intravaginally and intracervically, are associated with few, if any, systemic effects and appear to be the routes of choice. Extensive European experience with this mode of administration has demonstrated both efficacy and patient and physician acceptance for both induction of labor and cervical priming.

PGF_{2a} and PGE_1 have also been used successfully to induce labor. However, a high incidence of side effects is encountered, and PGE_2 seems more effective; therefore, these agents are not likely to see widespread clinical use in the future. They are mentioned here only for completeness.

The efficacy of orally administered PGE_2 has been reported to vary between 63 and 100 percent by Miller et al. [5], Murnaghan et al. [6], Visscher et al. [7], Friedman and Sachtelben [8], Friedman et al. [9], Gabert et al. [10], Kelly et al. [11], Lauersen and Wilson [12], and Thiery et al. [13].

As with oxytocin, the main determinant of success is the Bishop score at the onset. Other factors such as gravidity and the underlying medical and obstetrical condition(s) prompting the induction also appear to play a role. In my experience, the success rate in women with premature rupture of membranes has been approximately 95 percent with oral PGE_2 [14].

31

The success rates are also influenced by early amniotomy, escalating dosages, shorter intervals between dosages, continued intermittent dosages until delivery, and the use of oxytocin for augmentation of labor.

The characteristics of oral PGE_2-induced labor mimic those of normal spontaneous labor in many respects. The frequency and intensity of contractions are the same at comparable times in labor; the rise and fall times of contractions are identical, as is the tonus between contractions. The evolution of early labor is also similar in both. However, a major difference is identifiable when one compares the rate of cervical dilatation in the active phase of the first stage of labor. Patients undergoing induction of labor with oral PGE_2 dilate at a more rapid rate during the active phase of the first stage of labor, reaching nearly 3 cm per hour [14]. This rate of dilatation is equivalent to the ideal labor course reported by Friedman [15] and is achieved with normal uterine activity.

The forces of labor during the first stage are basically the contractions and the resistance of the cervix. With oral PGE_2, normal uterine contractions are achieved, but equally important there is also a marked softening of the cervix, which decreases its resistance to dilatation. It is the latter factor that is responsible for the rapid dilatation that is encountered in PGE_2-induced labors. The physical characteristics of the cervix were studied in our laboratory, and we found that the resistance to stretch was significantly less in women who were induced with PGE_2 at term than in those women undergoing spontaneous labor [16].

Table 2–4 lists the systemic side effects encountered in the author's experience with nearly 200 patients undergoing induction of labor with oral PGE_2. The incidence of hypertonus (2.5 percent) is similar to that encountered in patients in spontaneous labor. The incidence of fetal distress was exceedingly low, especially when one considers that over 50 percent of the patients were undergoing indicated induction of labor. The nausea or vomiting and diarrhea (or both) were usually self-limiting, most frequently occurring as one episode around the time of delivery. None was encountered in the early puerperium.

There are no extensive long-term follow-up studies in the literature of women that have undergone PGE_2 induction. However, the studies that have addressed the issue show no evidence of abnormal development in children, no problems with subsequent pregnancy and labor performance, and no identifiable gynecologic problems.

Table 2–4
Systemic Side Effects with Oral PGE_2

Diarrhea	13.1%
Vomiting	12.5%
Hypertonus	2.5%
Fetal distress	1.6%

The Future

In the past few years a large amount of data has appeared in the European literature regarding the use of PGE_2 intracervically and intravaginally: Shepherd et al. [17], Wingerup et al. [3], Gordon-Wright and Edler [18], and Pearce et al. [19]. With local application of small amounts of drug, the systemic effects are obviated, yet the efficacy is maintained. When the PGE_2 is applied in a gel into the cervix in a dose of only 0.5 mg, approximately 50% of patients will deliver after the primary induction [3]. In the remainder of patients there is a significant improvement in the cervix score. If the gel is confined only to the endocervical canal, frequently there is no increase in myometrial contractility, yet the priming of the cervix occurs. This local effect is useful for managing high-risk patients who need to be induced and have an unfavorable cervix.

Although the efficacy is similar between the intracervical and intravaginal application, there are more side effects with the vaginal route, and the dose is higher (3 to 5 mg versus 0.5 mg of PGE_2). Additionally, there is more pronounced myometrial stimulation. The intracervical application is a more sophisticated way of priming the cervix since the active substance reaches the target organ directly. This is also a more complicated mode of administration and will reduce the risk of overtreatment and self-administration.

The preliminary experience in Europe with the local PGE_2 administration (cervical, vaginal) has indicated that in women with an unfavorable cervix, the cesarean section rate is reduced substantially. Table 2–5 compares cesarean section rates in patients with or without cervical priming.

Preliminary investigation with the intracervical gel have been started in a few institutions in this country. However, much data needs to be accumulated before Food and Drug Administration approval can be realized; undoubtedly, this will take years. It is unfortunate that this ben-

Table 2–5
Effect of PGE_2 Cervical Priming on Cesarean Section Rates

Reference	No Priming	PGE_2 Gel Priming
Calder[a]	30%	<5%
Shepherd and Knuppel[b]	20%	2%
Wingerup et al[c]	25%	<10%

[a] SOURCE: Calder, A.A. The management of the unripe cervix. In Keirse, M.J.N.C., Anderson, A.B.M., Bennebroek Gravenhorse, J. (eds.), *Human Parturition*. Hingham, Mass.: Leiden University Press, pp. 201–217, 1979.

[b] SOURCE: Shepherd, J.H., Knuppel, R.A. The role of prostaglandins in ripening the cervix and inducing labor. *Clin. Perinatol.* 8:49–62, 1981.

[c] SOURCE: Ulmsten, U., Wingerup, L., Ekman, G. Local application of prostaglandin E_2 for cervical ripening or induction of term labor. *Clin. Obstet. Gynecol.* 26:95–105, 1983.

eficial mode of therapy cannot be instituted earlier. With intracervical PGE$_2$ gel we have essentially found the ideal cervical priming agent. It is safe, inexpensive, and practical and produces cervical change frequently without inducing contractions, systemic effects are infrequent (<1 percent), and there appear to be no long-term fetal, neonatal, or maternal sequelae.

References

1. Fuchs, A.R., Fuchs, F., Husslein, P., et al. Oxytocin receptors and human parturition: a dual role of oxytocin in the initiation of labor. *Science* 215:1396–98, 1982.
2. Bishop, E.H. Pelvic scoring for elective induction. *Obstet. Gynecol.* 24:266–68, 1964.
3. Ulmsten, U., Wingerup, L., Ekman, G. Local application of prostaglandin E$_2$ for cervical ripening or induction of term labor. *Clin. Obstet. Gynecol.* 26:95–105, 1983.
4. Friedman, E.A., Niswander, K.R., Bayonet-Rivera, N.P., Sachtleben, M.R. Relation of prelabor evaluation to inducibility and the course of labor. *Obstet. Gynecol.* 28:495–501, 1966.
5. Miller, J.F., Welply, G.A., Elstein, M. Prostaglandin E$_2$ tablets compared with intravenous oxytocin in induction of labor. *Br. Med. J.* 1:14, 1975.
6. Murnaghan, G.A., Lamki, H., Rashid, S., Pinkerton, J.H.M. Induction of labor with oral prostaglandin E$_2$. *J. Obstet. Gynaecol. Br. Commonw.* 81:141, 1974.
7. Visscher, R.D., Struyk, C.D., Visscher, H.C. Guidelines for elective induction of labor with oral prostaglandin E$_2$. *Obstet. Gynecol.* 49:15, 1977.
8. Friedman, E.A., Sachtleben, M.R. Oral prostaglandin E$_2$ for induction of labor at term. *Obstet. Gynecol.* 43:178, 1974.
9. Friedman, E.A., Sachtleben, M.R., Green, W. Oral prostaglandin E$_2$ for induction of labor at term. II. Comparison of two low-dosage regimens. *Am. J. Obstet. Gynecol.* 123:671, 1975.
10. Gabert, H.A., Brinton, J., Brown, B. Induction of labor with oral prostaglandin E$_2$. *Am. J. Obstet. Gynecol.* 125:333, 1976.
11. Kelly, J., Flynn, A.M., Bertrand, P.V. A comparison of oral prostaglandin E$_2$ and intravenous oxytocin in the induction of labor. *J. Obstet. Gynaecol. Br. Commonw.* 80:923, 1974.
12. Lauersen, N.H., Wilson, K.H. Induction of labor with oral prostaglandin E$_2$. *Obstet. Gynecol.* 44:793, 1974.
13. Thiery, M., YoLeslan, A., de Hemptinne, D., et al. Induction of labor with prostaglandin E$_2$ tablets. *J. Obstet. Gynaecol. Br. Commonw.* 81:303, 1974.
14. Ueland, K., Conrad, J. Characteristics of oral prostaglandin E$_2$ induced labor. *Clin. Obstet. Gynecol.* 26:87–94, 1983.
15. Friedman, E.A. *Labor: Clinical Evaluation & Management,* 2nd ed. East Norwalk, Conn.: Appleton-Century-Crofts, 1978.

16. Conrad, J.T., Ueland, K. The stretch modulus of human cervical tissue in spontaneous, oxytocin-induced, and prostaglandin E$_2$ induced labor. *Am. J. Obstet. Gynecol.* 133:11, 1979.

17. Shepherd, J.H., Bennett, M.J., Laurence, D., et al. Prostaglandin vaginal suppositories: a simple and safe approach to the induction of labor. *Obstet. Gynecol.* 58:596–600, 1981.

18. Gordon-Wright, A.P., Edler, M.G. Prostaglandin E$_2$ tablets used intravaginally for the induction of labor. *Br. J. Obstet. Gynaecol.* 87:32, 1979.

19. Pearce, J.M.F., Shepherd, J.H., and Sims, C.D. Prostaglandin pessaries for the induction of labor. *Lancet* 1:572, 1979.

20. Calder, A.A. *The management of the unripe cervix.* In Keirse, M.J.N.C., Anderson, A.B.M., Bennebroek Gravenhorse, J. (eds.), *Human Parturition.* Hingham, Mass.: Leiden University Press, pp. 201–217, 1979.

21. Shepherd, J.H., Knuppel, R.A. The role of prostaglandins in ripening the cervix and inducing labor. *Clin. Perinatol.* 8:49–62, 1981.

3

Management of Preterm Labor

Charles J. Ingardia, M.D.

Definition

One of the first problems that is encountered in the discussion of premature labor is one of definitions. If the basis of the definition is that of gestational age (i.e., less than 37 weeks), diagnosis has to be made through historical dating information, or neonatal assessment, or both. Dating information may be absent or inaccurate, and neonatal (Dubowitz) assessment may only give an approximation of gestational age. Another approach would be to delineate a birth weight (i.e., less than, 2,500 g) as a way of deciding what constitutes a premature birth. Of course it has become evident that there is a great range of birth weight and that the concept of the growth-retarded term infant and the preterm infant who is large for gestational age makes this approach less than ideal. As a working diagnosis a reasonable approach would be to say that preterm labor exists with the onset of regular uterine activity associated with evidence of progressive changes in cervical dilatation, effacement, or both in a gestation of less than 37 weeks.

Prenatal Assessment

Since only one-third of preterm labor patients are candidates for tocolysis, it is obvious that attention should center on proper identification of patients at risk when they present as routine obstetrical outpatients.

Data from the Obstetrical Statistical Cooperative reviewed by Kaltreider and Kohe [1] indicates historical, obstetrical, and medical complications that can be associated with preterm labor. Prepregnancy historical data associated with an increased risk of preterm delivery include maternal age less than 15 and greater than 40 years, previous preterm delivery, repetitive second-trimester abortions, uterine anomalies, history of pyelonephritis, and low socioeconomic class.

Pregnancy factors leading to an increased risk of preterm labor include multiple gestation, hydramnios, abruption, abdominal surgery, preeclampsia or eclampsia, poor weight gain, bacteria, and pyelonephritis (Table 3–1).

This assessment of risk factors needs to be ongoing. Several symptoms have been proposed to assigned risks to patients both by Kaminski and Papiernik [2] and Fredrick [3]. Creasy et al. [4] proposed a system in which the medium- and high-risk group together comprised 32 percent of their clinic population who delivered 80 percent of the preterm deliveries at their institutions. If the high-risk group were followed singularly, 10 to 12 percent of the population would lead to 70 percent of the preterm deliveries. These selected groups of patients may at least be followed more intensively and alerted for the signs of early labor. They can be instructed to palpate uterine activity and to detect increasing amounts of discharge or suprapubic pressure or low backache. Any increase would warrant further evaluation. On an outpatient basis, these patients may have weekly cervical assessments and be monitored very closely for any changes. Cervical changes detected in this way would warrant fetal monitoring for several hours to document any uterine activity. Observation or tocolysis could be instituted if uterine activity is noted. Prophylactically, patients who are at risk of premature labor should have nutritional counseling, anemias corrected, and refrain from smoking and possibly coitus, or, if that is not possible, use condoms to prevent the deposition of seminal prostaglandins in the vaginal vault. Urinary infections should be treated aggressively, and increased bed rest is advised, particularly with multiple gestations. Whether this group of high-risk patients benefits from prophylactic tocolysis is unclear, but Johnson et al. [5] have shown that in women with high risk of preterm delivery, weekly 17α-OH progesterone was associated with longer gestation than in untreated patients.

Candidates for Tocolysis

At the present time all patients with gestations of 20 to 37 weeks who demonstrate evidence of preterm labor that do not demonstrate the following contraindications are candidates for tocolysis: 1) fetal death, 2) chorioamniotis, 3) severe preeclampsia or eclampsia, 4) abruption or significant hemorrhage for an unknown source, 5) fetal distress except for

Table 3-1
Risk of Preterm Delivery*

Points	Socioeconomic status	Past history	Daily habits	Current pregnancy
1	2 children at home Low socioeconomic status	1 abortion Less than 1 year since last birth	Work outside home	Unusual fatigue
2	Younger than 20 years Older than 40 years Single parent	2 abortions	More than 10 cigarettes per day	Less than 13 kg gain by 32 weeks' gestation Albuminuria Hypertension Bacteriuria
3	Very low socioeconomic status Shorter than 150 cm Lighter than 45 kg	3 abortions	Heavy work Long tiring trip	Breech at 32 weeks Weight loss of 2 kg Head engaged Febrile illness
4	Younger than 18 years	Pyelonephritis		Metrorrhagia after 12 weeks' gestation Effacement Dilatation Uterine irritability
5		Uterine anomaly Second-trimester abortion DES exposure		Placenta previa Hydramnios
10		Premature delivery Repeated second-trimester abortion		Twins Abdominal surgery

* Score is computed by addition of the number of points given any item. 0–5 = low risk; 6–9 = medium risk; ≥ 10 = high risk. From Creasy, R.K., Gummer, B.A., Liggins, G.C. System for predicting spontaneous preterm birth. *Obstet. Gynecol.* 55:692–695, 1980. Reprinted with permission from the American College of Obstetricians and Gynecologists.

temporary intrauterine resuscitation from uterine hyperstimulation, and 6) congenital anomalies incompatible with life (i.e., anencephaly, renal agenesis).

Agents

There are several agents that are available for the control of uterine activity. They include the beta-agonists, magnesium sulfate, diazoxide, prostaglandin inhibitors, ethanol, and some newly tested calcium antagonists. The following discussion will be limited to the use of beta-agonist drugs and magnesium sulfate.

BETA-AGONIST DRUGS

Mechanism of Action   Beta-adrenergic agonists bind to receptors on the smooth muscle surface and activate formation of adenyl cyclase, the precursor of cyclic adenosine monophosphate. The resultant increase in intracellular cyclic adenosine monophosphate has several effects. It phosphorylates (inactivates) myosin kinase, the key enzyme in fusion of actin and myosin molecules. It also appears to decrease intracellular calcium by promoting storage in the sarcoplasmic reticulum. Cyclic adenosine monophosphate may also act by decreasing the number of gap junctions, which interferes with spread of electrical potential from muscle cell to muscle cell.

Beta-agonists work on two types of receptors (beta$_1$ and beta$_2$), which have different effects on metabolic function. The beta$_1$ receptors are primarily responsible for cardiac stimulation, increased bowel motility, and lipolysis.

Beta$_2$-receptors are primarily responsible for bronchodilatation, vasodilatation, decreased uterine contractility, increased renin, and increased glycogenolysis and insulin release. Associated effects also include increased antidiuretic hormone and aldosterone levels.

Toxicology   The side effects associated with the use of beta-agonists revolve around their many biochemical and metabolic effects. This may translate into clinical problems that may range from minimal maternal tachycardia and anxiousness to maternal death. The side effects that are of clinical importance are listed below: for beta$_1$, increased heart rate, increased stroke volume, and increased free fatty acids; for beta$_2$, decreased vascular tone, decreased detrusor tone, increased renin release, increased insulin, increased glucose, and increased water retention.

Kubli [6] has reported on over 55 cases of severe maternal morbidity with at least six deaths worldwide associated with the utilization of these drugs as tocolytics. The most common serious side effect is pulmonary edema, particularly with the adjuvant use of glucocorticoids to enhance fetal pulmonary lung maturity. this problem usually starts within hours of initiating tocolysis, but has occasionally been seen postpartum. The risk factors associated with the side effects of pulmonary edema include multiple gestation, positive fluid balance (ranging from 700 ml per 24 hours to 7,000 ml per 70 hours). It has been associated with all agents, and it has been associated with intravenous or subcutaneous administrtion. The etiology for the pulmonary edema is unclear, but it may involve increased water retention from increased antidiuretic hormone and aldosterone in these patients and may be exacerbated by the water-retaining properties of steroids. It may also result from exhaustion of the myocardium in a predamaged heart or from a rare case of beta-mimetic cardiomyopathy. Most of these patients respond to diuretics and conservative management. The six deaths reported so far have been in mothers with possible unsuspected underyling cardiac disease.

A widening of pulse pressures and slight hypotension can be noted. At the present time there have been no untoward fetal reactions with beta-agonist use. Occasionally, mild fetal tachycardia can be noted along with isolated reports of hypotension and hypoglycemia. Along with the general contraindications mentioned previously, specific contraindications to beta-agonist use include 1) uncontrolled diabetes mellitus, 2) severe hypovolemia, 3) hyperthyroidism, and 4) history of maternal cardiac disease or significant maternal arrhythmias.

Efficacy In almost all studies, the earlier the onset of treatment, the greater the success of achieving tocolysis. It is difficult to determine in some earlier reports whether the patient was in true or false labor, but recent data indicate that these drugs can be extremely successful, both in prevention of respiratory distress disease and perinatal death and promoting continuation of the pregnancy until term. Most series report a 80 to 90 percent success rate in postponing labor at least 48 to 72 hours, and Merkatz et al. [7] reported a 50 to 60 percent success rate in continuing the pregnancy to term.

Types Although several drugs are available worldwide, (salbutamol, fenoterol, orciprenaline, hexoprenaline), the drugs utilized most often in the United States are terbutaline and ritodrine hydrochloride. Ritodrine hydrochloride is approved by the Food and Drug Administration (1980) for use in suppression of preterm labor. Other drugs will undoubtedly emerge from some of the clinical trials that are presently being conducted in this country. The tocolytic differences among beta-agonist drugs have not been adequately studied to recommend one agent over the other. Hexoprenaline may be somewhat more beta$_2$ specific, but its superiority in a clinical study has not been demonstrated.

Administration   The initial clinical assessment of the patient who arrives for tocolysis involves a period of observation with recording the fetal heart tones and uterine activity. Vital signs are recorded frequently, and urine analysis, complete blood cell count, electrolytes, and glucose are obtained. This period allows time for proper evaluation to assure no contraindications exist and to determine whether true labor is present. In patients with uterine activity, but minimal or absent dilatation and effacement, this period of time may last for an hour or so. In many patients, uterine activity becomes irregular, no cervical change is noted, and the diagnosis of false labor is made. As a routine, this author hydrates patients with 500 to 700 cc of dextrose 5%/Ringer's lactate during this period of observation. This serves several functions. It may help correct dehydration and cause cessation of uterine activity (posterior pituitary effect?). It may act as a preload to these patients who may undergo sudden vasodilatation with expanded vascular capacity when beta-agonists are utilized. The patient who has advanced or progressive cervical dilatation and effacement (greater than 2 cm dilation or greater than 80 percent effacement or both) can be assumed to be in labor, and the assessment period may be eliminated except for hydration.

Dosages   Ritodrine hydrochloride (150 mg) is administered with an Imed or Ivac pump; three ampules of ritodrine hydrochloride are added to 485 cc of D5W (concentration = 0.3 mg/cc). The initial infusion is 15 μg/minute with increases of 50 μg/10 minutes until adequate uterine relaxation occurs (1 contraction every 30 minutes). This effective dose is continued for 12 hours. Maximum dosage level is 350 μg/minute and should be maintained for only 30 minutes. One tablet (10 mg) is given 30 minutes before termination of effective dose and then every 2 hours for 24 hours (12 doses). At this point in time, 20 mg four times a day followed by 10 mg four times a day can be given. Treatment is continued until 37 weeks.

Monitoring Side Effects   1) A thorough history is taken and a physical examination is made to detect any evidence or suspicion of maternal cardiac disease. 2) A maternal electrocardiogram is performed if arrhythmias are noted. 3) Vital signs are taken every 10 minutes during the infusion to detect any significant hypotension or significant tachycardia. 4) K^+ is determined because of the association of hypokalemia with use of the beta-agonists. 5) Blood glucose is determined initially and serially to note any change that may occur. With diabetic patients if the beta-agonists are utilized the blood glucose should be monitored frequently (every 2 hours) until glucose stabilizes. 6) Careful fluid management is essential, positive fluid balance is avoided, particularly after glucocorticoid use.

Routine use of central venous pressure monitoring has been suggested in these patients, but is mandatory with excessive volume expansion (i.e., blood transfusion or extreme positive fluid balance). With evidence of elevated central venous pressure (greater than 12 cm) cessation of fluid and beta-agonist should occur until the central venous pressure returns to normal range (less than 6 cm). With evidence of pulmonary edema, diuretics and oxygen supplementation should be utilized. The presence of chest pain should lead to the cessation of all beta-agonists, and an electrocardiogram should be obtained.

MAGNESIUM SULFATE

Mechanism of Action   Although the mechanism by which tocolysis is achieved with magnesium sulfate is not precisely known, it is unlikely that the effect is mediated at neural muscular junction with inhibition of acetylcholine release, as occurs with striated muscle. The effect on smooth muscle is a direct effect on the myometrial cell itself. Magnesium is most probably related to calcium antagonism and may make it less available at an intracellular level.

Toxicology   Magnesium sulfate is almost entirely eliminated through the kidneys. If no renal impairment exists, the kidneys can easily handle the dosages of the medication utilized for tocolysis. With renal impairment, toxic levels greater than 10 μg/ml can be achieved. These side effects include loss of deep tendon reflexes and respiratory depression. Cardiac arrest can be seen with high magnesium levels (>15 to 20 μg/ml). $MgSO_4$ can also potentiate the effects of succinylcholine, and this should be kept in mind if the patient must undergo general anesthesia. Pulmonary edema has been reported with its use. Fetal side effects include decreased variability on fetal heart tracing that can lead to misinterpretation. Neonatal effects include hypotonia, decreased gut motility, and hypocalcemia.

Efficacy   In one study by Steer and Petrie [8] with success defined as 24 hours of tocolysis, $MgSO_4$ was 77 percent successful. Nochimson et al. [9] and Kiss and Szöke [10] have reported success rates of 70 to 90 percent, depending on when tocolysis was initiated in relation to cervical dilatation and effacement and the status of the membranes (intact or ruptured).

Administration Assessment   As with beta-agonist drugs a period of observation with hydration should be utilized if the diagnosis of preterm labor is in question. Baseline information regarding maternal blood pressure, pulse, and uterine activity and fetal heart rate variability should be obtained before the initiation of tocolysis with magnesium sulfate. Baseline laboratory work should include blood urea nitrogen, creatinine, urine analysis, complete blood cell count, and electrolytes.

Dosage   The loading dose is 6 g (60 ml of a 10% $MgSO_4$ solution) over a 20-minute interval. The titration dose is 2 g (200 ml of a 10 percent solution added to 800 cc of Ringers lactate) at 100 cc/hour. Maintenance, once contractions are reduced in frequency and intensity (less than 1/30 minutes) to 1 g/hour. To achieve this, 10 ml of a 10 percent MgSO$_4$ solution is added to 800 cc of fluid at 100 cc/hour. The duration of treatment is affective; tocolysis is continued to 48 to 72 hours.

Monitoring Side Effects 1) Check magnesium levels. 2) Check vital signs every 15 minutes. 3) Discontinue drug if cervical dilatation is greater than 5 cm because it is usually ineffective in this advanced stage of labor. This discontinuance at this point will also allow fetal blood levels to diminish so that neonatal side effects will be minimized. 4) Watch for pulmonary edema. 5) Reduce dosage of succinylcholine. 6) Neonatal hypocalcemia and hypermagnemia may be reversed with calcium gluconate.

Special Considerations: IUGR Versus the Preterm Low-Birth-Weight Infant In the diagnosis of preterm gestation the determination of gestational age is believed to be less than 37 weeks. Pregnancy dating information such as last menstrual period, last normal menstrual period, uterine size on the first visit, date of positive pregnancy test, fetoscopic detection of fetal heart tones, and uterine fundal growth, and ultrasound (crown rump, length, femur length, BPD, and so on), can be extremely helpful in the determination of gestational age. If early data are not available or the patient presents late in prenatal care or in labor and delivery, determination of gestational age is more difficult. A woman with little dating information who presents in labor with a fundal height of 30 cm may represent a preterm gestation of 28 to 32 weeks or a growth-retarded 37-week gestation. Distinguishing between the two conditions becomes important in management decisions (i.e., tocolysis or no tocolysis). In these cases it is better to halt labor if possible until more thorough ultrasound can be performed utilizing head circumference, abdominal circumference, and so on to answer the question. The use of a lecithin/sphingomyelin ratio to assess the status of pulmonary lung maturity may also be entertained. Occasionally the issue of symmetrical growth retardation versus early gestation arises. Under these circumstances, unless serial ultrasound is performed, it is very difficult to determine whether one is dealing with a preterm low-birth-weight infant or a symmetrically growth-retarded infant.

Labor Patterns In Preterm Gestation

Data from Friedman [11] suggest that there are two populations of patients with regard to labor patterns in preterm gestation: those with an accelerative active phase (primarily nulliparous) and those with dysfunctional labor patterns (most commonly multiparous). The dysfunctional pattern seen most often with preterm labor is prolonged latent phase, protraction, or arrest disorders. These dysfunctional patterns are 12 times more likely in these preterm multiparous patients than in term gestation and are related to birth weight. Whether these disorders are secondary for relative cervical unripeness is unclear. Despite these dysfunctional patterns no greater ill effects can be seen in these infants as long as no evidence of fetal hypoxia with direct fetal monitoring exists, and patience is key in management. Although the issue of oxytocin augmentation and its role in increasing neonatal hyperbilirubinemia is not resolved, oxytocin is not contraindicated as long as a uterine pressure catheter is in place preventing hyperstimulation. If, however, inadequate uterine activity does not resolve with augmentation over 2 to 3 hours or if despite adequate uterine activity no progress in labor is noted over several hours, it seems prudent to move to cesarean section.

The Preterm Breech

The problem of breech presentation in preterm labor is a common one since up to 25 to 33 percent of gestations less than 32 weeks present at breech.

The increased mortality and morbidity for the preterm breech is due to several factors, including an added risk of perinatal asphyxia from birth trauma, prolapsed cord, or both as well as an increased likelihood of congenital anomalies. The issue of importance of mode of delivery and whether it can alter outcome is not resolved.

Several retrospective analyses including those of DeCrespigny and Pepperell [12] and Goldenberg and Nelson [13], indicate a three to fourfold increase in perinatal mortality in vaginal preterm breech delivery when compared with either vaginal preterm vertex delivery or preterm breech delivery via cesarean section. In a paired controlled study, Duenhoelter et al. [14] found a significant increase in morbidity and mortality associated with preterm breech vaginal delivery. Gimovsky and Petrie [15], in an attempt to see whether application of selective criteria for vaginal preterm breech delivery could alter the poorer outcome, found no significant differences between protocol and nonprotocol groups and recommended more liberal use of cesarean section. Karp et al. [16] could only substantiate the benefit of abdominal delivery in low-birth-weight infants (1,000 to 1,500 g) that presented as footling breeches.

Although the definitive answer from a carefully controlled prospective study is not yet available, the weight of retrospective analysis is in favor of abdominal delivery in the preterm breech infant.

The Preterm Vertex

Even more controversial is the issue of method of delivery when the preterm infant presents as a vertex. Smith et al. [17], studying the effect of mode of delivery on low-birth-weight infants (750 to 1,000 g) survival found a 35 percent survival rate in the vaginal delivery group compared with 80 percent in the abdominal delivery group. Unfortunately, this was not a well-controlled retrospective analysis. Similar data were reported by Bowes [18] in his analysis of perinatal outcome at the University of Colorado. Bejar et al. [19] have reported that the incidence of intraventricular hemorrhage was significantly higher in low-birth-weight infants whether breech or vertex when labor had occurred than when elective abdominal delivery was the mode of delivery.

Despite this indication of the possibility of improved outcome with abdominal delivery, no-well controlled prospective study utilizing intensive fetal monitoring and liberal use of cesarean section when signs of hypoxia occur, has been done. Until there are more definitive answers as to the role of delivery method, the preterm vertex infant can be continued to be delivered vaginally with direct fetal monitoring and avoidance of hypoxia.

Fetal Monitoring

Fetal monitoring of preterm infants has been shown to be predictive of fetal hypoxia, and continuous fetal monitoring appears to increase the likelihood of more favorable outcome. In a review of 61 preterm infants, Bowes et al. [20] suggested that decreased variability and late decelerations can be utilized as indexes of perinatal asphyxia.

Conduct of Labor

The choice of proper analgesia and anesthesia depends not only on the issue of the preterm gestation, but also any associated obstetrical conditions that may be associated with the preterm labor (i.e., abruptio placenta, eclampsia, and so on). The preterm fetus or neonate is more susceptible to the depressant effects of transplacental acquired anesthesia and analgesia agents because of 1) less protein available for drug binding, 2) higher bilirubin levels that compete for drug-binding protein, 3) poorly developed blood-brain barrier with increasing central nervous system concentrations of drugs, 4) greater body water content with decreased body fat, and 5) decreased ability to metabolize and excrete drugs. These factors can augment the drug effect on the fetus or neonate. Analgesic drugs, therefore, should be utilized at the least effective dose. Timing of analgesic administration may be important since intravenous injection at the upward slope of a contraction (decreased placental perfusion) probably leads to decreased initial first-pass uptake by the fetus. Analgesic drugs may be used in moderation when necessary.

The choice of anesthesia (epidural, spinal pudendal or local) depends on the clinical situation as well as concerns about reducing trauma to the preterm vertex. In a normovolemic, healthy gravida, epidural anesthesia offers the advantages of relief of first-stage pain (therefore less systemic analgesia) as well as providing for a relaxed perineum for the prevention of fetal head trauma.

Artificial rupture of the membranes should probably be delayed until the vertex is presenting to help cushion the fetal head and help out as an effective dilating wedge for cervical dilatation. The use of low forceps has been advocated by Bishop et al. [21], but probably offers no real advantage if delivery of the head can be controlled.

References

1. Kaltreider, D.F., Kohe, S. Epidemiology of preterm delivery. *Clin. Obstet. Gynecol.* 23:17, 1980.
2. Kaminski, M., Papiernik, E. Multifactorial study of the risk of prematurity at 32 weeks of gestation. II. A comparison between an empirical prediction and a discriminant. *J. Perinat. Med.* 2:30–36, 1974.
3. Fredrick, J. Antenatal identification of women at high risk of spontaneous preterm labor. *Br. J. Obstet. Gynaecol.* 83:351, 1976.
4. Creasy, R.K., Gummer, B.A., Liggins, G.C. System for predicting spontaneous preterm birth. *Obstet. Gynecol.* 55:692–695, 1980.
5. Johnson, J.W.C., Austin, K.L., Jones, G.C., et al. Efficacy of 17 hydroxy progesterone caprate in the prevention of premature labor. *N. Engl. J. Med.* 293:675, 1981.
6. Kubli, F. Data presented at symposium of perinatal medicine—San Francisco, Calif. August, 1981.
7. Merkatz, I.R., Peter, J.B., Barden, T.P. Ritodrine hydrochloride. A beta–mimetic agent for use in preterm labor. II. Evidence of Efficacy. *Obstet. Gynecol.* 56:7, 1980.
8. Steer, C.M., Petrie, R.H. A comparison of magnesium sulfate and alcohol for the prevention of premature labor. *Am. J. Obstet. Gynecol.* 129:1, 1977.
9. Nochimson, D.J., Petrie, R.H., Shah, B.L., et al. Comparison of conservative and dynamic management of premature rupture of membranes/premature labor syndrome: new approaches to the delivery of infants which may minimize the need for intensive care. *Clin. Perinatol.* 7:17–31, 1980.
10. Kiss, V.D., Szoke, B. Rolle Des Magnesiums Bei der Verhutung der Fruhgeburt. *Zentralbl. Gunakol.* 97:924, 1975.
11. Friedman, E.A. Fetal factors in labor: clinical evaluation and management, 2nd ed. New York: Appleton-Century–Crofts, 1978, p. 160.
12. DeCrespigny, L.S., Pepperell, R.J. Perinatal mortality and morbidity in breech presentation. *Obstet. Gynecol.* 53:141, 1976.
13. Goldenberg, R.L., Nelson, K.G. The premature breech. *Am. J. Obstet. Gynecol.* 127:240, 1977.
14. Duenhoelter, J.H., Wells, E., Reisch, J.S., et al. A paired controlled study of vaginal and abdominal delivery of the low birth weight breech fetus. *Obstet. Gynecol.* 54:310, 1979.

15. Gimovsky, M.L., Petrie, R.H. The intrapartum and neonatal performance of the low birth weight vaginal breech delivery. *J. Reprod. Med.* 27:451–454, 1982.

16. Karp, L.E., Doney, J.R., McCarthy, T., et al. The premature breech. Trial of labor or ceserean section. *Obstet. Gynecol.* 53:88, 1979.

17. Smith, M.L., Spence, S.A., Hull, D. Mode of delivery and survival in babies weighing less than 2000 gms at birth. *Br. Med. J.* 281:118, 1980.

18. Bowes, W.A. Delivery of the very low birth weight infant. *Clin. Perinatol.* 8:183–193, 1981.

19. Bejar, R., Curbelo, V., Coen, R., et al. Large intraventricular hemorrhage (IVH) and labor in infants ≥ 1000 gm. *Pediatr. Res.* 1:649, 1981.

20. Bowes, W.A., Gabbe, S.G., Bowes, C. Fetal heart rate monitoring in premature infants weighing 1500 gm. or less. *Am. J. Obstet. Gynecol.* 137:791, 1980.

21. Bishop, E.H., Israel, S.L., Briscoe, C.C. Obstetrics influence on the preterm infant's first year of development. *Obstet. Gynecol.* 26:628, 1965.

4

Which Position in Labor?

Joyce Roberts, C.N.M., Ph.D., F.A.A.N., and Carlos
Mendez-Bauer, M.D., Ph.D.

The issue of which position to use during labor has captured renewed interest within the last 15 years. However, it is an old issue in the practice of obstetrics. Before the development of obstetrical aids to assist with difficult labor or birth, and currently where obstetrical interventions are not readily available, maternal postures and delivery positions are important considerations. Englemann [1], Naroll et al. [2], and Atwood [3] describe the wide variety of positions used during labor and for delivery. They emphasize the predominant use of upright positions in more primitive and non-Western societies before obstetrical techniques were developed that can be accomplished more easily with women in a recumbent position. Upright positions include standing or walking, sitting, squatting, and kneeling. Neutral or recumbent positions include lateral, prone, semirecumbent, dorsal, lithotomy, exaggerated lithotomy, and hanging leg (or Walcher's) position.

Presumably, the factors influencing the selection of particular positions were those related to maternal comfort and accomplishment of delivery. Russell describes the dimensions of the birth canal that are altered (enlarged) with maternal posture [4–6]. For example, the uncomfortable, and essentially intolerable, Walcher's position pulls the pelvic girdle forward from the sacrum and increases the anteroposterior diameter of the inlet. The squatting position is accompanied by an increase in both the transverse and anteroposterior diameter of the outlet, as documented by several clinical investigators [7–10]. The exaggerated lithotomy position achieves this advantage of squatting when the parturient's legs are flexed toward her abdomen [11]. Although squatting is generally associated with birth, it is also advocated during labor to aid in fetal alignment with the pelvis and descent [10,12].

Although there is a valid basis for some of the positions used in the past to promote labor or accomplish delivery, it would be inappropriate to advocate a return to primitive practices. Some, in fact, were quite barbaric. These included suspending the pregnant woman from trees, posts, or an upright table, tossing her in a blanket, standing on her back, and, to a lesser extreme, fundal massage. A 1891 review of the various positions used during labor by Clarke [13] included this observation:

> Inquiry into the purpose for which any of the positions which women have from time to time assumed while in labor will show that the choice has been made more from the force of custom, from caprice, ignorance, and from a blind submission to authority exercised by those who make unwarrantable pretensions to skill in midwifery than from knowledge deducted from facts gained by careful study and close observation.

To a certain extent this might also be said about some of our contemporary practices.

During the early part of this century there was another clinician who expressed concern about maternal position during labor. This physician also sounds like a contemporary practitioner because his criticisms are directed toward the increasing use of recumbency at that time. In a paper published in the *New York Medical Journal* in 1909, King [12] states:

> My chief contention is that the recumbent posture during labor is much overdone, that it is often persisted in either by custom or by direct order of the obstetrician when it does positive harm by prolonging labor, by exhausting the woman, and sometimes leading to the persistence of faulty presentations as well as increasing the duration and the intensity of the woman's sufferings [12].

Englemann [1], King [12], Clarke [13], Jarcho [11], and many contemporary practitioners [13–23] have advocated changing positions or moving about during labor. It is often thought that a woman will naturally select the best position for her labor [24,25]. It has also been proposed that we study the influence of various positions on labor by just letting women do what they want to do and observe the result. This "natural experiment," however, has already been conducted. It is reported in the *Medical Times and Gazette* of 1857. Rigby [26] recorded his review of historical documents, travels to various countries, and observations of labors where unassisted women could take any positions they chose. This is his conclusion: a woman's behavior and position "will, in great measure be guided by the arrangements which are made for her confinement, and she will assume that posture for which they are specially adapted."

49

This is essentially where we are today. Modern obstetrical interventions, such as sedation, analgesia, intravenous fluid administration, and electronic fetal monitoring along with hospitalization have contributed to the care of laboring women in bed [27–30]. More recent changes in the arrangements made for birth reflected in the development of birth rooms or birthing centers allow greater flexibility in the conduct of labor and delivery. In response to consumers' and professionals' complaints that obstetrical intervention and, more specially, confinement to bed were adversely affecting the birth process, birth rooms or alternative birthing centers allow women who do not require obstetrical intervention to labor in a place that permits freedom of movement as well as access to care as needed. The questions remain: ''How can maternal position be used to facilitate labor?'' and, ''Which position is best?''

Clinical Phenomena Related to Maternal Position

As indicated above, the initial studies about maternal position and childbirth were cross-cultural and historical analyses describing the wide variation of positions used as well as a preference for upright positions [1,3,4,29,30]. In addition, individual clinicians have described the merits of specific positions based on their own experience. For example, King [12] advocated squatting, kneeling, and sitting in a rocking chair; Markoe [31] endorsed sitting and designed a special obstetric chair; Leak [32] and, more recently, Irwin [33] favored the left lateral position in opposition to the lithotomy position; McAuliffe [34] made a case for the prone position, maintaining that it increased the anteroposterior diameter of the abdomen and was more comfortable for women; and Blankfield [35] proposed that the dorsal recumbent position with raised head and shoulders facilitated engagement of the fetal head.

It was not until technology permitted the measurement of physiologic parameters that the effects of maternal position on maternal hemodynamics, uterine contractions, and fetal oxygenation were recognized. The clinical studies since the middle of the twentieth century have used this modern technology to describe the influence of maternal position on cardiac output [36,37] and intraabdominal pressure [38] and compare the effects of different positions, particularly lateral recumbency with supine recumbency. Next, maternal position was shown to influence the nature of uterine contractions; most recently, the upright and recumbent positions have been contrasted during labor.

MATERNAL HEMODYNAMICS

The main criticism regarding recumbent positions in labor has been directed toward the adverse hemodynamic effects of supine recumbency.

Fainting in the supine position was first described by Hanssen in 1942 [39]. Since then, several investigators have documented the compression of the inferior vena cava [40–43] and the descending aorta [44,45] by the gravid uterus. Vena caval recompression is accompanied by reduced venous return and cardiac output and subsequent blood pressure, pulse, and symptomatic changes in the woman. These are relieved with uterine contractions as the uterus lifts off the vena cava [45–47]. In contrast, aortic compression is not accompanied by brachial blood pressure or pulse changes or any maternal symptoms, and it is augmented by uterine contractions as well as by maternal bearing down efforts [44,47,48]. In the absence of maternal signs or symptoms, uterine perfusion may be reduced as a result of aortic compression and not be recognized until the fetus is in distress. Simply turning onto her side alleviates these adverse hemodynamic alterations for the expectant mother.

Positions other than the supine and lateral are also accompanied by significant hemodynamic changes. It is thought by some that the lithotomy position with the legs elevated overcomes the reduction in venous return in the supine position by promoting return of blood from the lower extremities. However, in contrast to an expected increase in cardiac output in the lithotomy position, Vorys et al. [37] consistently found a decrease. They attributed this to an increased dorsal direction of force by the gravid uterus on the inferior vena cava. Therefore, the lithotomy position augments and does not overcome the adverse hemodynamic effects of supine recumbency. In addition, the 45 degree Trendelenburg position was accompanied by a decrease in cardiac output that was similar to that in the lithotomy position. It is still common practice to elevate the lower extremities of people in shock. This is believed to increase venous return and cardiac output. This objective, however, will not be accomplished for a woman who is pregnant. In full-term pregnancy the opposite, a reduction in cardiac output, will result unless the gravida is turned on her side. In the left lateral Trendelenburg inclination cardiac output increased to the same extent as in the left side positions [37]. Therefore, when there is a need to increase cardiac output, as in shock or fetal distress, the lateral position will accomplish that effect, whereas the supine, lithotomy, or supine Trendelenburg position will result in a decrease.

FETAL CONDITION

These hemodynamic changes are accompanied by altered placental perfusion [44,49]. Compromised fetal status manifested by fetal heart rate deceleration, bradycardia, or acidosis [50–52] may occur in the supine and lithotomy positions. For this reason, it has become standard practice to encourage the pregnant woman to lie on her side rather than on her back [51].

51

UTERINE CONTRACTIONS

It is also well recognized that maternal position influences the quality of uterine contractions. This was first documented by Williams [53] in 1952, who also described earlier work by Stallworthy. They developed a simple method of internal tocography, and noticed that when the parturient sat up the contractions were more intense than when she had been on her back. They attributed this change to a better application of the fetal presenting part to the cervix. In 1957 Turnbull [54] noticed that when the parturient was on either her right or left side contractions were stronger, but less frequent, than when she lay flat on her back. Since then, this effect of lateral versus supine recumbency on uterine contractions has been documented by several clinical investigators [55–58]. Therefore, the lateral recumbent position seems advantageous not only because of the avoidance of maternal hemodynamic and fetal compromise, but also because of the improved quality of uterine contractions that may be a result of more adequate uterine perfusion. It is also thought that women are more comfortable resting on their sides rather than on their backs, although this variable was not systematically addressed in these initial studies that focused on hemodynamics or uterine contractility.

LABOR PROGRESS

Along with maternal comfort and, more recently, fetal condition, labor progression has been the major consideration in the use of a particular maternal position. Those practitioners who have advocated a specific position have thought that it favored good uterine action and improved or promoted desirable labor progress. Until recently the assessment of labor progress had been a subjective comparison among alternative approaches. More specific criteria included the incidence of spontaneous versus operative births [31] and the duration of the stages of labor. Most recently, standards have been developed to quantify the efficiency of uterine action and make more objective comparisons among maternal positions [59–69].

Although birth outcome is the major overall consideration, especially in conjunction with the conduct of the second stage of labor, labor progression is the critical dimension of the first stage of labor. The more recent research that is reviewed and reported here focuses on the first stage of labor and how it is influenced by maternal position.

Clinical Studies of Maternal Position During Labor

The cross-cultural and descriptive studies done before controlled clinical comparisons indicated that upright positions were more favorable for "hastening" dilatation and promoting fetal descent. Contemporary researchers have examined the benefits of upright positions further.

CONTROLLED COMPARISONS

In accordance with the standard research design for clinical trials, the initial experimental studies established control and experimental groups using random assignment. The earliest experimental studies were a comparison of the general categories of upright versus recumbent positions followed by those that compared ambulation with recumbency. The specific features of those studies are reviewed elsewhere [59] and will be summarized here.

Upright Versus Recumbent   The upright positions used in several studies comparing any upright position with lateral or supine recumbency included a semirecumbent ("proposed" or "semiupright") position in bed along with walking and sitting [60–63]. The results are mixed, with Chan [60] and McManus and Calder [63] reporting "no difference" between the groups and "no advantage" to the upright positions. In contrast Liu [61] and Mitre [62] found significantly shorter labors in their semiupright groups. The difference in these results may be attributed to the variation in the positions that were compared. Whereas Mitre and Liu required that the women in the recumbent groups remain in a supine position, Chan allowed the women in the recumbent group to lie in either a lateral or supine position, and McManus and Calder required the women in their recumbent group to lie on their sides. Thus, there was a combination of recumbent as well as upright positions used.

Ambulation Versus Recumbency   Other studies have specifically compared walking and periods of standing or sitting with recumbency in bed [64–67]. Diaz et al. [64] and Flynn et al. [66,67] reported significant advantages for the fetus, increased comfort for the women, and a shorter duration of labor. In addition, Flynn et al. [66,67] incorporated telemetry to combined continuous fetal monitoring with ambulation. In contrast, Williams et al. [65] found no difference in the length of the stages of labor, mode of delivery, or the incidence of fetal distress. However, 87.5 percent of the ambulant patients in their study asked to return to bed in the early active phase of labor, which may have minimized the benefits of ambulation.

Another recent randomized trial by Read et al. [68] compared ambulation with recumbency and the use of oxytocin for augmenting dysfunctional labor. Women with arrested active labor were randomly assigned to either an ambulation or a recumbent, oxytocin group. Labor progress was slightly, but not significantly, better in the ambulatory group. Therefore, ambulation may be an alternative to oxytocin to promote adequate labor progress.

53

The lack of agreement among these studies reflects the influence of confounding variables, such as the use of oxytocin or anesthesia [63], in some of the groups. It also reflects the variation in the maternal positions used. In addition, some of the investigators reported that it was difficult for women to maintain a constant position throughout labor or even to remain consistently upright [60,65]. For these reasons, another approach was used by us to examine and compare the effect of specific maternal positions.

Subject as Own Control   A research design with the subject as her own control overcomes some of the limitations of the control-experimental group research design by controlling the individual obstetrical variables that can influence the dependent outcome variables that are affected by maternal position. By asking women to alternate, at 30-minute intervals, between two specific positions, the resulting changes in the quality of contractions, labor progress, comfort, and fetal status may be interpreted as an effect of the position used, since all of the other individual and obstetrical variables remain the same in women in both positions. In addition, the parturient was not required to maintain one position but, instead, offered her impression of the two positions she was using. This design required fewer subjects to achieve statistically valid results since the variability within subjects was controlled.

The single-subject design was first used by Mendez-Bauer et al. [69,70] with 20 subjects to compare standing with the supine position. This study was the first in a series of studies contrasting specific maternal positions during the first stage of labor.

Comparisons of Specific Positions

Several institutions have participated in a collaborative study to provide comparable scientific data regarding the advantages and disadvantages of different positions during labor. The single-subject research design described above was used in all of the study sites, which included maternity centers in Madrid; Freiburg, Germany; and Chicago [70].

The purpose of this series of contrasts was to compare the influence of the following pairs of positions on uterine contractions, labor progress, maternal comfort and fetal heart rate: standing versus supine, standing versus sitting, supine versus sitting, side versus sitting, and side versus supine.

SUBJECTS

The five contrasts included a total of 93 essentially healthy nullipara, with 11 to 23 subjects in each contrast. They were invited to participate in the study when they were admitted to the hospital in early spontaneous labor at term. The first position used was determined by random assignment. The women were asked to alternate between two positions at 30-minute intervals throughout the first stage of labor. They were allowed to discontinue alternating between positions when it was no longer comfortable for them to do so or when any medications or care was indicated. No drugs were administered to the participants before or during the period of data collection.

MONITORING

The dependent variables of uterine contractions, fetal heart rate, labor progress, and maternal comfort were assessed continuously or with each position change.

Intrauterine pressure was measured by means of transcervical open-ended, water-filled catheter introduced into the uterus. The catheter was attached to a pressure transducer placed on the highest part of the fundus to ensure a stable and valid intrauterine pressure baseline as the woman changed positions (Figure 4–1). An extra long transducer cord was used to enable the woman to easily move from the bed to sit in a chair and change positions. The advantages of this technique are published elsewhere [71].

Figure 4–1

Monitoring of Intrauterine Pressure with Abdominal Placement of Pressure Transducer. (*From Roberts, J., Malasanos, L., Mendez-Bauer, C. Maternal positions in labor: Analysis in relation to comfort and efficiency. In: Lederman, P., Raff, B. (eds.)* Perinatal Parental Behavior: Nursing Research and Implications for Newborn Health, New York: Alan R. Liss, 1981. Copyright 1981 by the March of Dimes Birth Defects Foundation and reprinted with permission.)

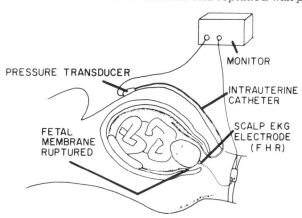

Table 4–1

Measurements of Uterine Contractions

Variable	Unit	Measure
Intensity	mmHg	From baseline tonus to peak pressure
Frequency	Number of contractions per 10 minutes	From peak to peak of contractions, calculated for 10 minutes
Uterine activity	Montevideo units	Intensity $\times$ frequency
Uterine efficiency	Madrid units[a] [73,74]	$\dfrac{\Delta \text{ dilatation (cm)}}{\text{uterine work}^{b}} \times 10^{5}$

[a] Formula from references 73 and 74.
[b] Uterine work is the sum of the intensities of all uterine contractions for a given period of time.

Cervical dilatation was assessed at the onset of the study and after each 30-minute period by vaginal examination done by the same clinical investigator. This clinical assessment was simultaneously verified with calibrated measuring forces. This procedure proved to greatly enhance the accuracy of the routine clinical evaluation of cervical dilatation.

Data collection began after uterine and fetal monitoring was established. The units and measurement of the variables related to uterine contractility are summarized in Table 4–1.

Fetal heart rate was determined from an electrocardiogram signal that was obtained by placing an electrode on the fetal scalp when the membranes were ruptured.

The woman's perception of contractions, comfort and discomfort, location of sensation with contractions, and fatigue were assessed with each position change. Two raters independently recorded the woman's responses on a rating check list. The percent agreement between the two ratings were greater than 88 percent on all the items.

RESULTS

The results are summarized for uterine contractility and efficiency, maternal comfort, and position preference in Table 4–2. Means were compared by either paired t-tests or two-way analysis of variance. Position preference was compared by contingency analysis.

Uterine Contractions The contraction frequency and intensity for a specific position were relatively similar among the contrasted positions. For example, the intensity of contractions in the sitting position was 31.75 mmHg when contrasted with the side position, and 31.06 mmHg when

Table 4-2

Influence of Different Positions on Uterine Contractions and Labor[a]

	Supine-Standing n = 20		Supine-Sitting n = 23		Standing-Sitting n = 20		Sitting-Side n = 19		Supine-Side n = 11	
Intensity (mmHg)	31[b]	41	30	34	35	31	32[b]	39	38[b]	47
Frequency (n/10 min)	4.4	4.2	4.2	4.1	4.3	4.4	3.4[b]	2.9	4.2[b]	3.6
Uterine Activity (Montevideo Units)	129[b]	160	122	129	146	123	98[b]	108	153	160
Uterine Efficiency (Madrid Units; n = times in each position	160[b] 274 (n = 17)[c] n = 65[d] n = 64		122 227 (n = 20)		364 285 (n = 20) n = 41 n = 39		175[b] 311 (n = 18) n = 37 n = 42		309 234 (n = 11) n = 22 n = 25	
Duration (3 to 10 cm)	3 h 55 min		5 h 30 min		3 h 31 min		7 h 21 min		5 h 24 min	
Most comfort or preferred position	+		+		+		+ (early 1st stage) + (late 1st stage)		No significant difference	

[a] Numbers are mean values.
[b] P < 0.05.
[c] Number of subjects per study.
[d] Number of times the subject was in each position.

contrasted with standing. The intensity of contractions was greastest in the standing and side positions and lowest in the supine and sitting positions. In contrast, contraction frequency was greatest in the supine and sitting positions and least on the side. Contraction intensity and frequency were significantly different $(P < 0.05)$ in the comparisons of the sitting and side positions and of the supine position with the side. Contractions on the side were stronger and less frequent. When standing, contractions were significantly more intense than supine, but there was no difference in contraction frequency. There was no difference in contraction frequency and intensity between the supine and sitting positions or between the sitting and standing positions (Table 4–2).

Labor Progress When subjects serve as their own control and alternate between positions it is not possible to compare the overall duration of labor. In looking at the mean duration of labor from 3 to 10 cm in the contrasted positions, none exceeded the mean duration reported by Cibils [72] for the active portion of labor for nullipara. However, the mean duration of labor in these contrasts, which included the standing position, was more similar to that for multipara, by Cibil's standard, than to that for nullipara.

This design enabled the comparison of the ability of the uterine contractions to accomplish cervical dilatation in the contrasted positions. Uterine efficiency was determined for each 30-minute period, and the mean efficiency was calculated for each position (Table 4–2). Uterine efficiency is a numerical evaluation of the ability of uterine contractions to dilate the cervix for a given period of time. The modified formula [73–75] used to calculate uterine efficiency is shown in Table 4–1. Uterine efficiency is greatest in the standing position and least in the supine position. However, the efficiency of a specific position seemed to be related to the position with which it was compared. For example, the efficiency of the sitting position is significantly less than that of the side position. In the contrast with the supine position, the efficiency of the sittting position was greater (Figure 4–2). It was also noted that the efficiency of uterine contractions was greater in late labor (from 6 to 10 cm) than in early labor (2 to 5.5 cm) in all comparisons. Significant differences $(P < 0.01)$ were found in uterine efficiency between the side and sitting, sitting and supine, and standing and supine positions (Figure 4–2). Contractions were most efficient standing and on the side. Uterine efficiency was least in the supine and sitting positions in early labor.

Fetal Heart Rate The fetal heart rate was examined for the incidence of decelerations with uterine contractions. The decelerations were classified as early decelerations (type I dips), late decelerations (type II dips), and variable decelerations (type I + II). The question addressed in these studies was whether the incidence of fetal heart rate decelerations (number

Figure 4–2

Uterine Efficiency in Different Positions.

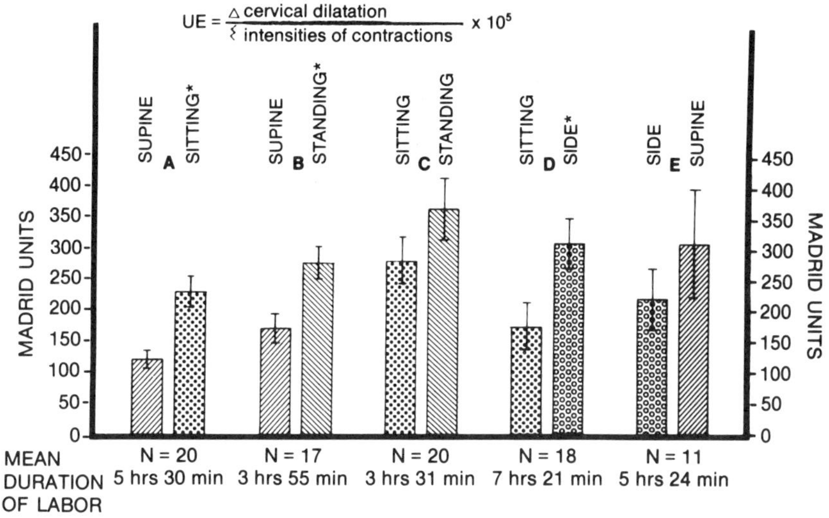

$$UE = \frac{\triangle \text{ cervical dilatation}}{\text{⨋ intensities of contractions}} \times 10^5$$

MEAN
DURATION
OF LABOR

	N = 20	N = 17	N = 20	N = 18	N = 11
	5 hrs 30 min	3 hrs 55 min	3 hrs 31 min	7 hrs 21 min	5 hrs 24 min

*p < 0.01 (paired t test)

of decelerations per number of contractions) was associated with maternal position.

The results showed no association, since similar incidences of early, late, and variable decelerations were recorded in any position.

Maternal Comfort   The reports of the women indicated that they were more comfortable standing or sitting then lying on their back, and they preferred sitting to standing. In the contrast between the side position and sitting there was a significant change in the parturient's preference from early to late labor (Table 4–3). In early labor most of the women preferred sitting. In late labor, after 5.5 cm, they preferred to lie on their sides. For the entire first stage of labor there was no significant difference in the women's preference for lying on their sides, compared to their backs when they alternated between these two positions.

Discussion and Conclusion

The purpose of the series of five studies was to contrast the effects of different maternal positons on major aspects of the first stage of labor [59,70]. In addition, we sought to identify which positions provided advantages or disadvantages to the laboring woman. Based on historical and

59

Table 4–3
Contingency Analysis of Maternal Position
Preference in Early and Late Labor

Preferred position	Early Labor ($<$ 6 cm)	Late Labor ($\geq$ 6 cm)	Totals
Side	7 (10.5)[a]	14 (10.5)	21
Sitting	12 (10.5)	5 (8.5)	17
Totals	19	19	38

[a] Numbers within parentheses are expected values.
$P < 0.05$, $\chi^2_{(1)} = 5.22$.

cross-cultural analyses, upright positions were favored, although clinical studies have not been consistent in their endorsement of the upright positions.

In this series, the standing position and the lateral recumbent position were accompanied by the most intense, least frequent, and most efficient uterine contractions. The lateral recumbent position was found to be more efficient than the upright sitting position, particularly in early labor. This may explain the results of the studies of McManus and Calder [63], Chan [60], and Williams et al. [65], who reported no advantage to the upright position. In those studies the recumbent position used was the lateral position.

The standing position is accompanied by mechanical and gravitational and hemodynamic advantages that may augment uterine contractions and cervical dilatation [73]. The lateral position is also accompanied by hemodynamic advantages that are conducive to optimal uterine blood flow. The pattern of uterine contractions in the sitting position is similar to that in the supine position in contrast to lateral recumbency. Contractions in both the sitting and supine positions are more frequent and less intense than on the side. In addition, the sitting and supine positions share similar hemodynamic properties. Ueland et al. in 1969 [36] reported that during pregnancy the cardiac output in the sitting position declines in a pattern that is similar to that in the supine position, in contrast to that in the side position. Further studies are needed to establish the underlying mechanism(s) of altered uterine contractions in various positions during labor.

Not only are specific maternal positions accompanied by a fairly consistent pattern of uterine contractions, but also the efficiency of contractions is influenced by the position [59,70]. For example, the sitting position increased the efficiency in dilating the cervix when it was alternated with walking rather than with lying on the back. In addition, the supine position was accompanied by contractions as efficient as those on the side when women alternated between lying on their sides and on their backs. It may be that the adverse effects of supine recumbency do not develop when this position is not retained for prolonged periods of time. In the side and supine positions the same pattern of contractions was seen as has been reported by others, i.e., contractions were more intense and less frequent on the side. However, the efficiency of the contractions on the back was essentially the same as on the side. Three factors may account for this: an "efficient" position (the side) was combined with a less efficient position (supine) and improved the quality of the contraction in the alternated position; the increased frequency of contractions on the back, combined with an adequate intensity (greater than 30 mmHg mean intensity), yielded efficient contractions that accomplished cervical dilatation; and changing or alternating between positions may have enhanced the quality of uterine contractions.

In this series, there was not a significant increase in the incidence of fetal heart rate decelerations in any position. This may be because essentially healthy, low-risk women were included in the studies. This is consistent, however, with the superior fetal outcome reported by Flynn et al. [67], who allowed their subjects to ambulate, and the absence of adverse fetal consequences in the other studies that assessed fetal outcome in conjunction with maternal position [61–65].

Preliminary observations by us had suggested that the presence of a nuchal cord was accompanied by an early appearance and a higher incidence of decelerations in the sitting position. In the comparison of the side with the sitting position there was no greater incidence of decelerations in the presence of a nuchal cord (26 percent of labors) in the sitting position than on the side. Therefore, we concluded that fetal status, as reflected by fetal heart rate, was not adversely affected by a sitting position, even in cases of nuchal cord, as was suspected from earlier observations. Even in the standing position there were no harmful effects on the fetus in terms of head or umbilical cord compression [73]. According to these results it can be concluded that sitting, standing, or lying on the back for 30-minute periods had no adverse fetal effects. The lateral recumbent position offers the advantage of longer intervals between contractions, which may be of benefit to the fetus that is becoming compromised from the stress of labor.

In consideration of the differences in the efficiency of contraction in various positions, Geoffrey Dawes' opinion seems appropriate. He said, "Nothing could be worse, it would seem, for the fetus in utero, than to be subjected repeatedly to ineffective uterine contractions" [76]. Therefore women should be allowed, and encouraged, to stand and walk in early labor and lie on their side if confinement to bed is indicated.

When the women alternated between two positions they were able to distinguish differences in comfort [59,70]. They preferred standing to lying on their back, even though contractions were more intense. They preferred sitting to the supine position and to standing up. However, as labor progressed and they became more uncomfortable and tired, the side position was preferred. Many of the subjects also liked being able to change their position. Therefore, even though a specific position may be preferred, moving and changing positions may be important in achieving comfort as well as uterine efficiency.

One concern emerged from these contrasts in conjunction with maternal preference and the efficiency of contraction: it was the significant preference of women to sit in a chair in early labor when, in contrast to the side or standing position, contractions are least efficient. In addition, in late labor, 50 percent of the women who were sitting developed obstetrical difficulties with rotation of the fetal head in the pelvis [73]. The data suggested that the parturients preferred this position because it was accompanied by less back pain. However, if a woman maintains this position her labor may not progress as well.

One alternative to retaining a sitting position would be to combine walking and standing with short, 10 to 15-minute periods of sitting. Another alternative may be the use of a rocking chair rather than a straight-backed chair. Rocking may overcome the dependent circulatory stasis in the lower extremities, if that is a significant contribution to the reduced efficiency of contractions in the sitting position.

In conclusion, upright positions, standing and sitting, are efficient for labor, particularly if they are combined [59,70]. The lateral recumbent position is an efficient recumbent position. The efficiency of the supine position is not reduced if it is combined with periods of lying on the side. Although mechanical and hemodynamic mechanisms seem to mediate the effect of specific positions on labor, the underlying basis remain to be confirmed. The contribution of movement and position change also need to be explored as important factors.

References

1. Englemann, G.J. *Labor Among Primitive Peoples* (2nd ed.). St. Louis: J.H. Chambers, 1883, p. 148.
2. Naroll, F., Naroll, R., Howard, F.H. Positions of women in childbirth. *Am. J. Obstet. Gynecol.* 82:943–954, 1961.
3. Atwood, R.J. Parturitional posture and related birth behavior. *Acta Obstet. Gynecol. Scand.* Supplement 57:1–25, 1976.
4. Russell, J.G.B Moulding of the pelvic outlet. *J. Obstet, Gynaecol. Br. Commonw.* 76:817–820, 1969.
5. Russell, J.G.B. *Radiology in Obstetrics and Antenatal Paediatrics*. London: Butterworth, 1973, p. 169.
6. Russell, J.G.B. The rationale of primitive delivery positions. *Br. J. Obstet. Gynaecol.* 89:712–715, 1982.

7. Young, J. Relaxation of the pelvic joints in pregnancy: pelvic arthropathy of pregnancy. *J. Obstet. Gynaecol. Br. Emp.* 47:493–524, 1940.

8. Borell, U., Fernstrom, I. The mechanism of labour. *Radiol. Clin. N. Am.* 5:73–85, 1967.

9. Ehrstrom, C., Personal correspondence quoted in McKay, S. (ed.), Maternal position during labor and birth. *ICEA Rev.* 2:1, 1978.

10. Vaughan, K.D. *Safe Childbirth: The Three Essentials.* London: Bailliere, Tindall and Cox, 1937.

11. Jarcho, J. The role of posture in obstetrics. *Surg. Gynecol. Obstet.* 48:257–264, 1929.

12. King, A.F.A. The significance of posture in obstetrics. *N.Y. Med. J.* 90:1054–1058, 1909.

13. Clarke, A.P. The influence of the position of the patient in labor in causing uterine inertia and pelvic disturbances. *J. Am. Med. Assoc.* 16:433–435, 1891.

14. Brookmiller, M.M., Bowen, G.L., Carpenter, D. *Textbook of Obstetric and Gynecologic Nursing* (5th ed.) Philadelphia: The W.B. Saunders Co., 1965, p. 192.

15. Davis, M.F., Rubin, R. *DeLee's Obstetrics for Nurses* (17th ed.). Philadelphia: The W.B. Saunders Co., 1963, p. 160.

16. Eastman, N.J. *Williams Obstetrics* (10th ed.). New York: Appleton-Century-Crofts, 1950, p. 391.

17. Fitzhugh, M.L., Newton, M. Muscle action during childbirth. *Phys. Ther. Rev.* 36:805–809, 1957.

18. Moir, J.C. *Munro Kerr's Operative Obstetrics* (7th ed.). Baltimore: The Williams & Wilkins Co., 1964, p. 38.

19. Moore, M.L. *Realities in Childbearing.* Philadelphia: The W.B. Saunders Co., 1978, pp. 388–394.

20. Myles, M.F. *Textbook for midwives* (7th ed.). London: Churchill Livingstone, 1971, p. 282.

21. Rhodes, P. Posture in obstetrics. *Physiotherapy* 53:158–163, 1967.

22. Sturrock, W., Yoemans, S. Childbearing and the nursing process. In Clanson, J.P., Flook, M.H., Ford, B., et al. (eds.), *Maternity Nursing Today.* New York: McGraw-Hill Book Co., 1973, pp. 468–470.

23. Wilson, J.R., Beecham, C.T., Carrington, E.R. *Obstetrics and Gynecology* (5th ed.). St. Louis: The C.V. Mosby Co., 1975, p. 399.

24. Edgar, J.C. *The Practice of Obstetrics* (3rd ed.). Philadelphia: P. Blakiston's Sons & Co., 1907, p. 868.

25. Liu, Y.C. Position during labor and delivery: history and perspective. *J. Nurse-Midwifery* 24:23–26, 1979.

26. Rigby, E. What is the natural position of women during labor? *Med. Times Gaz.* 15:345–346, 1857.

27. Lieberman, J.J. Childbirth practices: from darkness to light. *J. Obstet. Gynecol. Neonat. Nurs.* 5:41–45, 1976.

28. Roberts, J.E. Maternal positions for childbirth: a historical review of nursing care practices. *J. Obstet. Gynecol. Neonat. Nurs.* 8:24–32, 1979.

29. Roberts, J. Alternative positions for childbirth. I. First stage of labor. *J. Nurse-Midwifery* 25:11–18, 1980.

30. Roberts, J., Mendez-Bauer, C. A perspective of maternal position during labor. *J. Perinat. Med.* 8:255–264, 1980.
31. Markoe, J.W. Posture in obstetrics. *Bull. Lying-In Hosp. N.Y.* 11:11–26, 1917.
32. Leak, W.N. Position for delivery. *Br. Med. J.* 2:735–736, 1955.
33. Irwin, H.W. Practical considerations for the routine application of left lateral Sims' position for vaginal delivery. *Am. J. Obstet. Gynecol.* 131:129–133, 1978.
34. McAuliffe, P. The prone position in obstetrics. *Med. J. Aust.* (August 1):182–183, 1964.
35. Blankfield, A. The optimum position for childbirth. *Med. J. Aust.* (October 16):666–688, 1965.
36. Ueland, K., Novy, M.J., Peterson, E.N., Metcalf, J. Maternal cardiovascular dynamics. IV. The influence of gestational age on the maternal cardiovascular response to posture and exercise. *Am. J. Obstet. Gynecol.* 104:856–864, 1969.
37. Vorys, N., Ullery, J.C., Hanusek, G.E. The cardiac output changes in various positions in pregnancy. *Am. J. Obstet. Gynecol.* 82:1312–1321, 1961.
38. Mengert, W., Murphy, D. Intra-abdominal pressures created by voluntary muscular effort. *Surg. Gynecol. Obstet.* 57:745–751, 1933.
39. Hanssen, R. Ohnmacht und schwangerschaft (fainting and pregnancy). *Klin. Wschr.* 21:241–253, 1942.
40. Howard, B., Goodson, J., Mengert, W.F. Supine hypotensive syndrome in late pregnancy. *Obstet. Gynecol.* 1:371–377, 1953.
41. Quilligan, E.J., Tyler, C. Postural effects on the cardiovascular status in pregnancy: a comparison of the lateral and supine postures. *Am. J. Obstet. Gynecol.* 78:465–471, 1959.
42. Kerr, M.G. The mechanical effects of the gravid uterus in late pregnancy. *J. Obstet. Gynecol.* 72:513–529, 1965.
43. Lees, M.M., Scott, D.B., Kerr, M.G. Hemodynamic changes associated with labour. *J. Obstet. Gynaecol. Br. Commonw.* 77:29–36, 1970.
44. Bieniarz, J., Crottogini, J.J., Curuchet, E., et al. Aortocaval compression by the uterus in late human pregnancy. *Am. J. Obstet. Gynecol.* 100:203–217, 1968.
45. Eckstein, K.L., Marx, G.F. Aortocaval compression and uterine displacement. *Anesthesiology* 40:92–96, 1974.
46. Bonica, J.J. *Principles and Practice of Obstetric Analgesia and Anesthesia.* Philadelphia: F.A. Davis, 1967, p. 32.
47. Bassell, G.M., Humayun, S.G., Marx, G.F. Maternal bearing-down efforts—another fetal risk? *Obstet. Gynecol.* 56:39–41, 1980.
48. Marx, G.F., Husain, F.J., Shiau, H.F. Brachial and femoral blood pressures during the prenatal period. *Am. J. Obstet. Gynecol.* 136:11–13, 1980.
49. Kauppila, A., Koskinen, M., Puolakka, J., et al. Decreased intervillous and unchanged myometrial blood flow in supine recumbency. *Obstet. Gynecol.* 55:203–205, 1980.
50. Adamsons, K. Factors influencing the acid-base state of the fetus during labor. In *Perinatal Factors Affecting Human Development.* Pan American Health Organization Scientific Publication no. 185, 1969, p. 175.
51. Goodlin, R. Importance of the lateral position during labor. *Obstet. Gynecol.* 1:698–701, 1971.

52. Humphrey, M.D., Chang, A., Wood, C.J., et al. A decrease in fetal pH during the second stage of labour, when conducted in the dorsal position. *J. Obstet. Gynaecol. Br. Commonw.* 81:600–602, 1974.

53. Williams, E.A. Abnormal uterine action in labour. *J. Obstet. Gynaecol. Br. Emp.* 59:635–641, 1952.

54. Turnbull, A.C. Uterine contractions in normal and abnormal labour. *J. Obstet. Gynaecol. Br. Emp.* 64:321–333, 1957.

55. Caldeyro-Barcia, R., Noriega-Guerra, L., Cibils, L.A., et al. Effect of position changes on the intensity and frequency of uterine contractions during labor. *Am. J. Obstet. Gynecol.* 80:284–290, 1960.

56. Hendricks, C.H. Amniotic fluid pressure recording. *Clin. Obstet. Gynecol.* 9:535–553, 1966.

57. Paul, R.H., Petrie, R.H. *Fetal Intensive Care: Current Concepts.* Los Angeles: University of Southern California Press, 1973, p. 73.

58. Pontonnier, G., Puech, F., Grandjean, H., Rolland, M. Some physical and biochemical parameters during normal labour. *Biol. Neonate* 26:159–173, 1975.

59. Roberts, J., Mendez-Bauer, C., Wodell, D. The effects of maternal position on uterine contractility and efficiency. *Birth* 10:243–249, 1983.

60. Chan, D. Positions in labor. *Br. Med. J.* 5323:100–102, 1963.

61. Liu, Y.C. Effects of an upright position during labor. *Am. J. Nurs.* 74:2202–2205, 1974.

62. Mitre, I.N. The influence of maternal position on duration of the active phase of labor. *Int. J. Gynaecol. Obstet.* 12:181–183, 1974.

63. McManus, T.J., Calder, A.A. Upright posture and efficiency of labour. *Lancet* 1:72–74, 1978.

64. Diaz, A.G., Schwarcz, R., Fescina, Y.R. Caldeyro-Barcia, R. Efectos de la posicion vertical materna sobre la evolucion del parto. *Separata de la Rev. Clin. Invest. Ginecol. Obstet.* 5:101–109, 1978.

65. Williams, R.M., Thom, M.H., Studd, J.W. A study of the benefits and acceptability of ambulation in spontaneous labour. *Br. J. Obstet. Gynaecol.* 87:122–126, 1980.

66. Flynn, A., Kelly, J. Continuous fetal monitoring in the ambulant patient in labour. *Br. Med. J.* 2:842–843, 1976.

67. Flynn, A.M., Kelly, J., Hollins, G., Lynch, P.F. Ambulation in labour. *Br. Med. J.* 2:591–593, 1978.

68. Read, J.A., Miller, F.C., Paul, R.H. Randomized trial of ambulation versus oxytocin for labor enhancement: a preliminary report. *Am. J. Obstet. Gynecol.* 139:669–673, 1981.

69. Mendez-Bauer, C., Arroyo, J., Garcia-Ramos, C., et al. Effects of standing position on spontaneous uterine contractility and other aspects of labor. *J. Perinat. Med.* 3:89–100, 1975.

70. Mendez-Bauer, C., Newton, M. Maternal position during labor and second stage. In: Philipp, E., Barnes, J., Newton, M. (eds). *Scientific Foundations of Obstetrics and Gynecology,* 3rd ed. London: William Heinemann, in press.

71. Arroyo, J., Mendez-Bauer, C. The maintenance of a stable baseline in intra-uterine pressure with varying maternal position—a practical approach. *J. Perinat. Med.* 3:129–131, 1975.

72. Cibils, L.A. Enhancement and induction of labor. In Aladjam, S. (ed.), *Risks in the Practice of Modern Obstetrics* (2nd ed.). St. Louis: C.V. Mosby Co., 1975, pp. 187–188.
73. Mendez-Bauer, C., Arroyo, J., Mendez, A., et al. Effects of different maternal positions during labour. In *5th European Congress of Perinatal Medicine*, Uppsala, Sweden, 1976, pp. 9–12.
74. Mendez-Bauer, C., Arroyo, J., Zamarriego, J. Maternal standing position in first stage of labor. In Scarpelli, E.M., Cosmi, E.V. (eds.), *Reviews in Perinatal Medicine*, vol. 1 Baltimore: University Park Press, 1976.
75. Mendez-Bauer, C., Arroyo, J., Reina, L., et al. Monitoring and maternal posture. In: *Sixth European Congress of Parinatal Medicine, Vienna 1978*. Stuttgart: Georg Thieme Publishers, 1979, pp. 294–296.
76. Dawes, G. *The fetus and birth*. Ciba Found. Symp. 47:3, 1977.

5

Cesarean Section: Enough is Enough

Paul R. Meier, M.D.

Introduction

In 1965, 1 in 20 deliveries was accomplished by cesarean section; this year the number will be 1 in 6. This phenomenal change has been the subject of much lively debate in the obstetrical literature, among various consumer groups, and even in governmental agencies. In October of 1981 the National Institute of Child Health and Human Development issued a Consensus Development Statement on cesarean childbirth [1]. It concluded:

> The rising cesarean birth rate is a matter of concern. The consensus statement reflects the judgement that this trend of rising cesarean birth rates may be stopped and perhaps reversed, while continuing to make improvements in maternal and fetal outcomes, the goal of clinical obstetrics today.

The following discussion is a reflection on this general statement. Beginning with the four diagnoses that have contributed most to the increased cesarean delivery rates, alternative management options are considered, and a clinical scheme is developed that may lead to a realization of the sentiment expressed by the study task force in their concluding statement.

Discussion

Two fundamental beliefs underlie obstetricians' increased reliance on cesarean delivery. They are the belief that cesarean section is a safe and relatively benign procedure and the belief that cesarean section will improve either maternal or perinatal outcome. These beliefs are so pervasive that in some hospitals the cesarean section rate now exceeds 25 percent. It is surprising that beliefs so strongly held are based on so little hard evidence.

Cesarean section is a relatively safe procedure. The availability of blood products for transfusion, effective antibiotics, and safer anesthetic techniques have combined to make maternal mortality exceedingly rare. In one series over 10,000 cesarean deliveries were performed without a maternal death [2]. Nevertheless, the likelihood of a maternal death after cesarean section is two to three times greater than it is after vaginal delivery [3]. Maternal morbidity is also greater after cesarean section than after vaginal delivery. Evrard et al. found that nearly one in five patients sustained some morbidity after cesarean section; three-fourths of it was infectious in nature [4]. Clearly, although cesarean section is a very safe procedure, it is associated with a greater likelihood of maternal death or significant morbidity than is a vaginal delivery. It follows that, given equal perinatal outcome, vaginal delivery is preferred over cesarean section to minimize maternal risks.

Cesarean delivery is believed to improve maternal or perinatal outcome in a variety of obstetrical situations. The graphic comparison of both maternal outcome and perinatal outcome compared with the cesarean delivery rate seems to suggest a direct correlation between these variables [5]. If cesarean section is so strongly related to improved perinatal outcome, it would seem reasonable to expect that this relationship should be apparent in other geographic areas. This is not the case. At the National Maternity Hospital in Dublin, Ireland, the cesarean section rate has been relatively constant at about 5 percent over the years 1965 through 1980. Perinatal mortality has decreased over those years to the same degree

Table 5–1

Indication	96 of All Cesareans Done in 1978
Dystocia	31
Repeat	31
Breech	12
Fetal distress	5

SOURCE: Cesarean Childbirth, Department of Health and Human Services, National Institute of Health Publication no. 82–2067, 1981.

and to the same low level as in the United States [6]. Since decreasing perinatal mortality rates may be quite independent of increasing cesarean section rates, attempts to stabilize or reverse the rise in cesarean deliveries are at least permissable as long as perinatal outcome is closely monitored.

Eight of every 10 cesarean deliveries are performed for one of four diagnoses. Table 5-1 lists these diagnoses and the percentage of all cesarean deliveries they represent. Clearly any attempt to modify the present cesarean section rate must focus on these four diagnostic groups.

DYSTOCIA

Dystocia is a term of low specificity. Meaning simply "difficult childbirth," this diagnosis accounts for approximately 30 percent of the increase in the cesarean birth rate seen during the decade of the 1970s. The vast majority of cesarean deliveries performed because of dystocia are in pregnancies with infants of normal size and in the vertex presentation. Thus, the dramatic increase in cesarean deliveries in this category is difficult to understand. Several intriguing studies suggest that the number of cesarean deliveries performed for this indication may, in fact, be excessive.

O'Driscoll and Foley [6] observed that during the same time period that the cesarean section rate increased by over 300 percent in the United States, it remained constant in their institution (National Maternity Hospital, Dublin). When they compared the number of cesarean sections performed for dystocia in the United States with those performed for the same indication in Dublin, the ratio was 7:1. They attributed this difference to their aggressive management of labor, which is the standard of practice at the National Maternity Hospital. This management focuses on "the correct initial diagnosis of labor, regular assessment of early progress, and effective stimulation with oxytocin whenever the pace of dilatation of the cervix is slow in the nulliparous patient." They conclude that "with the same medical approach to management of labor, it is difficult to see why cesarean birth rates in the United States could not be reduced sharply with equally satisfactory results [6,7].

In this country Seitchik and Rao reported on the obstetrical experience of 58 women whose first pregnancy was delivered by cesarean section for cephalopelvic disproportion and "failure to progress" in labor [8]. All of the primary cesarean sections were performed after what was deemed a satisfactory trial of labor including a trial of oxytocin therapy. In a subsequent pregnancy all 58 women were given a trial of labor, and 40 achieved a vaginal delivery. When the records of these women were reviewed to assess the adequacy of the initial trial of labor, a number of errors or management faults were identified. These included inadequate duration of oxytocin therapy, diagnosis of labor not established before artificial rupture of membranes, failure to recognize latent-phase labor, and technical errors that probably prevented adequate oxytocin therapy from being delivered. In 11 patients no source of potential management errors could be identified; in this group, 6 women gave birth vaginally after a subsequent trial of labor.

Taken together, these two articles demonstrate how little we know about the components of effective labor. Perhaps greater attention paid to the diagnosis of true labor and the aggressive management of active labor could result in a decrease in the number of primary cesarean sections done for dystocia.

REPEAT CESAREAN

Approximately 150,000 babies are delivered by cesarean section each year in this country because their mothers had a prior cesarean delivery. This represents approximately one-third of all cesarean sections performed each year in the United States. It is in this group that a clear alternative to current management practices exists. Before 1978, a trial of labor after cesarean delivery was virtually unknown. More recently numerous articles have appeared documenting the safety, the high rate of subsequent vaginal delivery, and the acceptability of a trial of labor after a prior low transverse cesarean section [8–10]. Although some controversy exists as to the conditions required to safely conduct a trial of labor, no controversy exists as to the clear reduction in the number of cesareans performed when labor is expected after a prior cesarean delivery [9]. When the dictum "once a cesarean, always a cesarean" is abandoned and labor is allowed to occur naturally, the result will be a decrease in the total cesarean section rate.

BREECH PRESENTATION

At term a breech presentation is encountered in 3 to 4 percent of all pregnancies. The current management of the term breech fetus follows one of two general patterns; either cesarean section for all breech infants or labor in selected breeches with cesarean section reserved for those who fail labor or in whom labor is not deemed to be safe. In either case the incidence of cesarean delivery is high. Again, an alternative to these two traditional plans of management may result in a lower cesarean delivery rate without jeopardizing perinatal outcome. In 1973 Brooks Ranney offered such an alternative when he presented his paper "The Gentle Art of External Cephalic Version" [11]. In his practice he was able to diminish the incidence of breech presentation at term from the expected 4 percent to less than 1 percent by means of external cephalic version. Although often discussed, this paper made little apparent impact in actual clinical practice. In 1974 Saling and Muller-Holve suggested that external cephalic version should be performed while using tocolytic drugs to relax the uterus. They were successful in their version attempts 75 percent of the time and reduced the incidence of breech presentation at term by one-half [12]. Finally Van Dorsten and his colleagues reported a small prospective controlled trial of external cephalic version. Practiced under a specific protocol, there was a significant reduction in the incidence of breech presentation at term and in the incidence of cesarean sections [13].

FETAL DISTRESS

The diagnosis of fetal distress has accounted for about 10 to 15 percent of the increase in the cesarean section rate. There is a lingering suspicion that some of this increase can be attributed to the widespread use of continuous electronic fetal monitoring during labor. Prospective studies by Haverkamp et al. suggested that fetal distress and consequent cesarean section was much more common in patients monitored by continuous electronic means than in patients monitored by periodic auscultation [14]. Even the use of fetal scalp pH assessment in cases of suspected fetal distress did not lower the cesarean section rate to that of the group managed by periodic auscultation alone [15].

Zalar and Quilligan assessed the impact of electronic monitoring and fetal scalp pH evaluation on the cesarean delivery rate [16]. They concluded that utilization of fetal scalp pH determinations did prevent cesarean sections that may have been done on the basis of fetal heart rate tracings alone. They admitted, however, that ''continuous fetal heart monitoring, even with the assistance of scalp sampling in this study, 'overpredicts' neonatal depression based on the 5 minute Apgar score.'' It is likely that fetal distress will continue to be overcalled during labor. Certainly it is more reasonable to err in this direction than to err by undercalling fetal distress. To admit this possibility does not negate the need to utilize every possible means to assess fetal health when fetal distress is suspected. Although not perfect, fetal scalp pH assessment is a useful evaluation that should be used on a regular basis.

The distressed fetus will often respond favorably to oxygen therapy, changes in maternal position, normalization of maternal blood pressure, or cessation of oxytocin therapy. If a specific cause for the distress is found and treated, and the fetus promptly responds to these manipulations, cesarean delivery may often be avoided.

Finally, it may be that fetal distress is in some way related to maternal anxiety and stress. Less fetal distress and lower cesarean delivery rates have been reported in mothers who had experienced some form of child-

71

birth education [17]. Haverkamp et al. have speculated that the lower incidence of fetal distress in the group monitored by auscultation may have been related to the constant presence of a nurturing labor nurse [14]. Certainly the available evidence is sufficient to suggest the need for more study in this area.

Summary

A concerted effort to halt and perhaps reverse the increasing cesarean delivery rate seems warranted. Any such effort requires that there be careful, simultaneous monitoring of perinatal morbidity and mortality as well as monitoring of maternal morbidity. Such an endeavor should stress the following points: 1) careful attention paid to the accurate diagnosis of labor; 2) aggressive management of active labor including the appropriate use of oxytocin; 3) anticipation of a trial of labor in patients with one previous low transverse cesarean section without new or recurrent indication; 4) management of the term breech by attempted external cephalic version under tocolysis or a trial of labor (or both) in selected cases of breech presentation; 5) regular use of fetal scalp pH assessment to enhance the reliability of the diagnosis of fetal distress detected by electronic fetal monitoring; 6) more intensive effort to educate expectant parents in the antepartum period concerning labor and delivery; 7) provision of constant supportive care during the intrapartum period to minimize maternal anxiety and fear.

What might be the outcome of such an effort? If cesarean deliveries for dystocia were decreased or were diminished to the level currently found in Ireland, the present cesarean section rate would fall from over 15 percent to about 11 percent. Since one repeat cesarean is developed for every two primary cesarean deliveries done, an additional fall to 9 percent would ultimately occur. If all patients with one prior low transverse cesarean section and no recurrent or new indication for cesarean delivery were allowed to labor, a further reduction to the range of 6 to 7 percent might occur. If breech presentation decreased and the diagnosis of fetal distress remained constant, a final reduction of one to two percentage points might be realized, yielding a cesarean section rate of about 5 percent. All of this could be accomplished without compromising either perinatal or maternal well-being. Is such a thing possible?

References

1. Cesarean Childbirth, U.S. Department of Health and Human Services, National Institutes of Health Publication no. 82-2067, 1981.

2. Frigoletto, F.D., Ryan, K.J., Phillippe, M. Maternal mortality rate associated with cesarean section: an appraisal. *Am. J. Obstet. Gynecol.* 136:969, 1980.
3. Petitti, D., Olson, R.O., Williams, R.L. Cesarean section in California 1960 through 1975. *Am. J. Obstet. Gynecol.* 133:391, 1979.
4. Evrard, J.R., Gold, E.M., Cahill, T.F. Cesarean section: a contemporary assessment. *J. Reprod. Med.* 24:147, 1980.
5. Bottoms, S.F., Rosen, M.G., Sohol, R.J. The increase in the cesarean birth rate. *N. Engl. J. Med.* 302:559, 1980.
6. O'Driscoll, K., Foley, M. Correlation of decrease in perinatal mortality and increase in cesarean section rates. *Obstet. Gynecol.* 61:1, 1983.
7. O'Driscoll, K., Stronge, J.M., Minoque, M. Active management of labour. *Br. Med. J.* 3:135, 1973.
8. Seitchik, T., Rao, V.R.R. Cesarean delivery in nulliparous women for failed oxytocin-augmented labor: route of delivery in subsequent pregnancy. *Am. J. Obstet. Gynecol.* 143:393, 1982.
9. Meier, P.R., Porreco, R.P. Trial of labor following cesarean section: a two year experience. *Am. J. Obstet. Gynecol.* 144:671, 1982.
10. Lavin, J.P., Stephens, R.J., Mrodovnik, M.: Vaginal delivery in patients with a prior cesarean section. *Obstet. Gynecol.* 59:135, 1982.
11. Ranney, B. The gentle art of external cephalic version. *Am. J. Obstet. Gynecol.* 116:239, 1973.
12. Saling, E., Muller-Holve, W. External cephalic version under tocolysis. *J. Perinat. Med.* 3:115, 1975.
13. Van Dorsten, J.P., Schifrin, B.S., Wallace, R.L. Randomized control trial of external cephalic version with tocolysis in later pregnancy. *Am. J. Obstet. Gynecol.* 141:417, 1981.
14. Haverkamp, A.D., Thompson, H.E., McFee, J.G., et al. The evaluation of continuous fetal heart rate monitoring in high-risk pregnancy. *Am. J. Obstet. Gynecol.* 125:310, 1976.
15. Haverkamp, A.D., Orleans, M., Langendoerfer, S., et al. A controlled trial of the differential effects of intrapartum fetal monitoring. *Am. J. Obstet. Gynecol.* 134:399, 1979.
16. Zalar, R.W., Quilligan, E.J. The influence of scalp sampling on the cesarean section rate for fetal distress. *Am. J. Obstet, Gynecol.* 135:239, 1979.
17. Hughey, M.J., McElin, T.W., Young, T. Maternal and fetal outcome of lamaze-prepared patients. *Obstet. Gynecol.* 51:643, 1978.

6

Autoimmune Thrombocytopenia and Pregnancy

Russell K. Laros, Jr., M.D.

It has been 20 years since Harrington et al. carried out his classical experiment aimed at delineating the cause of autoimmune thrombocytopenia (ATP) [1]. Harrington was stimulated by the observation that a significant percentage of infants whose mothers had ATP were themselves thrombocytopenic. This suggested that the causative factor was a circulating humoral substance of a sufficiently small molecular weight to cross the placenta. To prove this hypothesis he infused plasma from patients with ATP into several normal recipients, including himself. All of the recipients immediately became thrombocytopenic. More recently, Shulman et al. [2] and Karpatkin et al. [3] have further delineated the idiologic factor in ATP and demonstrated that it is an immunoglobular (IgG) antibody that attaches itself to human lymphocyte antigen sites on the surface of platelets.

In the past decade a great deal of work has gone into better defining and being able to measure the antibody responsible for ATP. Several laboratory techniques have been developed which allow reliable identification of the platelet-associated IgG (PA-IgG). The majority of patients with ATP are found to have an increased level of PA-IgG. However, another group of patients exist where both an elevated level of PA-IgG and platelet-associated C_3 can be identified. A third group of patients has normal levels of

PA-IgG, but elevated levels of platelet-associated C_3. Finally a group exists with no apparent circulating antiplatelet antibodies; it is this group that Karpatkin identifies as having idiopathic thrombocytopenic purpura [7].

When significant amounts of PA-IgG exist on the surface of platelets the reticuloendothelial system (which includes the spleen, liver, and bone marrow) is responsible for platelet destruction. Additionally, the spleen is the primary site of antibody production. However, in patients who have undergone splenectomy the bone marrow becomes the major site of antibody production and also a significant site of platelet destruction.

The direct PA-IgG detects antibody on the surface of the patient's platelets. This assay generally correlates well with the clinical picture and shows an inverse relationship with the patient's platelet count. The indirect method measures PA-IgG in the platelet serum by reacting it with donor platelets from a normal individual. Because the indirect assay has not correlated well with clinical status, it is of limited use. However, Cines et al. recently reported a correlation between circulating antiplatelet antibody (indirect tests) and the presence and extent of neonatal thrombocytopenia [5].

The obstetrician-gynecologist is often the first physician to see patients with newly acquired ATP [6,7]. Most patients give a history of easy bruisability or bleeding from mucous membranes (or both). Physical examination is normal, except for ecchymoses, petechiae, and mucosal bleeding. The clinical course of ATP may be classified as either acute or chronic. The acute disorder, which mostly affects children, generally follows a viral illness. Boys and girls are affected in equal numbers and the disease is generally self-limited. However, approximately 10 to 20 percent of children will go on to develop the chronic form of the disease. The chronic variety is long lasting without definitive therapy. The platelet count usually remains low, and the remission refers to the absence of symptoms rather than a normal platelet level. The chronic ATP is more common in women in a ratio of 2:1 to 4:1. Laboratory evaluation should include a complete blood count, bone marrow examination, a coagulation screen including a prothrombin time and activated partial thromboplastin time, and antiplatelet antibody studies. In ATP one anticipates an entirely normal blood count with the exception of thrombocytopenia. The bone marrow is also normal with an increased number of megakaryocytes. The platelets that are observed on the peripheral smear are frequently large, which is simply an expression of their premature release from the bone marrow. The prothrombin time and activated partial thromboplastin time are normal. If the patient has an elevated antinucleus antibody she must be evaluated for lupus. From a practical point of view, the thrombocytopenia observed in lupus is identical in pathophysiology with that in ATP; however, one must be cognizant that other systems may be involved in lupus and thoroughly explore for such involvement.

The two major modalities of therapy are corticosteroids and sple-nectomy [8]. In the occasional patient who fails these standard therapeutic regimens, immunosuppression therapy, gamma globulin, and danazol may be considered [9–11]. Prednisone is begun in a dose of 1 ml/kg per day. When a response occurs, the dose is gradually tapered to the lowest pos-sible level, which will maintain a reasonable platelet count and clinical remission. Because long-term usage of corticosteroids is fraught with complications, treatment should not be continued for more than 6 to 8 months.

Splenectomy is indicated in patients refractory to corticosteroid ther-apy. Splenectomy removes both the major site of antibody production and, more importantly, the major site of platelet destruction [5]. In essence one is creating a reasonable balance between platelet production and de-struction even though the patient may not achieve a total immunologic remission and may still produce a substantial amount of antiplatelet an-tibody.

The immunosuppressive agents most widely used have included cy-clophosphamide, vincristine and azathioprine [7,9]. Obviously these would only be considered during pregnancy in a most desperate situation. The same consideration would hold for danazol [10], and there is as yet no specific experience with gamma globulin administration for ATP during pregnancy.

Most authors consider that pregnancy has no influence on the clinical course of ATP [12–16]. However two series have reported an exacerbation of thrombocytopenia during pregnancy [17,18]. There are a number of reports of splenectomy carried out successfully during pregnancy [17,19–21]. If splenectomy is contemplated, ideally it should be performed during the second trimester.

Postpartum hemorrhage from the placental site is an unusual com-plication of ATP. Undoubtedly, this is because the major hemostatic mechanism after placental separation is myometrial contraction. It is im-portant that meticulous mechanical hemostasis be obtained if any traumatic lacerations occur or if surgical intervention is required. If cesarean section is carried out and the platelet count is less than 550×10^9 per 1, platelet transfusions are recommended to minimize hemorrhage at the time of sur-gery [22].

The most controversial issue relates to the mode of delivery [22,23]. Based on the observation that approximately 50 percent of infants of mothers with ATP will themselves be thrombocytopenic and the obser-vation that a few of these infants have experienced central nervous system bleeding, and on the premise that cesarean section will protect these infants from central nervous system bleeding, Territo et al. [24] and later Murray and Harris [25], suggested that cesarean section is the preferred mode of delivery. Our evaluation of the literature and our own experience do not lead us to the same conclusion [23].

During the past 15 years we have managed 19 pregnancies in women with immune thrombocytopenia; sixteen cases were ATP, and 3 were associated with lupus. Initial treatment included steroids for 11 patients, steroids and splenectomy for 6 patients, splenectomy, and chemotherapy for 1 patient, and no treatment for 1 patient. In every instance the use of cesarean section was dictated only by obstetrical indications. There were eight cases of spontaneous vaginal delivery, five cases of forceps or vacuum delivery, and six cesarean sections. The indications for cesarean section were four repeat procedures, one because of failed induction, and one for breech presentation. Seventeen of the infants are living and well, and two were stillborn. Seven of the liveborn infants were thrombocytopenic at delivery or later developed thrombocytopenia (platelet counts less than $100 \times 10^9/L$), and three developed platelet counts lower than $30 \times 10^9/L$. All of the liveborn infants had Apgar scores greater than or equal to 8; although two of the infants developed ecchymoses, none had significant morbidity relating to their thrombocytopenia.

Obviously it would be inappropriate to draw conclusions from such limited data. However, if one reviews the literature dealing with immune thrombocytopenia and pregnancy from 1953 on, there have been 134 infants delivered by the vaginal route and 31 delivered by cesarean section [23]. Table 6–1 details the platelet counts of this population, and Table 6–2 shows the incidence of hemorrhage in those cases where the fetal platelet count was less than $100 \times 10^9/L$. Obviously, it is only these latter infants who are actually at risk and might benefit from cesarean section. The incidence of hemorrhage is no less when the route of delivery is cesarean section.

In view of the controversy there are really three courses one can take in choosing the route of delivery for patients with ATP: cesarean section for all, selected cesarean section based on some laboratory study that indicates which infants are really at risk, and finally vaginal delivery for all unless an obstetrical indication for cesarean section supervenes. Because we are not convinced that cesarean section is beneficial for the infant and because it undoubtedly adds to the chances of morbidity for the mother, we have chosen the third approach. If one wishes to use selective cesarean section, a fetal platelet count should be obtained during labor as described by Scott and associates [26], and then cesarean section should be performed only on those infants found to have platelet counts less than $30 \times 10^9/L$.

Karpatkin et al. [27] have recently stressed the value of maternal treatment with corticosteroids during pregnancy. Previous studies by Heys [15] and Jones et al. [19] and as our own experience [23] have not confirmed any correlation between the fetal platelet count and maternal treatment with prednisone. After ingestion, prednisone is converted to prednisolone, only 10 percent of which crosses the placenta because of inactivation by 11-β-ol dehydrogenase. However, because corticosteroids are effective

Table 6-1
Cases of ATP Delivered Vaginally (Stillbirths Excluded)

Study, Year	Reference	Number of Cases	Neonates with Lowest Platelet Count ($\times 10^9$/L)			Hemorrhage	Any Neonatal	
			<100	<50	<30		Serious Hemorrhage	Treatment
Territo et al.	1973 [24]	1	1	0	0	0	0	0
Jones et al.	1977 [17]	42	10	7	6	4	1	3
O'Reilly and Taber et al.	1978 [20]	8[a]	6	5	5	3	0	3
Noriega-Guerra et al.	1979 [21]	18	9	7	4	8	0	8
Scott et al.	1980 [26]	8	3	0	0	0	0	0
Karpatkin et al.	1981 [27]	18	12	11	7	1	0	?
Kelton et al.	1982 [28]	27	4	4	3	3	0	3
Laros and Kagan	1983 [23]	12	5	4	2	2	0	1
Total		134	50	38	28	21	1	?

[a] One set of triplets.

78

Table 6-2

Cases of ATP Delivered by Cesarean Section (Stillbirths Excluded)

Study, Year	Reference	Number of Cases	Neonates with Lowest Platelet Count ($\times 10^9$/L)			Hemorrhage	Any Neonatal	
			<100	<50	<30		Serious Hemorrhage	Treatment
Territo et al.	1973 [24]	5	3	3	3	3	3	2
Jones et al.	1974 [17]	2	2	2	2	1	0	1
Murray and Harris	1975 [25]	2	2	2	0	0	0	0
Scott et al.	1980 [26]	4	3	3	3	3	0	?
Karpatkin et al.	1981 [27]	1	1	0	0	0	0	?
Kelton et al.	1982 [28]	12	4	3	1	0	0	1
Laros and Kagan	1983 [23]	5	2	2	0	0	0	0
Total		31	17	15	9	6	3	?

Figure 6–1

Scheme of Management for Immune Thrombocytopenic Purpura During Pregnancy.

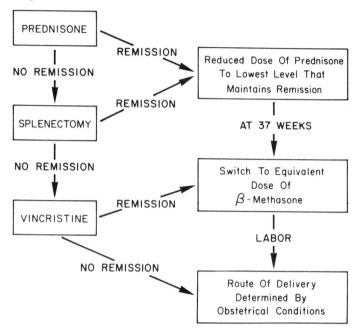

in treating neonatal, passively acquired ATP, one might hypothesize the benefit of switching to an equivalent dose of a corticosteroid that crosses the placenta, such as beta-methasone or dexamethasone in the final few weeks before delivery [17]. We stress that there are no data documenting the validity of this hypothesis.

Our current scheme of management is outlined in Figure 6-1. We define a remission as a platelet count of 50×10^9 to 100×10^9/L without any bleeding manifestations. At 37 weeks beta-methasone is substituted for prednisone in a dosage ratio of 0.6:5. In instances where splenectomy is required it should be performed before the 32nd week of gestation because of the technical difficulties encountered thereafter. In view of the data available, we are not willing to base our decision on the route of delivery on either the maternal PA-IgG or the fetal scalp platelet count.

References

1. Harrington, W.J., Minnich, V., Arimura, G. The autoimmune thrombocytopenia. *Prog. Hematol.* 1:166–173, 1956.
2. Shulman, N.R., Marder, V.J., Weinrach, R.S. Similarities between known antiplatelet antibodies and the factor responsible for thrombocytopenia in idi-

opathic purpura. Physiologic, serologic and isotopic studies. *Ann. N.Y. Acad. Sci.* 124:499–504, 1965.

3. Karpatkin, S., Ascher, P.H., Strick, N., et al. Heavy chain subclass of human antiplatelet antibodies. *Clin. Immunol. Immunopathol.* 261:127–130, 1973.

4. Cines, D.B., Schreiber, A.D. Immune thrombocytopenia: use of a Coombs antiglobulin test to detect IgG and C_3 on platelets. *N. Engl. J. Med.* 300:106–111, 1979.

5. Cines, D., Dussk, B., Tomaski, A., et al. Immune thrombocytopenic purpura and pregnancy. *N. Engl. J. Med.* 306:826–831, 1982.

6. Baldini, M. Idiopathic thrombocytopenic purpura and the ITP syndrome. *Med. Clin. North Am.* 56:47–58, 1972.

7. Karpatkin, S. Autoimmune thrombocytopenic purpura. *Blood* 56:329–343, 1980.

8. Ahn, Y.S., Harrington, W.J. Treatment of idiopathic thrombocytopenic purpura (ITP). *Annu. Rev. Med.* 28:299–309, 1977.

9. McMillan, R. Chronic idiopathic thrombocytopenic purpura. *N. Engl. J. Med.* 304:1135–1139, 1981.

10. Ahn, Y.S., Harrington, W.J., Simon, S.R., et al. Danazol for the treatment of idiopathic thrombocytopenic purpura. *N. Engl. J. Med.* 308:1396, 1983.

11. Fehr, J., Hofman, V., Kappeler, V. Transient reversal of thrombocytopenia in idiopathic thrombocytopenic purpura by high-dose intravenous gamma globulin. *N. Engl. J. Med.* 306:1254–1258, 1982.

12. Peterson, O.H., Larson, D. Thrombocytopenic purpura in pregnancy. *Obstet. Gynecol.* 4:454–461, 1954.

13. Tancer, M.L. Idiopathic thrombocytopenic purpura and pregnancy. *Am. J. Obstet. Gynecol.* 79:148, 1960.

14. Carloss, H.W., McMillan, R., Crosby, W.H. Management of pregnancy in women with immune thrombocytopenic purpura. *J. Am. Med. Assoc.* 244:2756–2758, 1980.

15. Heys, R.F. Childbearing and idiopathic thrombocytopenic purpura. *J. Obstet. Gynaecol. Br. Commonw.* 73:205–214, 1966.

16. Goodhue, P.A., Evans, T.S. Idiopathic thrombocytopenic purpura in pregnancy. *Obstet. Gynecol. Surv.* 18:671–683, 1963.

17. Laros, R.K., Sweet, R.L. Management of idiopathic thrombocytopenic purpura during pregnancy. *Am. J. Obstet. Gynecol.* 122:182–191, 1975.

18. Zilliacus, H. Thrombocytopenia in pregnancy. *Clin. Obstet. Gynecol.* 2:404–425, 1964.

19. Jones, R.W., Asher, M.I., Rutherford, C.J., Munro, H.M. Autoimmune (idiopathic) thrombocytopenic purpura in pregnancy and the newborn. *Br. J. Obstet. Gynaecol.* 84:679–683, 1977.

20. O'Reilly, R.A., Taber, B.Z. Immunologic thrombocytopenic purpura and pregnancy: six new cases. *Obstet. Gynecol.* 51:590–597, 1978.

21. Noriega-Guerra, L., Aviles-Miranda, A., de la Cadena, O.A., et al. Pregnancy in patients with autoimmune thrombocytopenic purpura. *Am. J. Obstet. Gynecol.* 133:439–440, 1979.

22. Kagan, R., Laros, R.K. Immune thrombocytopenia. *Clin. Obstet. Gynecol.* 26:537–546, 1983.

23. Laros, R.K., Kagan, R. Route of delivery for patients with immune thrombocytopenia purpura. *Am. J. Obstet. Gynecol.* 148:901–908, 1984.

24. Territo, M., Finklestein, J., Oh, W., et al. Management of autoimmune thrombocytopenia in pregnancy and in the neonate. *Obstet. Gynecol.* 41:579–584, 1973.
25. Murray, J.M., Harris, R.E. The management of the pregnant patient with idiopathic thrombocytopenic purpura. *Am. J. Obstet. Gynecol.* 126:449–451, 1976.
26. Scott, J.R., Cruikshank, D.P., Kochenour, N.K., et al. Fetal platelet counts in the obstetric management of immunologic thrombocytopenic purpura. *Am. J. Obstet. Gynecol.* 136:495–499, 1980.
27. Karpatkin, M., Porges, R., Karpatkin, S. Platelet counts in infants of women with autoimmune thrombocytopenia. *N. Engl. J. Med.* 305:936–939, 1981.
28. Kelton, J.C., Inwood, M.J., et al. The prenatal prediction of thrombocytopenia in infants of mothers with clinically diagnosed immune thrombocytopenia. *Am. J. Obstet. Gynecol.* 144:449–454, 1982.

7

Thromboembolic Disease in Obstetrics and Gynecology

Russell K. Laros, Jr., M.D.

The incidence of thromboembolic disease (TED) has been reported in from 1 per 100 to 1 per 1,000 pregnancies. Additionally, TED can produce significant morbidity after a variety of gynecologic surgical procedures. Many years ago, Virchow defined a triad of pathophysiologic events that predisposed to TED. These are 1) injury to vessel wall, 2) stasis, and 3) a hypercoagulable state. Each is present to a greater or lesser degree during pregnancy and also after pelvic surgery.

It has been estimated that, untreated, approximately 25 percent of patients with TED will go on to have a pulmonary embolus (PE) [1]. Again, without proper therapy, 15 percent will die. In contrast, treatment reduces the occurrence of PE to only 5 percent with a mortality rate of less than 1 percent [2]. Thus, because TED occurs relatively frequently in an obstetric-gynecologic practice and because appropriate diagnosis and treatment has a substantial effect on outcome, it behooves the obstetrician-gynecologist to be facile in both diagnosis and treatment of the disease [3].

Diagnosis

The classic signs and symptoms of deep vein thrombosis (DVT) include muscle pain, tenderness, and swelling of the affected extremity. The Homan's sign (pain on dorsiflection) is often positive. Laboratory aids that have been advocated to establish the diagnosis include venography, ^{125}I scanning, sonography, and impedance plethysmography. Venography is clearly the reference standard against which other studies are compared. [125]I fibrinogen scanning is an excellent technique that correlates well with venography for thrombi located in the lower extremity from the midthigh down. Unfortunately, the technique is relatively insensitive in the area of the upper thigh and pelvis [4]. Impedance plethysmography has the advantage of being noninvasive and without radiation risk. Although the combination of ^{125}I scanning and impedance plethysmography allows diagnosis in the majority of nonpregnant patients without resorting to venography, similar data are not available during pregnancy.

Unfortunately, the clinician is often left with either having to proceed with venography or initiate treatment on the basis of clinical diagnosis alone. Because anticoagulant therapy is only required for three to four weeks after an acute episode of DVT, we have been willing to proceed on the basis of strong clinical evidence without a confirmatory venogram during pregnancy. Where the symptoms are less clear, a venogram is obtained. We realize that reliance on clinical signs and symptoms alone may be attended by as high as a 50 percent diagnostic error, and we look forward to improved, noninvasive techniques that will provide a higher degree of diagnostic accuracy. In nonpregnant patients, we follow the scheme of Hirsch, et al. [5] utilizing a combination of ^{125}I scanning and impedance plethysmography.

The symptoms of PE include tachypnea, dyspnea, pleuritic pain, apprehension, cough, tachycardia, hemoptysis, and fever [6]. Unfortunately, with the exception of pleuritic pain and hemoptysis, these symptoms are seen in postoperative patients who do not suffer from PE. Confirmatory physical findings relate to acute right heart failure and include jugular vein distension, an enlarged liver, a left parasternal heave, and fixed splitting of the second heart sound.

Laboratory studies useful in the diagnosis of PE include the electrocardiogram, chest X-ray, fibrinopeptide A level, lung scan, and pulmonary arteriograph. Although the electrocardiogram is abnormal in 90 percent of patients with PE, the most common abnormalities are nonspecific T-wave inversions and tachycardia. The classic findings of acute right heart failure, including right axis deviation, an $S_1Q_3T_3$ pattern, complete right bundle branch block, and p-pulmonale, are relatively unusual.

When the physician suspects a PE the first study done should be an arterial pO_2. If this is normal (greater than 90 mmHg while breathing room air) the patient absolutely does not have a PE. If the pO_2 is abnormal a chest film and lung scan should be performed. Angiography is indicated only if surgical intervention is contemplated or when it is necessary to prove anticoagulant failures requiring venocaval interruption [7].

Treatment

Ancillary treatment of DVT includes bed rest, elevation, heat, analgesic drugs, and elastic stockings. Bed rest with elevation of the involved extremity is valuable initially because it promotes venous return and decreases edema. However, as soon as conditions permit the patient should be encouraged to ambulate since bed rest itself may enhance venous stasis, and there is no evidence that prolonged bed rest prevents embolus detachment. Application of moist heat to the involved areas can cause symptomatic improvement. Analgesic drugs may be required, but those affecting platelet function should be avoided. When correctly designed elastic stockings are used, there is significant increase in the velocity of venous blood flow.

The symptomatic treatment of PE includes oxygen, analgesia, bed rest, vasoactive means, and aminopylline. Oxygen therapy is particularly important during pregnancy, and the maternal pO_2 should be maintained above 70 mmHg. Positive pressure therapy may be required if pulmonary edema is present. Analgesics can be used if the patient experiences significant pain or apprehension (or both).

A vasoactive amine such as isoproterenol or dopamine is indicated for treatment of shock. Isoproterenol (1 mg in 500 ml of normal saline yielding 2 μg/ml) is given a dose of 2 to 8 μg/minute. Dopamine (200 mg in 500 ml of normal saline yielding 400 μg/ml) is begun at 200 μg/minute and increased to a maximum dose of 3,000 μg/minute. If shock is present, the patient should be monitored via a central line measuring eithr the pulmonary wedge pressure or central venous pressure.

Aminophylline is useful in decreasing bronchospasm and additionally has a diuretic action that is particularly beneficial when pulmonary edema is present. The initial dose should be 4 to 5 mg/k of body weight infused over 20 minutes followed by 12 to 15 μg/kg per minute (250 mg in 500 ml of normal saline yielding 500 μg/ml). The dosage should be adjusted to achieve a serum of 10 to 20 μg/ml.

While the above-mentioned symptomatic treatments are important, the backbone of treatment of DVT and PE is anticoagulation. Three major types of therapeutic agents are available, each directed at a different portion of the coagulation process. They consist of agents that interfere with platelet adhesion and aggregation, agents that interfere with fibrin formation, and agents that facilitate clot lysis. In the United States, the most widely used agents are those interfering with fibrin formation, more specifically heparin and the coumarin derivatives. When treating an established DVT, full anticoagulating doses of heparin are utilized with the objective of completely blocking fibrin formation. Heparin should be initiated by the intravenous route utilizing a loading dose of 5,000 U for DVT and 10 to 15,000 U for PE. The patient then is given 15 to 20 U/kg per hour with the dose adjusted to achieve an activated partial thromboplastin time of 2.5 to 3 times normal. It is clear that both the incidence of complications and recurrent TED can be minimized using this approach to therapy. When the patient has been stabilized and the symptoms are improving, the route of administration may be switched to intermittent subcutaneous heparin; if the patient is not pregnant, an oral coumarin agent can be used.

We prefer to instruct the patients in self-injection with heparin utilizing a 25-gauge needle and alternating injection sites on the abdomen. A heparin concentration of 40,000 U/ml is used, and the patient is taught to ice the injection site before each injection, thereby minimizing the occurence of ecchymoses. When conversion is begun, the total daily dose required for intravenous anticoagulation is divided by 3, and the appropriate aliquot of heparin is administered every 8 hours.

The major complication of heparin therapy is hemorrhage; however, careful monitoring can minimize this risk [8,9]. Heparin can cause osteoporosis when administered in doses of greater than 15,000 U per day for more than 6 months [10]. However, this is rarely a problem in obstetrics and gynecology as our patients do not require long-term therapy. Other rare effects of heparin include alopecia, allergic reactions, hypotension, pain at the injection site, and thrombocytopenia. Thrombocytopenia is characterized by a decline in platelet count between the third and eighth day of therapy, with recovery usually following within five days of discontinuation of heparin [11].

When the treatment modality has been converted to intermittent subcutaneous heparin therapy, blood samples should be obtained 6 hours after a dose, and the next dose adjusted so as to achieve an activated partial-thromboplastin time of approximately 1.5 times normal. Once a steady state is achieved, monitoring can be decreased to every other day and ultimately to weekly.

Indications for anticoagulant therapy beyond the acute episode include the occurrence of a PE. We usually treat uncomplicated DVT for 3 to 6 weeks and institute prophylaxis during labor, delivery, and the immediate post partum period. If PE has occurred, therapy should be extended to 6 months. Similarly, therapy should be extended for patients with iliofemoral thrombosis or recurrent venous thrombosis [12].

Although the coumarin agents are widely used to treat TED in nonpregnant persons, they are contraindicated during pregnancy [13]. If administered during the first trimester a syndrome which phenotypically resembles Conradi-Hunermann chondrodysplasia punctata may result. These children are born with multiple congenital anomalies including nasal cartilage hypoplasia, stippling of the bones, growth retardation, microcephaly, and optic atrophy. In a collected series of 214 patients, there were 25 fetal deaths, yielding a mortality of 11.7 percent [14]. In this series, the great majority of such events appeared to be secondary to the trauma of delivery itself. However, in a prospective study of 23 women with heart valve prosthesis who conceived 40 times while receiving coumarin agents, fetal wastage exceeded 80 percent [15].

For nonpregnant patients and the occasional pregnant patient where the balance of risk allows utilization of coumarin therapy the usual anticoagulating dose is 10 to 15 mg of warfarin daily until the prothrombin time is increased to 1.5 to 2.5 times normal. Thereafter, maintenance of 3 to 20 mg daily is utilized, and the prothrombin time is reevaluated once or twice weekly. During conversion from heparin to warfarin, the heparin therapy should be continued until adequate anticoagulation is achieved. Because heparin can prolong the prothrombin time by 2 to 4 seconds, the prothrombin time should be at least 2.5 times normal before heparin is discontinued.

Selected patients such as those with recent pulmonary embolization, recent iliofemoral DVT, and heart valve prostheses should be continued on full heparin anticoagulation during delivery or surgery. These patients should be hospitalized in anticipation of the surgical event, and the regimen should be converted to continuous intravenous heparin. The dosage should be adjusted to achieve an activated partial thromboplastin time of 1.25 to 1.5 times normal during labor and delivery or surgery. Such a regimen does not increase postpartum hemorrhage; however, there is an increase in the incidence of wound hematoma. Conduction anesthesia is contraindicated in a fully anticoagulated patient [12].

DVT Prophylaxis

A variety of agents have proven to be effective in prevention and include the vitamin K antagonist, heparin, dextran, aspirin, and dipyridamole. Currently, low-dose heparin is the most widely used therapeutic modality. The prophylactic effect of "minidose" heparin relates to the fact that a critical concentration of factor X_a (activated factor X) is required for thrombosis formation. Small doses of heparin markedly enhance the activity of antithrombin III, the major plasma inhibitor of factor X_a. Standard regimens employ only 5,000 U of heparin administered subcutaneously every 8 to 12 hours. This dose is sufficient to more than minimally prolong the activated partial thromboplastin time and it is not necessary to monitor the clotting time. The only adverse effect reported is a slight increase in the occurrence of wound hematomas. Multiple studies have confirmed that minidose heparin prophylaxis in patients undergoing abdominal surgery markedly decreases the incidences of DVT and fatal PE [16–19]. Patients should have a baseline hematologic evaluation before initiating prophylactic therapy, and the platelet count should be repeated several times during the first week of therapy. We believe that prophylactic doses of heparin should be used at the time of labor and delivery under the following circumstances: 1) previous PE, 2) previous DVT, 3) patients at high risk for phlebitis such as those with severe varicosities undergoing cesarean section. In gynecologic surgery we believe that prophylaxis is indicated for patients 1) over the age of 40 undergoing major pelvic procedures and 2) undergoing radical pelvic surgery.

When conduction anestheisa is planned the regimen is changed so that the first dose is given at least 6 hours before anesthesia will be required. An activated partial thromboplastin time is obtained before initiating anesthesia, and the second dose of heparin is not given until immediately after the operation.

References

1. Wessler, S. Medical management of venous thrombosis. *Annu. Rev. Med.* 27:313–324, 1976.
2. Villasanta, U. Thromboembolic disease in pregnancy. *Am. J. Obstet. Gynecol.* 93:142–160, 1965.
3. Laros, R.K., Alger, L.S. Thromboembolism and pregnancy. *Clin. Obstet. Gynecol.* 22:871–888, 1979.
4. Gallus, A.S. 125-I fibrinogen leg scanning. In Fratantoni, J., Wessler, S. (eds.), *Prophylactic Therapy of Deep Vein Thrombosis and Pulmonary Embolism.* Bethesda, Md.: National Institutes of Health, 1975, pp. 62–76.
5. Hull, R., Hirsch, J., Sackett, D.L., et al. Cost effectiveness of clinical diagnosis, venography, and noninvasive testing in patients with symptomatic deep-vein thrombosis. *N. Engl. J. Med.* 304:1561–1567, 1981.
6. Sasahara, A.A. The diagnosis of pulmonary embolism: current status. In Fratantoni, J., Wessler, S. (eds.), *Prophylactic Therapy of Deep Vein thrombosis and Pulmonary Embolism.* Bethesda, Md.: National Institutes of Health, 1975, pp. 114–122.
7. Sasahara, A.A. Therapy for pulmonary embolism. *J. Am. Med. Assoc.* 229:1795–1798, 1974.
8. Gervin, A.S. Complications of heparin therapy. *Surg. Gynecol. Obstet.* 140:789–795, 1975.
9. Basu, D., Gallus, A., Hirsh, J., et al. A prospective study of the value of monitoring heparin treatment with the activated partial thromboplastin time. *N. Engl. J. Med.* 287:324–327, 1972.
10. Griffith, G.C., Nichols, G., J., Asher, I.D., et al. Heparin osteoporosis. *J. Am. Med. Assoc.* 193:185–190, 1965.
11. Babcock, R.B., Dumper, C.M., Scharkman, W.B. Heparin-induced immune thrombocytopenia. *N. Engl. J. Med.* 295:237–246, 1976.
12. Laros, R.K. Venous thromboembolism. In Quilligan, F.J. (ed.), *Current Therapy in Obstetrics and Gynecology.* Philadelphia: The W. B. Saunders Co., 1982, pp. 21–239.

13. Shaul, W.L., Hall, J.G. Multiple congenital anomalies associated with oral anticoagulants. *Am. J. Obstet. Gynecol.* 127:191–198, 1977.
14. Laros, R.K. Anticoagulants: indications and use. *Contemp. Obstet. Gynecol.* 5:67–71, 1975.
15. Lutz, D.J., Noller, K.L., Spittell, J.A., Jr., et al. Pregnancy and its complications following cardiac valve prostheses. *Am. J. Obstet. Gynecol.* 131:460–468, 1978.
16. Gallus, A.S., Hirsch, J., Tuttle, R.J., et al. Small subcutaneous doses of heparin in prevention of venous thrombosis. *N. Engl. J. Med.* 288:545–552, 1973.
17. Kakkar, V.V., Nicolaides, A.N., Field, E.S., et al. Low doses of heparin in prevention of deep vein thrombosis. *Lancet* 2:669–671, 1971.
18. Nicolaides, A.N., Hirsch, J., Tuttle, R.J., et al. Small doses of subcutneous sodium heparin in preventing deep venous thrombosis after major surgery. *Lancet* 2:890, 1972.
19. Wessler, S. Heparin as an antithrombotic agent: low dose prophylaxis. *J. Am. Med. Assoc.* 236:389–394, 1976.

8

Pregnancy-Induced Hypertension: New Perspectives on an Old Disorder

John Patrick O'Grady, M.D.

Life is short, the art long, opportunity fleeting, experience treacherous, judgment difficult.
Hippocrates, Aphorisms, I.I., 350 B.C.

Introduction

Hypertension, occurring in 5 to 7 percent of all pregnancies, is a complex and serious disorder with the potential for both fetal and maternal injury [1–6]. Hypertension coexists with pregnancy by serendipity, by preceding the gravid state, or as a primary disease process arising during the course of gestation. Hypertension arising de novo in pregnancy is frequently (and often inaccurately) termed preeclampsia. Hypertensive states noted in pregnant women may also be designated as pregnancy-aggravated hypertension, gestational hypertension, toxemia of pregnancy, chronic hypertension with superimposed preeclampsia, or several other descriptive titles depending upon the presentation, past history, and the clinician involved in establishing the diagnosis. Part of the interest in the hypertensive disorders of pregnancy is that the distinction between the disorders is difficult, theories of etiology are multiple, and therapeutic plans are many.

Although much is known of hypertensive states in pregnant women, many controversies persist. Much of the published material is anecdotal, contradictory, and repetitive. A clearer focus on the diagnosis and treatment of this complex disorder based on an understanding of its pathophysiology is necessary. This chapter focuses on errors in establishing the correct diagnosis in hypertensive women and the dilemmas inherent in therapeutic choices.

Hypertension in Pregnancy: Definitions

Preeclampsia of pregnancy is often termed a disease of theories. It is also a disease of therapies and of descriptive titles. Toxemia of pregnancy and preeclampsia are commonly used interchangeably to mean a syndrome involving specified hypertension ($\geqslant 140/90$ or a rise of $\geqslant 30$/mmHg systolic or $\geqslant 15$ mmHg diastolic) with proteinuria (> 300 mg/24 hours) and edema occurring in pregnant women after the 20th week of gestation with a return to normal values within 10 days after delivery [7]. Toxemia as a textbook term dates from the early 20th century. The word initially was used to describe hypertension in pregnancy, implying that the etiology was due to a toxic fetal product absorbed into the maternal circulation. Despite efforts to remove the term "toxemia" from medical use, it still aggressively persists in clinical obstetrics. Preeclampsia implies that the syndrome may progress into convulsions. Pregnancy-induced hypertension (PIH) also recently has emerged as a clinical term for hypertension first observed during pregnancy [6].

The disease may present occasionally with atypical symptoms including blindness, coagulopathy, nephrotic syndrome, or seemingly isolated hepatic dysfunction [5,8–10]. Accurate clinical diagnosis of "true" preeclampsia as separated from other disorders capable of producing hypertension is notoriously difficult. As Chesley [11] observes, a hypertensive, pregnant woman diagnosed as preeclamptic may have preeclampsia, chronic hypertension with superimposed preeclampsia, chronic "hypertension" that has abated with the usual decline in the middle trimester, or another disease process altogether (i.e., chronic glomerulonephritis). Therefore, the establishment of an accurate diagnosis in this disorder is difficult and all too often retrospective.

Biopsy studies indicate that even when the diagnosis is clinically assigned by experienced observers, it is substantiated by a specific lesion "glomerular endotheliosis" on renal biopsy in only 60 to 80 percent of cases [12,13] (Table 8–1).

Table 8–1
Renal Pathology in 176 Hypertensive Gravidas

Diagnosis	Number of Patients	Primigavidas	Multiparas
Preeclampsia[a]	96	79	17
With nephrosclerosis	13	6	7
With renal disease	3	1	2
With both	2	1	1
Nephrosclerosis	19	3	16
With renal disease	4	2	2
Renal disease	31	12	19
Normal histology	8	0	8

[a] Only glomerular endotheliosis on biopsy [12].

91

The specificity of glomerular endotheliosis for preeclampsia [14] is not universally accepted. However, a number of biopsy studies (see Fisher et al. [12] for review) support glomerular endotheliosis as distinctive for preeclampsia. Fisher et al. [12] note that this abnormality is present in a minority of hypertensive multiparas, but in 60 to 80 percent of nulliparous, hypertensive women. The specificity of the lesion is supported by studies of patients biopsied in the puerperium and then subsequently followed with careful attention to the eventual development of chronic hypertension. Women with glomerular endotheliosis on renal biopsy proved to have the same prevalence of hypertension as the reference population. In contrast, 74 percent of those with evidence of nephrosclerosis had developed fixed hypertension by a mean of 79 months (range 4 to 199 months) after the initial biopsy. Epidemiologic studies supported by the biopsy data previously reviewed have at length clarified the long-term implications of preeclampsia and eclampsia as opposed to the other hypertensive disorders with which it may be confused. The unique, long-term studies of Chesley show that "classic" eclampsia and proteinuric preeclampsia carry no implication for the eventual development of chronic hypertension [11]. However, gestational hypertension without proteinuria or abnormal edema is frequently a sign of latent hypertension that has been revealed during pregnancy and carries a much different prognosis. Therefore, pregnancy serves as a screening test for eventual chronic hypertension. Development of gestational hypertension (not preeclampsia or eclampsia) indicates that a woman is at high risk for the eventual development of chronic hypertension. Finally, women with normotensive pregnancies prove to have a low incidence of hypertension. Also, if hypertension occurs, it has a later onset.

Concepts of the possible etiology of preeclampsia are many and therapeutic plans variable [15,16]. Discussion of these points is beyond the scope of this chapter. However, recent interest has centered on immunologic abnormalities [17,18], prostaglandin deficiency syndromes [19], abnormalities of Ca^{++} metabolism [20], or genetic disorders [11] as likely etiologies. However, as in the past, no current, single explanation for preeclampsia adequately explains the clinical and laboratory features of the disease.

Clinical Blood Pressure Measurement

The inconsistencies between reports of the prognosis and treatment of hypertensive pregnant patients relate to different populations, various criteria for evaluation and screening, and partially to variations in the clinical recording of arterial blood pressure. The inexactitude and complexity of the clinical measurement of arterial pressure are often overlooked, and the definitions of normal arterial pressure are frequently incompletely understood. In 1904, Korotkoff described a series of five phases or sounds heard by clinical auscultation as peripheral arterial pressure was measured with a sphygmomanometer [21]. These sounds depend upon the passage of blood through arterial vessels with and without external cuff compression. It has long been recognized that end zero bias, variation between observers, patient position and emotional state, and the technique used (cuff size, auscultating ability of operator, and so on) affect results. Additionally, care must be taken that the appropriate sound of Korotkoff is used to designate the diastolic blood pressure [21]. Most clinicians report the diastolic pressure at Korotkoff's phase IV (muffling of the arterial sound as the mercury column in the manometer falls). But in some studies the fifth phase (disappearance of the muffled sound) is accepted as the diastolic measurement. The fifth Korotkoff phase gives a reading below simultaneously measured intraarterial pressure, whereas the fourth phase gives a reading too high. However, clinically, the fifth phase is often not useful in pregnant patients, as no disappearance of the arterial sound may occur as the mercury column drops.

In recognition of these inherent inaccuracies, the definitions for the diagnosis of hypertension require documentation of repeated pressure elevations six hours apart [7]. End zero bias, the recording of arterial pressure by clinicians in 10-mmHg segments, and the inherent errors in routine pressure ascertainment are partially overcome in clinical studies by the use of a "random zero" sphygmomanometer. These devices vary the height of the mercury column during pressure determinations in a random fashion not controlled by the operator. After a pressure is recorded, the artifactual, additional pressure elevation is released, and the true pressure is calculated [22].

When careful attention to these and other variables of technique and recording have been used, diastolic blood pressures are found to be surprisingly low, especially if ascertained in young nulliparas resting in lateral recumbancy [23,24]. As Table 8–2 indicates, the resting diastolic pressure early in the third trimester averages less than 50 mmHg (torr) in normal, young nulliparas.

However, the emphasis on diastolic pressure levels as critical in pa-

Table 8–2
Diastolic Arterial Blood Pressure (mmHg)[a]

Gestational age (weeks)	29	30	31	32
Mean mmHg ± SEM	49.2 ± 1.25	48.8 ± 1.11	49.0 ± 1.11	50.8 ± 1.08

[a] Korotkoff phase IV, by Doppler ultrasound following left lateral recumbancy for 30 minutes; ages, 14 to 20 years; $n = 40$.

tient evaluation obscures the fact that mean arterial pressure (MAP) may be a better reflection of the true effect of pressure on hemodynamics [3]. As normally calculated, MAP equals the diastolic pressure added to one-third of the pulse pressure. Using this calculation applied to data derived from 14,833 pregnancies, Page and Christianson [3] have shown that perinatal mortality increases progressively with each 5-torr rise in MAP. With an MAP of >90 torr after the 18th week of gestation there was a significant increase in stillborn rates, growth-retarded infants, and third-trimester proteinuria, hypertension, and diagnosed preeclampsia. These effects were more marked in black women than in white women. For many clinicians arterial pressures when reported as MAPs hold surprises. For example, a MAP of 90 torr occurs when the arterial pressure is recorded as 130/70 or at 110/80, neither of which, on casual review, would be interpreted as elevated. Friedman's analysis of arterial blood pressure in pregnant women indicates that elevated pressure (in this study, diastolic blood pressure) and proteinuria are additive in their adverse effects on pregnancy. In collaborative study data involving 38,636 gravidas, fetal death rates increased proportionately to diastolic pressure, with a fourfold rise if diastolic pressure reached or exceeded 95 torr. Sustained diastolic pressures as low as 75 torr were associated with excess fetal loss if accompanied by proteinuria. In fact, when analyzed by gestational age, fetal mortality was significantly increased if diastolic pressure reached or exceeded 75 torr before the 27th week of gestation.

Therefore, in epidemologic studies of arterial pressure in pregnancy, pressure elevations that appear moderate, especially if commencing early in gestation, have a significant impact on fetal mortality [25]. This data and the data of Page and Christianson indicate that apparent mild elevations in pressure are not benign. Further, the linear increase in perinatal complications suggests that if there is a threshold pressure below which demonstrable damage does not occur, it is much lower in pregnancy than commonly appreciated.

Hypertension and Cardiovascular Physiology

Discussion of the pathophysiology of PIH implies specific understanding of the cardiovascular alterations in normal gestation and how these are deranged in the hypertensive state. Changes in cardiovascular function in pregnancy include alterations in stroke volume, peripheral resistance, and vascular volume. The etiology of these changes is not understood, but is felt to be due to the hormonal alterations coincident with pregnancy [26].

In normal pregnancy vascular volume expands to 140 to 150 percent of the normal state before pregnancy, with detectable change by the sixth week of gestation (Figure 8–1). Mean plasma volume reaches a maximum

Figure 8–1

Measured Plasma Volumes in 453 Normal Pregnant Women. The shaded segment indicates the 80th through 20th percentile. Solid lines indicate the lowest and highest recorded values (milligrams per kilogram). *(Modified from Lund, C. J., Donovan, J. C. Blood volume during pregnancy: significance of plasma and red cell volumes.* Am. J. Obstet. Gynecol. 98:393–403, 1967).

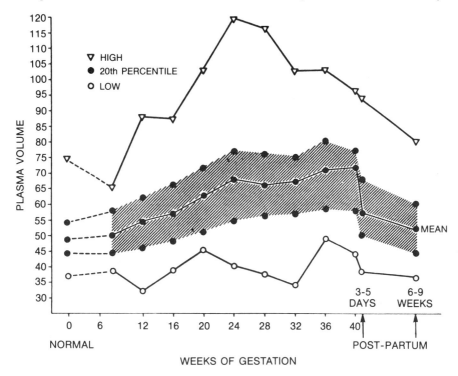

by the 26th week and then remains essentially stable until term. There is, however, substantial variation in measurements of individual patients with a wide range of normal for plasma volumes [27].

Adequate vascular expansion is correlated with infant birth weight and is a sign of normal compensation to the pregnant state [28]. Fluid retention and the development of dependent edema are common to both normal gestation and preeclampsia. Peripheral edema is no longer considered a reliable sign of PIH and simply reflects a normal expansion of extracellular volume [29,30]. Preeclampsia may occur (and even be more severe) in the absence of peripheral edema [5,29]. Despite edema, it is clear that dietary sodium restriction or diuretic treatment (or both) has no beneficial effects in avoidance of preeclampsia [31]. Sodium metabolism is deranged in PIH; however, the mechanism is unknown, as neither changes in glomerular filtration rate nor alterations in aldosterone secretion

Figure 8–2

Plasma Volume in Pregnancy. Plasma volume (milliliters per centimeter of height) (mean ± SD) sequentially in normal pregnant women (■, n = 189) and in women who developed hypertension (☐, n = 40). At 33 to 36 weeks of amenorrhoea, only data from the 29 women whose blood pressure had not yet risen are shown (*** = p < 0.001). *(From Gallery, E.D. M., Hunyor, S.N., Gyory, A.Z. Plasma volume contraction: a significant factor in both pregnancy-associated hypertension and pregnancy. Q. J. Med. 48:593–602, 1979).*

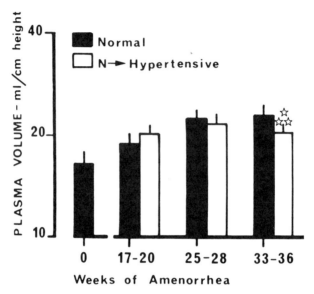

appear to be an adequate explanation. Lindeheimer and Katz [9] make the interesting suggestion that desoxycorticosterone, possibly of fetal origin, may play a role in abnormal edema formation.

In established PIH, intravascular volume is reduced [30–33]. Also, when followed serially, patients with chronic hypertension who eventually develop PIH fail to show the vascular expansion expected for normal pregnancy [33]. Gallery et al. [30] have studied vascular volume as measured by Evans blue dye in clinically normal patients. In patients eventually developing elevated blood pressure, volume reductions preceded clinical hypertension by one to four weeks (Figure 8–2).

Vasospasm and changes in vascular permeability shift fluid entering the vascular system from the intravascular to the extravascular compartment [23]. This fluid shift reduces the circulating blood volume and leads to increased blood viscosity, which may accelerate and contribute to the placental dysfunction often present in PIH [34,35]. There is no consensus of opinion on the plasma volume of pregnant patients with mild to moderate hypertension. In this setting, vascular volume has been reported to be the same as for normal, pregnant patients [30,36] or reduced [29,32,37]. These differences in the chronically hypertensive woman likely relate to the populations tested, the type and severity of the underlying disease, and where in the clinical course patients were evaluated. It is a paradox of physiology that vascular volume appropriate for the normal adult woman is distinctly abnormal in the pregnant state. Gallery [29] and others [32,37–39] suggest that the failure of vascular expansion is a marker for the severity and course of PIH and a valuable tool for studying the disorder.

The vascular volume research data are difficult to translate into clinical management. The current therapeutic debate is whether diminished volume is a contributing cause of preeclampsia and thus deserves treatment or is merely a physiologic marker reflecting the severity of the underlying process [29,31,39–43]. Or, better put, whether if reduced vascular volume can be detected, reexpansion is likely to improve the patient's clinical status and permit pregnancy to continue. Assali, and Vaughn, for example [40] argue that the observed reductions in volume are hemodynamically insignificant, representing a mean decrease of only about 9 percent.

Treatment for the reexpansion of diminished volume is not new. Chesley [5] reviewed case reports going back to the early 1930s reporting treatment of eclamptics with intravenous solutions of acacia, resulting in apparent clinical improvement. Subsequent studies have involved the infusion of blood, plasma, serum, or plasma expanders such as dextran or mannitol to treat preeclamptics with variable reports of hemodilution, diuresis, and reduction of arterial pressure [31,39,41]. The physiologic reasons behind these reported improvements are uncertain. Some patients may have been seriously volume depleted by prolonged disease or inappropriate treatment, thus, for them, acute volume replacement constituted appropriate therapy. In other cases, the patients were treated with a number of agents with vascular expansion simply part of complex polypharmacy, and it is impossible to clearly identify the agent(s) responsible for the reported clinical response. The best recent work on vascular expansion therapy is by Gallery [29]. Fourteen women with "pregnancy-associated" hypertension who failed to respond to 48 hours of simple hospital bed rest were infused with 500 cc of a plasma protein extract. Significant declines in arterial pressure in 12 of 14 cases were reported, with the arterial pressure remaining down for a mean duration of 48 hours. (Figure 8–3).

Gallery et al. [43] have also reported the reversal of plasma volume constriction during treatment of PIH patients with a beta blocker, oxyprenolol, but not with methyldopa, despite adequate pressure control with both. Pressure control with the beta blocker was accompanied by improved fetal growth in utero as expressed in fetal and placental weights at birth

Figure 8–3

Blood pressure response of 14 patients to the intravenous infusion of stable protein substrate (SPPS). Note that the effect is variable, and one patient had increases in pressure in response to protein infusion. The period of response was both brief and unpredictable. *(From Gallery, E.D.M. Pregnancy-associated hypertension: interrelationships of volume and blood pressure changes. Clin. Exper. Hypertension 1: 39–47, 1982, by courtesy of Marcel Dekker, Inc.)*

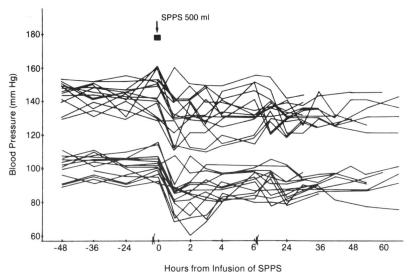

Hours from Infusion of SPPS

as compared with methyldopa. Perhaps newer pharmacologic agents can promote vascular reexpansion by relieving vasospasm and other circulatory abnormalities and lead to improved fetal outcomes. However, more clinical studies need to be performed in various categories of patients before any firm conclusions can be reached.

It is clear that changes in peripheral resistance and shifts in circulating volume from intravascular to extravascular sites characterize many, but not all, patients with gestational hypertension. Although vascular volume expansion has not been harmful in the most reported instances when used [39], it is still not clear how treatment of this sign of PIH is therapeutically helpful in clinical management as long as the basic feature, increased vascular resistance, persists. Assali and Vaughn [40] and Morris and O'Grady [42] have been particularly critical of the vascular expansion school. Basing their critique on cardiovascular physiology, they forcefully argue that volume fits itself to the space provided within the vascular system. Therefore, alterations in volume are not the cause, but the effect of changes in peripheral resistance. Viewed in this light, it is irrational to treat volume alone without concomitant therapy for vasospasm. Reports such as Gallery's of apparent return of measured volume toward expected pregnancy norms with control of hypertension is what should be expected if the peripheral resistance of PIH is relieved. Moreover, if rapid vascular expansion is administered in the face of renal dysfunction it may simply result in vascular overload and serious complications [6].

At present, there is limited applicability of the vascular data to clinical obstetrics. In the experience of most clinicians, selected patients with PIH will be found to have marked oliguria and hypovolemia. With pharmacologic reductions in peripheral resistance these women will profit from judicious vascular reexpansion in the process of preparing them for delivery. If treatment for volume depletion has any other applications, except as a research tool, it must at present be considered.

Hypertension: Clinical Management

The problem in management of the hypertensive pregnant patient is how to convert theories of pathophysiology into rational therapy. The principal reason that therapeutics have changed little in recent years is that the choice of a management plan is of trivial concern in the majority of pregnant patients with hypertension. The disorder (in the classic sense of preeclampsia) is most common in young nulliparas. The onset is frequently in the end of the third trimester, but may rarely first occur before 20 weeks of gestation or even postpartum. Treatment consists of documenting the diagnosis, preventing convulsions, dampening severe elevations in blood pressure, and achieving delivery. These therapeutic maneuvers have been unchanged for many years and, when accompanied by close and experienced clinical observation, produce uniformly good fetal and maternal results [5,6,31,44,45]. The therapeutic challenge arises in management of patients who are chronically hypertensive throughout pregnancy or who develop acute, symptomatic hypertension remote from term.

Before considering therapy in PIH, it is essential to determine whether maternal or fetal indications exist for termination of pregnancy. If the parturient has documented evidence of coagulopathy with abnormalities of platelet count, fibrinogen, or basic coagulation profiles, termination is appropriate regardless of the period of gestation. Also, obstetricians terminate pregnancy in the face of serious maternal complications, abruptio placentae, eclamptic convulsions or other major neurologic signs, or significant hepatic enzyme elevations. Clinical maternal deterioration with rising blood pressure and increasing symptomology despite hospitalization or therapy (or both) is also an indication for delivery. Evidence of fetal compromise as evidenced by ultrasonic studies suggesting fetal growth retardation, especially if accompanied by marked oligohydramnios or fetal heart rate decelerations with uterine contractions (a positive contraction stress test), would also be considered a persuasive indication for termination. We need to narrow our view to therapeutic issues in patients who are discovered to have elevations in blood pressure when neither maternal nor fetal reasons demand immediate termination of pregnancy.

If we elect not to deliver a patient with hypertension we must face several questions. First, can pregnancy be safely prolonged despite hypertension? Second, does treatment of chronic or acute hypertension during pregnancy prevent maternal or fetal complications? Third, what level of blood pressure should be treated and how vigorously?

The general training given obstetricians is that preeclampsia is a progressive, relentless disorder that, if left untreated, results in serious complications [6]. Thus, once a diagnosis is established, the only effective treatment is delivery. Therapeutics in this view are for the acute control of symptoms. Continuation of pregnancy is permissible only if the hypertension is in the mildest and the earliest phases or responds promptly to restriction of activity, or hospitalization, or both [46]. Conversely, if hypertension is felt to be chronic without acute exacerbation, the common view is that pregnancy may continue and that only acute deterioration needs prompt intervention.

The desirability of treating hypertension in pregnancy, unless severe, is controversial [31,45,47–50]. Several major authors believe that control of other than serious hypertension cannot be supported by the available data [6,31,45,48,50]. This argument is based on several premises. For example, Berkowitz [48], Chesley [31], and Sibai et al. [50] argue that improvement in maternal and fetal well-being cannot be documented in patients treated for mild to moderate chronic pressure elevations. It is also argued that hypertensive therapy reduces effective uterine blood flow [6]. According to this view, currently available pharmacologic control of hypertension necessarily compromises either fetal or maternal interests. Thus, only moderate to severe hypertension would be considered for treatment where clear maternal indications exist and the avoidance of serious complications outweighs the potential fetal risks.

There are some aspects of this controversy where the majority of clinicians would find agreement. There is a general consensus that hypertensive pregnant patients with elevations of diastolic pressure greater than 110 torr need prompt therapy to reduce arterial tension. The potential deleterious effects of such advanced hypertension are well established by both clinical and research studies [1,47,48]. Experiments indicate surprisingly rapid and extensive microscopic damage to vascular beds in the face of hypertension [51,52] corresponding to levels of 180/120 torr in humans. Severe hypertension also predisposes to hypertensive encephalopathy and retinopathy [53] due to gross dysfunction in the autoregulatory control of the central nervous system [54]. Elevated arterial pressure and severe vasospasm may also lead to convulsions, blindness, or other central nervous system symptoms. Under these circumstances, pressure elevations are in all senses malignant and must be promptly treated to avoid major complications. However, most cases are found beyond these extremes. Although there will be little discussion among clinicians about the necessity for control of severely elevated maternal arterial pressure, there is little consensus about treatment and its goals in cases of less profound pressure elevations where the maternal risk is not so clear or the clinical circumstances are not so urgent.

Depending upon the patient pool selected and the type of analysis performed, one either can [47,55] or cannot [31,48,50] support treatment of moderate hypertension in chronically hypertensive women.

The situation with regard to preeclamptic, and not chronically hypertensive, patients with elevations of arterial pressure over previously normal values is unsettled and is often only indirectly addressed in the various reviews of PIH treatment. The grouping of patients with acute and chronic hypertension implies that the same arguments for or against established treatment goals have equal validity for both. Although this may be true in the most florid and acute stages in which maternal considerations necessitate prompt intervention and termination, it is not necessarily true in less urgent circumstances. Whether the patients with preeclampsia should be treated like patients with chronic hypertension is conjectural. Physiologically, the preeclamptic patients are different. They are more frequently found to have glomerular endotheliosis rather than nephrosclerosis by biopsy [12,13]. Gallery et al. [30] and Lund and Donovan [27] note that the vascular volume of preeclamptic patients is usually different from that of chronically hypertensive patients. The onset of hypertension may be more acute and commonly begins from a physiologically lower MAP. Finally, the population involved is usually younger, and excellent results have been reported from clinical series where antihypertensive drugs are not commonly used [6,46].

Therapeutic nihilism in the treatment of preeclampsia arises from a series of beliefs. Gant and Worley [6], Pritchard [45], and Gilstrap et al. [46] are opponents of pharmacologic therapeutics, arguing that treatment is simply unnecessary in all but the most severe cases, as excellent results can be obtained in most cases without their use. There is also the widely held, but unsupported (and incorrect), belief that there exists a given diastolic blood pressure below which convulsions do not occur. A decision not to treat also is tied to the concept that reductions in MAP necessarily imply worsening of uteroplacental blood flow and thus fetal compromise.

Pressure and Placental Perfusion

There is an established clinical belief that elevated blood pressure either should not be treated during pregnancy or that, if treated, it should not be dropped below a specified level because of the need to maintain a

101

certain (but unspecified) pressure head to assure placental perfusion. This pervasive concept implies that reductions in MAP inevitably reduce placental perfusion and worsen fetoplacental function. The control of placental perfusion is as yet incompletely understood [56], and the current belief is that uteroplacental blood flow is diminished in preeclampsia [9,31,57]. The situation is complicated by the anatomic changes that occur due to trophoblastic invasion of the muscular coats surrounding uterine spiral arteries [58]. If this process produces lead pipe-like vessels with anatomically restricted lumens, then it is possible that the characteristics of human uterine blood flow might be principally pressure related and similar to flow characteristics of the ovine placenta. If this were strictly true, any reductions in perfusion pressure would necessarily diminish placental blood flow. Many clinicians believe and teach that the diastolic blood pressure of hypertensive pregnant patients should not be allowed to fall below 90 torr under treatment, regardless of what the prehypertensive or predicted diastolic pressure was or should be. However, there are no data substantiating this particular level of pressure control as demonstrably more desirable than 75, 85, or even 95 torr. The 90-torr limit is more defensible if suggested as a therapeutic goal for patients with chronic hypertension. Under these circumstances, holding pressures at 90 torr may either mimic the resting, nonpregnant pressure or represent at best a moderate increase in diastolic arterial blood pressure. However, this logic is less persuasive in preeclampsia. In these usually younger and often nulliparous patients a fixed diastolic arterial blood pressure of 90 torr may represent a 20 to 30-torr increase over basal pressure and thus be seriously elevated.

In the absence of conflicting or inconvenient data it is easy to make definite pronouncements about a desirable diastolic or mean arterial blood pressure as a therapeutic goal. In the chronically hypertensive, a reasonable goal may be to return the diastolic arterial pressure to the prepregnancy level, if known, or 90 torr, whichever is lower. If prepregnancy levels are not known, then 90 torr remains a reasonable goal at least by familiarity, but admittedly it is arbitrary. In preeclamptics remote from term, however, when normal or nearly normal pressures were documented early in gestation, pressure reductions to levels considered within the normal range for that patient's age and parity should be considered if she is not to be promptly delivered. Such a strategy is as arbitrary as the accepted 90-torr level. Yet, as stepwise reductions in mean arterial pressure are noted to improve fetal survival and perhaps reduce fetal morbidity, such an approach is equally defensible. However, such a strategy reflects a belief that "moderate" pressure elevations are not beneficial during pregnancy and deserve active treatment. Clearly, such a position is neither favored nor supported by many of the writers in this field. This discussion hinges on an important, but surprisingly poorly investigated, point: how elevated diastolic pressure in humans affects fetal and placental function. In normal pregnancy, the placental circulation must be able to function in the face of a range of changes in maternal MAP. Intermittent supine hypotension, the 15 percent reduction in MAP during sleep state, and the effects of uterine contractions both before and during labor are examples of stress with which the normal fetoplacental unit must inevitably contend (see discussions by Lindheimer and Kate [9] and Redman [47]).

Research studies on the control of uteroplacental blood flow are bedeviled by wide species variation and differing methodologies. As Rankin and McLaughlin [56] point out, the maternal placental vascular bed does not appear to be under maternal control, yet displays excellent matching of perfusion ratios indicating the function of a local control mechanism capable of circulating matching within the placental cotyledons. The strong implication is that the links between fetomaternal circulation matching are under humoral control, probably modulated by the fetus. Recent suspicion has suggested that abnormalities in prostacyclin production, noted in the umbilical vessels of fetuses from pregnancies complicated by PIH, intrauterine growth retardation, or both—two cases in which reduced placental perfusion is a recognized feature—may be critical. Recent uncertainty about the prostacyclin mechanism has focused attention toward other anachnodonic acid metabolites, particularly the leukotrienes in local control of placental flow (J.H.G. Rankin, personal communication.)

Animal studies provide species models for the study of placental perfusion, but are complicated by methodologic and species variation. In acute ovine experiments, uterine blood flow appears to have a direct relationship to pressure, and autoregulation is not noted. However, in rabbits autoregulation has been reported over a range of perfusion pressures [62]. The validity of these observations is strongly debated. Species differences may explain these discrepancies. However, it is also possible that autoregulation is operative over varied time periods in different species, a subtlety lost if only acute experimentation is performed. The efforts of Venuto et al. are strongly criticized by Gant and Worley [6] and Chesley [31], who are particularly critical of the fact the studies were performed in an anesthetized animal preparation. There are, however, compelling clinical grounds for the belief that the placenta in many hypertensive patients is capable of function and perhaps even improved function after pharmacologic reduction in arterial pressure. Longitudinal studies of the control of chronically elevated blood pressure in pregnant patients indicate improved fetal survival in threatened cases [63–67]. In treatment of acutely elevated blood pressure in gravid patients, Morris et al. [68] noted that 35 to 50 percent reductions in MAP induced rapidly by intravenous diazoxide were frequently tolerated without significant fetal heart rate changes or poor pregnancy outcomes. Obviously, there are limits to which such aggressive pressure treatment can reach before both placental and fetal reserves are exhausted. It does appear that acute and precipitous drops in arterial pressure may be associated with signs of fetal distress [44,68]. For example, fetal heart rate decelerations have been reported after aggressive administration of hydralazine and diazoxide to severely hypertensive women [45]. Yet we and others [69,70] have observed rapid fluctuations of MAP in hypertensive pregnant patients undergoing hemodialysis where acute pressure fluctuations of 20 to 50 torr are common with the commencement of machine function. These rapid fluctuations seem to be well tolerated by the fetus, at least as reflected in electronic fetal monitoring tracings of the fetal heart.

It is not true that reductions in elevated arterial pressure, especially in long-term treatment of hypertension, are necessarily deleterious to placental function. As a matter of fact, a case can be made that the reverse is true [43,47]. There exists substantial clinical evidence from trials of patients undergoing hypertensive therapy that reductions in arterial pressure improve fetal survival [63–67]. The case for pressure control having beneficial effects on fetal survival and growth is strengthened when patients are treated early in pregnancy. Redman et al. [65] and Leather et al. [63] both observed decreased middle trimester losses in chronically hypertensive patients who were under treatment. In the past, little attention has been directed at the possible adverse effects of even mild to moderate blood pressure elevations in the middle trimester. Silverstone et al. [55] studied arterial pressure in a series of 156 gestations in patients whose pregnancies were complicated by fetal death and spontaneously terminated between 16 and 27 weeks of gestation. The mean pressure in the loss group was 80 ± 14 torr, by standard view a minimal elevation. Although this pressure appears normal, it is clear from a number of clinical studies that this pressure is in fact significantly elevated for the middle trimester [3,25,42,55]. Thus, the general belief that "moderate" pressure elevations, at least that occurring early in gestation, are not associated with fetal risk is simply incorrect. Thus, although embarrassment of fetoplacental circulation is an important theoretical concern, clinical experience suggests that reductions in maternal MAP are benign in most cases, unless acute and extreme drops occur in the most severely ill patients. There is no overwhelming clinical evidence that aggressive treatment of hypertension is detrimental to fetus and mother, and there is substantial suggestion that the reverse is in fact true. As Redman aptly states [47], if placental perfusion can only be assured by serious sustained increases in maternal blood pressure, then prompt delivery is the appropriate treatment. This is rarely the case.

PIH: Therapeutic Agents

If hypertension is to be treated, which agents are appropriate? In American obstetrics, three agents, magnesium sulfate, methyldopa, and hydralazine, have achieved overwhelming popularity for the treatment of preeclampsia [31,45,48].

Magnesium sulfate is not properly an antihypertensive, but more accurately a sedative and anticonvulsant agent, and is by far the most popular. Principal reliance on $MgSO_4$ and prompt delivery in preeclampsia have resulted in extremely good statistics for maternal and fetal survival [45]. Most practicing obstetricians add parenteral hydralazine to $MgSO_4$ in more acute cases of acute PIH, again with great safety attested by years of experience [31]. In mild PIH, oral methyldopa in doses up to 2 g/day occasionally accompanied by hydralazine is administered [65]. European investigators have been substantially more aggressive in the use of newer agents, especially beta blockers, and new interest has been raised in calcium channel blockers. Interested readers are referred to the recent review of Berkowitz [48] for a discussion and review of available agents.

Conclusions

PIH is a complex syndrome involving patients of varied age, parity, and underlying disorders who are pregnant and have elevated arterial pressure. Exact diagnosis in many cases is impossible, except retrospectively. Acute elevations of arterial pressure, if accompanied by serious maternal or fetal signs, are best managed by prompt delivery. The onset of acute symptoms late in pregnancy usually presents no significant clinical dilemma or therapeutic problems. Control of acute pressure elevations, treatment with one or more antileptics, and prompt termination of pregnancy will result in uniformly good outcomes. The difficult patients are those remote from term with significant elevations of arterial pressure. The preponderance of clinical evidence suggests that reductions in arterial pressure are not detrimental to pregnancy. In fact, the contrary is more likely true. Therapeutic maneuvers for the control of elevated pressure are appropriate, and the best prospective studies suggest that the treatment of moderate elevations of arterial pressure improves fetal well-being. The claims that the newer beta blockers, or vascular expansion therapy ameliorate the fluid and pressure disorders in hypertensive pregnant women simply require additional study and verification. The choice of agent for blood pressure control is less critical than care in maintaining the reductions in arterial pressure, while carefully following parameters of fetal growth and maternal and fetal well-being.

References

1. Lin, C.C., Lindheimer, M.D., River, P., Moawad, A.H. Fetal outcome in hypertensive disorders of pregnancy. *Am. J. Obstet. Gynecol.* 142:255–260, 1982.

2. Naeye, R.L., Friedman, E.A. Causes of perinatal death associated with gestational hypertension and proteinuria. *Am. J. Obstet. Gynecol.* 133:8–10, 1979.

3. Page, E.W., Christianson, R. The impact of mean arterial pressure in the middle trimester upon the outcome of pregnancy. *Am. J. Obstet. Gynecol.* 125:740–746, 1975.

4. Pritchard, J.A., MacDonald, P.C. Hypertensive disorders in pregnancy. In: *Williams Obstetrics,* 16th ed. New York: Appleton-Century-Crofts, 1980, pp. 665–700.

5. Chesley, L.C. *Hypertensive Disorders in Pregnancy.* Norwalk, Conn.: Appleton-Century-Crofts, 1978, pp. 525.

6. Gant, N.F., Worley, R.J. *Hypertension in Pregnancy: Concepts and Management.* Norwalk, Conn.: Appleton-Century-Crofts, 1981, p. 211.

7. Hughes, E.C. (ed.) *Obstetric-Gynecologic Terminology.* Philadelphia: F.A. Davis, 1972, pp. 422–423.

8. Weinstein, L. Syndrome of hemolysis, elevated liver enzymes, and low platelet count: a severe consequence of hypertension in pregnancy. *Am. J. Obstet. Gynecol.* 142:159–167, 1982.

9. Lindheimer, M.D., Katz, A.I. pathophysiology of preeclampsia. *Annu. Rev. Med.* 32:273–289, 1981.

10. Schwartz, M.L., Brenner, W.E. Pregnancy-induced hypertension presenting with life threatening thrombocytopenia. *Am. J. Obstet. Gynecol.* 146:756–759, 1983.

11. Chesley, L.C. Hypertension in pregnancy: definitions, familial factor, and remote prognosis. *Kidney Int.* 18:234–240, 1980.

12. Fisher, K.A., Luger, A., Spargo, B.H., Lindheimer, M.D. Hypertension in pregnancy: clinical pathological correlations and remote prognosis. *Medicine* 60:4, 267–276, 1981.

13. Nochy, D., Biermaut, P., Hinglais, N., et al. Renal lesions in the hypertensive syndromes of pregnancy: immunomorphological and ultrastructural studies in 114 cases. *Clin. Nephrol.* 13:155–162, 1980.

14. Robson, J.S. Proteinuria and the renal lesion in preeclampsia and abruptio placentae. *Perspect. Nephrol. Hypertens.* 5:61–72, 1976.

15. Trudinger, B.J., Parik, I. Attitudes to the mangement of hypertension in pregnancy: a survey of Australian fellows. *Aust. NZ. J. Obstet. Gynaecol.* 22:191–197, 1982.

16. Pritchard, J.A., McDonald, P.C. Hypertensive disorders in pregnancy. In: *Williams Obstetrics,* 16th ed. Norwalk, Conn.: Appleton-Century-Crofts, 1980, pp. 678–679.

17. Need, J.A. Immunological phenomena and preeclamptic toxemia. *Clin. Obstet. Gynecol.* 6:443–460, 1979.

18. Dodson, M.G. Immunology of abortion and preeclampsia. *Compr. Ther.* 8:59–66, 1982.

19. Speroff, L., Dorfman, G.S. Prostaglandins and pregnancy hypertension. *Clin. Obstet. Gynecol.* 4:635–649, 1977.

20. Belizan, J.M., Villar, J., Zalazar, A., et al. Preliminary evidence of the effect of calcium supplementation on blood pressure in normal pregnant women. *Am. J. Obstet. Gynecol.* 146:175–180, 1983.

21. Moss, A.J. Criterion for diastolic pressure: revolution counter revolution and now a compromise. *Pediatrics* 71:854–855, 1983.

22. Wright, B.M., Dore, C.F. A random zero sphygmomanometer. *Lancet* 1:337–338, 1970.
23. Morris, J.A. Medical complications of pregnancy: the acute hypertensive disorders. *Hosp. Form.* 13:445–456, 1978.
24. Gallery, E.D.M., Hunyor, S.N., Ross, M., Gyory, A.Z. Predicting the development of pregnancy-associated hypertension: the place of standardized blood pressure measurements. *Lancet* 1:1273–1275, 1977.
25. Friedman, E.A., Neff, R.K. Pregnancy outcome as related to hypertension, edema and proteinuria. In Lindheimer, M.D., Katz, A.I., Zuspan, F.P. (ed.), *Hypertension in Pregnancy.* New York: John Wiley & Sons, Inc., 1976, pp. 13–22.
26. Walters, W.A.W., Lin, Y.L. Women receiving oral cardiovascular dynamics in contraceptive therapy. *Lancet* 2:879–881, 1969.
27. Lund, C.J., Donovan, J.C. Blood volume during pregnancy: significance of plasma and red cell volumes. *Am. J. Obstet. Gynecol.* 98:393–403, 1967.
28. Hytten, F., Paintin, D.B. Increase in plasma volume during normal pregnancy. *J. Obstet. Gynaecol. Br. Commonw.* 70:402–407, 1963.
29. Gallery, E.D.M. Pregnancy-associated hypertension: interrelationships of volume and blood pressure changes. *Clin. Exper. Hypertension* 1:39–47, 1982.
30. Gallery, E.D.M., Hunyor, S.N., Gyory, A.Z. Plasma volume contraction: a significant factor in both pregnancy-associated hypertension (preeclampsia) and chronic hypertension in pregnancy. *Q. J. Med.* 48:593–602, 1979.
31. Chesley, L.C. The control of hypertension in pregnancy. *Obstet. Gynecol. Ann.* 10:69–106, 1981.
32. Soffronoffi, E.C., Kaufmann, B.M., Connaughton, J.F. Intravascular volume determinations and fetal outcome in hypertensive diseases of pregnancy. *Am. J. Obstet. Gynecol.* 124:4–9, 1977.
33. Blekta M., Hlavaty, V., Trnkova, M., et al. Volume of whole blood and absolute amount of serum proteins in the early stage of late toxemia of pregnancy. *Am. J. Obstet. Gynecol.* 106:10–13, 1970.
34. Sagen, N., Koller, O., Haram, K. Haemoconcentration in severe preeclampsia. *Br. J. Obstet. Gynaecol.* 89:802–805, 1982.
35. Koller, O. The clinical significance of hemodilution during pregnancy. *Obstet. Gynecol. Surv.* 37:649–652, 1982.
36. Sibai, B.M., Abdella, T.N., Anderson, G.D., Ditts, P.V. Plasma volume findings in pregnant women with mild hypertension: therapeutic considerations. *Am. J. Obstet. Gynecol.* 145:539–544, 1983.
37. Arias, F. Expansion of intravascular volume and fetal outcome in patients with chronic hypertension and pregnancy. *Am. J. Obstet. Gynecol.* 123:610–616, 1975.
38. Goodlin, R.C., Dobry, C.A., Anderson, J.C., et al. Clinical signs of normal plasma volume expansion during pregnancy. *Am. J. Obstet. Gynecol.* 145:1001–1009, 1983.
39. Goodlin, R.C., Quaife, M.F., Dirksen, J.W. The significance, diagnosis and treatment of maternal hypovolemia as associated with fetal/maternal illness. *Semin. Perinatol.* 5:165, 1981.
40. Assali, N.S., Vaughn, D.L. Blood volume in preeclampsia: fantasy and reality. *Am. J. Obstet. Gynecol.* 129:355–359, 1977.

41. Goodlin, R.C., Cotton, D.M., Haesslein, H.C. Severe edema-proteinuria-hypertension gestosis. *Am. J. Obstet. Gynecol.* 132:595–598, 1978.
42. Morris, J.A., O'Grady, J.P. A critical approach to the treatment of severe gestational hypertension. *Urol. Health.* 7:34–38, 1978.
43. Gallery, E.D.M., Saunders, D.M., Hunyor, S.N., Gyory, A.Z. Randomized comparison of methyldopa and oxprenolol for treatment of hypertension in pregnancy. *Br. Med. J.* 1:1591–1594, 1979.
44. Zuspan, F.P. Problems encountered in the treatment of pregnancy induced hypertension: a point of view. *Am. J. Obstet. Gynecol.* 131:591–597, 1978.
45. Pritchard, J.A. Management of preeclampsia and eclampsia. *Kidney Int.* 18:259–266, 1980.
46. Gilstrap, L.C., Cunningham, F.G., Whalby, P.J. Management of pregnancy induced hypertension in the nulliparous patient remote from term. *Semin. Perinatol.* 2:73–81, 1978.
47. Redman, C.W.G. Treatment of hypertension in pregnancy. *Kidney Intern.* 18:267–278, 1980.
48. Berkowitz, R.L. Anti-hypertensive drugs in the pregnant patient. *Obstet. Gynecol. Surv.* 35:191–204, 1980.
49. Roberts, J.M. When the hypertensive patient becomes pregnant. *Contemp. Ob/Gyn.* 13:47–55, 1979.
50. Sibai, B.M., Abdella, T.N., Anderson, G.D. Pregnancy outcome in 211 patients with mild, chronic hypertension. *Obstet. Gynecol.* 61:571–576, 1983.
51. Byrom, F.B. The nature of malignancy in hypertensive disease, evidence from the retina of the rat. *Lancet* 1:516–520, 1963.
52. Sybulski, S., Toth, A., and Maughan, G.B. The influence of experimental renal hypertension on pregnancy in the rat. *Am. J. Obstet. Gynecol.* 110:314–317, 1978.
53. Keith, T.A. Hypertensive crisis: recognition and management. *J. Am. Med. Assoc.* 237:1570–1577, 1977.
54. Johansson, B., Strandgaard, S., Lassen, N.A. On the pathogenesis of hypertensive encephalopathy. *Circ. Res.* 3435(Suppl.): I:167–174, 1974.
55. Silverstone, A., Trudinger, B.J., Lewis, P.J., Bulpitt, C.J. Maternal hypertension and intrauterine fetal death in mid-pregnancy. *Br. J. Obstet. Gynaecol.* 87:457–461, 1980.
56. Rankin, J.H.G., McLaughlin, M.K. The regulation of the placental blood flow. *J. Dev. Physiol.* 1:3–30, 1979.
57. Landesman, R., McLarn, W.D., Ollstein, R.N., Mendelsohn, B. Reserpine in toxemia of pregnancy. *Obstet. Gynecol.* 9:377–383, 1957.
58. Brosens, I.A. Morphological changes in the uteroplacental bed in pregnancy. *Clin. Obstet. Gynecol.* 4:573–593, 1977.
59. Dadak, C., Kefalides, A., Sinzinger, H., Weber, G. Reduced umbilical artery prostacyclin formation in complicated pregnancies. *Am. J. Obstet. Gynecol.* 144:792–795, 1982.
60. Makila, U.M., Jouppila, P., Kirkinen, P., et al. Relation between umbilical prostaglandin production and blood flow in the fetus. *Lancet* 1:728–729, 1983.
61. Stewart, M.J., Clark, D.A., Dunderji, S.G., et al. Decreased prostacyclin production: a characteristic of chronic placental insufficiency syndromes. *Lancet* 1:1126–1128, 1981.

62. Venuto, R.C., Cox, J.W., Stein, J.H., Ferris, T.F. The effects of changes in perfusion pressure on uteroplacental blood flow in the pregnant rabbit. *J. Clin. Invest.* 57:938–944, 1976.

63. Leather, H.M., Humphreys, D.M., Baker, P., Chadd, M.A. A controlled trial of hypotensive agents in hypertension in pregnancy. *Lancet* 2:488–490, 1968.

64. Redmond, C.W.G., Beilin, L.J., Bonnar, J., Ounsted, M.K. Fetal outcome in trial of antihypertensive treatment in pregnancy. *Lancet* 2:753–756, 1976.

65. Redman, C.W.G., Beilin, L.J., Bonnar, J. Treatment of hypertension in pregnancy with methyldopa: blood pressure control and side effects. *Br. J. Obstet. Gynaecol.* 84:419–426, 1977.

66. Kincaid-Smith, P., Bullen, M., Mills, J. Prolonged use of methyldopa in severe hypertension in pregnancy. *Br. Med. J.* 1:274–276, 1966.

67. Eliahou, H.E., Silverberg, D.S., Reisin, E., et al. Propranolol for the treatment of hypertension in pregnancy. *Br. J. Obstet. Gynaecol.* 85:431–436, 1978.

68. Morris, J.A., Arce, J.J., Hamilton, C.J., et al. The management of severe preeclampsia and eclampsia with intravenous diazoxide. *Obstet. Gynecol.* 49:675–680, 1977.

69. Hensel, A., Pauls, A., vonHerrath, D., Schaefer, K. Successful hemodialysis for acute renal failure in late pregnancy. *Am. J. Nephrol.* 2:98–100, 1982.

70. Kobayashi, H., Matsumoto, Y., Otsubo, O., et al. Successful pregnancy in a patient undergoing chronic hemodialysis. *Obstet. Gynecol.* 57:382–386, 1981.

Management of Dangerous Cardiovascular Lesions During Pregnancy

Kent Ueland, M.D.

Introduction

Heart disease during pregnancy may have an effect on the health of two persons, the mother and the fetus. Although the incidence of heart disease has declined significantly during the past several decades, it is still encountered in approximately 0.5 to 1.5 percent of pregnancies [1,2]. During this time the relative incidence of congenital heart disease has increased, whereas that of rheumatic heart disease has declined. Advances in cardiovascular surgery certainly have contributed to this change, as we are now encountering an increasing number of women who reach reproductive age who have undergone either palliative or corrective surgery when young. In spite of the declining incidence of cardiovascular disease, it remains the leading nonobstetric cause of maternal mortality [3].

The outcome of pregnancy for both mother and fetus appears to be related to the functional capacity of the heart. The potential dangers to the mother are several. The hemodynamic burden imposed by pregnancy may result in significant disability and even death. The maternal risks from certain forms of cardiovascular diseases are substantial, and this is discussed in detail in this Chapter. Pregnancy may also aggravate preexisting maternal cardiovascular disease. Bacterial endocarditis may complicate labor and delivery in women with certain forms of high-risk heart diseases. It also appears that rheumatic fever, although now rare in this country, may be more likely to recur during pregnancy [4,5]. Last, pregnancy may cause heart disease. Peripartum cardiomyopathy is a primary myocardial disease that develops late in pregnancy or in the puerperium. The etiology is unknown, but recent data reported by Melvin et al. [6] suggest that viral myocarditis may at times be the cause.

As for the fetus, the risk may also be substantial. When maternal heart disease is severe, fetal wastage can be as high as 50 percent [2,7]. Additionally, the fetus has an increased likelihood of being born with heart disease if one of the parents or a sibling has congenital heart disease [8]. Finally, there is the increased risk that the child may lose its mother at an early age because of the heart disease.

Pregnancy and Cardiovascular Physiology

Cardiac output rises early in pregnancy, and a significant elevation has been demonstrated by 12 weeks of gestation [1,9]. It continues to rise until 28 to 32 weeks and then is maintained at a relatively high level until term, showing a significant fall late in pregnancy only when measured in the supine position [10].

The increasing influence of posture on maternal hemodynamics as pregnancy advances has been demonstrated in a serial study [10]. A change in maternal position from supine to lateral produced a rise in CO of only 8 percent at 20 to 24 weeks of gestation, 14 percent at 28 to 32 weeks, and 29 percent at term. Scott and Kerr [11] convincingly demonstrated by radiographic means that the posture-related hemodynamic changes were produced by uterine compression of the inferior vena cava, which resulted in marked diminution in venous return to the heart.

Heart rate increases by approximately 10 to 15 beats per minute during pregnancy. The peak change occurs in most maternal positions near term. Stroke volume, on the other hand, appears to be highest in early to middle pregnancy and then declines progressively to term, reaching levels at or below those of the nonpregnant person [10].

Blood pressure declines near the end of the first trimester and generally through the middle trimester of pregnancy. The diastolic fall is greater than the systolic fall and results in a rise in pulse pressure [12]. The change is accentuated in the supine position.

The increment in blood volume during gestation varies considerably in different women, ranging from 20 to 100 percent [13]. It increases most rapidly during the first 20 to 30 weeks of pregnancy, but it continues to rise gradually to term [13,14]. On occasion, the increase in plasma volume exceeds that of the red cell mass, and there is a slight decline in hemoglobin values. However, this phenomenon appears to be entirely dependent on the availability and utilization of iron. Patients treated prophylactically with oral iron do not have a significant decline in hemoglobin concentrations late in pregnancy [15].

Parturition and Maternal Hemodynamics

With the onset of labor, venous return is augmented by the blood squeezed out of the uterus during each contraction. The resultant increase in cardiac output is most dramatic when the woman is supine. The accompanying bradycardia is attributed to the rise in arterial blood pressure secondary to the increase in venous return and cardiac output. During uterine contractions, blood flow is diverted to the upper portion of the body because the contracting uterus partially obstructs the abdominal aorta. Cesarean section delivery avoids the intermittent hemodynamic changes of labor, but is associated with the hemodynamic effects of apprehension, anesthesia, and surgical manipulation. Subarachnoid block, epidural block using an anesthetic solution containing epinephrine, or balanced general anesthesia (pentothal, nitrous oxide, oxygen, and succinylcholine) are all associated with major, although transient, hemodynamic changes. Epidural anesthesia without epinephrine in the anesthetic solution is the most effective of the techniques explored so far in maintaining hemodynamic stability [16]. Balanced general anesthesia offers a reasonable alternative for surgical delivery. Hemodynamic stability is fairly well maintained, except at the times of endotracheal intubation and extubation [17]. In the postpartum period, relative bradycardia is common, and the resting cardiac output falls progressively to normal levels over the course of a few weeks. It is possible that these postpartum changes are affected by lactation, but the effects of lactation on maternal hemodynamics have not been studied in humans.

General Guidelines in Management

Fetal well-being must be considered as part of the diagnostic and management approaches, but the highest priority must be given to maternal health and well-being. If there are alternatives to the use of certain drugs, the one deemed safest for the fetus should be used, but not if there is an increased risk to the mother. However, if certain drugs, diagnostic studies, or surgery is required for the maximum safety of the mother, it should be used unhesitatingly.

The mainstay of medical management for the pregnant cardiac patient is rest and reassurance; the patient can rest in bed at home or may require prolonged hospitalization in some clinical conditions. Pregnancy increases cardiac work, and heart disease decreases cardiac capacity; therefore, one must attempt to limit other demands placed on the heart. Restriction of physical activity reduces the burden on the heart. Emotional support and reassurance have a similar effect by limiting the cardiac stress of fear and anxiety. Even in patients with milder forms of heart disease, limitation of physical activity seems important if one considers the fetus. Infants born to mothers with asymptomatic or mildly symptomatic heart disease are smaller than their normal counter-parts, and the prematurity rate is higher [18]. Perhaps this is a reflection of the inability of the diseased heart to meet the increased demands of pregnancy and normal physical activity.

To maintain venous return to the heart and prevent pooling of blood in the lower extremities, elastic support to the legs is recommended throughout pregnancy when the patient is ambulatory. This becomes increasingly important during late pregnancy. This will help maintain cardiovascular stability and prevent the occasional large fluctuations in hemodynamics associated with a sudden change in maternal position.

Prophylactic antibiotic therapy is recommended during pregnancy for all patients with rheumatic heart disease. Broad-spectrum systemic prophylaxis should be provided during all dental work and at the time of labor and delivery. This is especially important in patients undergoing some form of obstetric manipulation, i.e., manual removal of the placenta or cesarean section, as maternal bacteremia frequently accompanies these procedures. Ampicillin-gentamycin or similar broad-spectrum combinations are advised because of the diversity of organisms found in the maternal blood stream after delivery. During pregnancy, prompt antibiotic treatment of urinary tract infections and respiratory infections is important, as infection and fever can place an additional burden on the heart.

Moderate sodium restriction is indicated for most women with heart disease during pregnancy, but only under unusual circumstances is there a need to limit it to less than 2g/day. The sodium requirements of the fetus and the increased demands of the mother must both be met. More stringent limitations will also make it difficult for the pregnant woman to maintain an adequate protein intake. If the cardiac disability is severe and strict limitation is imperative, one must then weigh the potential risks of continuing the pregnancy, for both mother and fetus, against those of termination.

Supplemental oral iron is strongly recommended for all pregnant women. A minimum daily supplement of 60 mg of elemental iron should be provided. When taken regularly this will maintain a normal hemoglobin level throughout pregnancy [15]. Diet alone cannot provide enough iron to meet the demands of pregnancy. Anemia must be avoided in the pregnant cardiac patient because of the increased demands it places on the heart.

Frequent visits to both cardiologist and obstetrician are necessary throughout pregnancy. This serves a threefold purpose: it alleviates fear and anxiety by providing consistent and reassuring information and emotional support, it allows the cardiologist to make frequent checks on the patient's cardiorespiratory status, and it gives the obstetrician a chance to closely monitor fetal growth and development. Serial determinations of vital capacity can be useful in detecting early signs of pulmonary congestion, especially in the seriously ill cardiac patient who is at risk of developing pulmonary edema.

Careful obstetric surveillance of fetal growth and development is imperative. Frequent clinical estimation (measurement) of uterine fundal height and serial ultrasonography can provide valuable information about fetal growth. Later in pregnancy, weekly nonstress and contraction stress testing are useful parameters for defining fetal-placental relationships.

In women with serious cardiac disability, therapeutic abortion should be offered as an alternative measure. The abortion should be done vaginally within the first 12 weeks of pregnancy and is not recommended beyond 16 weeks of pregnancy because of its inherent risks.

Sterilization is recommended only for those women with severe cardiac disability who have surgically uncorrectable lesions. Mortensen and Ellsworth [19] clearly demonstrated in a series of patients that pregnancy is safe in women who have had corrective cardiovascular surgery. Postpartum sterilization should not be done in patients with serious cardiovascular disease. The procedure is better undertaken at a time when basal cardiovascular conditions prevail.

Advances in cardiovascular surgery during the past two decades have been remarkable. Improved functional results are due both to new surgical techniques and to improved supportive technology. Morbidity and mortality statistics have continued to decline. Cardiovascular surgery is also being performed more frequently during pregnancy, with increased safety for the mother. However, the risks to the fetus can be considerable. In my opinion, cardiovascular surgery during pregnancy should be limited to very few specific circumstances. It should be performed in the patient with severe cardiac disability who does not respond to intensive medical management and who refused therapeutic abortion, for whatever reason, or in the occasional patient with severe cardiovascular disease who is beyond the time in gestation when safe vaginal evacuation of the uterus is possible. This opinion is based on the following considerations: 1) basal cardiovascular conditions do not prevail during pregnancy; 2) there are documented histochemical changes in the walls of large blood vessels during pregnancy and no reassurance that the heart is not similarly involved, a phenomenon that may affect tissue strength and healing; 3) the fetus is at considerable risk from prolonged major anesthesia or hypotension (or both); and 4) the results of a large series showed that maternal and fetal mortality statistics are best when medical management is used primarily, and cardiovascular surgery is reserved for a small number of patients. Cardiovascular surgery is best done in the nonpregnant person; ideally, it should be carried out before the childbearing age.

Most Common Dangerous Cardiovascular Lesions

RHEUMATIC HEART DISEASE

Not only has the incidence of rheumatic heart disease declined significantly during the past 30 years, but also the severity of the disease has decreased. In a 25-year review of data from two large centers in England, Szekely et al. [20] found a decline in the incidence of rheumatic heart disease in pregnancy from 3.5 percent (1940s) to 0.7 percent (1960s). In the same study, they found a significant decline in the common major complications of rheumatic heart disease, incuding pulmonary edema, heart failure, atrial fibrillation, and systemic embolization. I attribute these trends not only to a change in the natural course of the disease, but also to improved medical management of the more severe cases and to cardiac surgery in selected cases. There is reason to assume that a similar trend has occurred in this country, because a pregnant woman with severe rheumatic heart disease is rarely encountered in most major centers.

MITRAL STENOSIS

Mitral stenosis with or without other rheumatic valvular involvement is by far the most common lesion encountered during pregnancy. Since the major hemodynamic changes accompanying pregnancy make this lesion particularly hazardous, it will be the only rheumatic valvular disease discussed in detail.

The primary hemodynamic defect in patients with mitral stenosis is obstruction to blood flow from the left atrium to the left ventricle. The major hemodynamic changes of pregnancy that are dangerous to patients include increased cardiac output, increased heart rate, increased atrial irritability, and increased pulmonary blood volume. The latter has been demonstrated in pregnant women with significant mitral stenosis [21]. The relative tachycardia is the single most important change since it limits the time for blood flow during diastole. Therapy is basically aimed at limiting the demands placed on the heart. Physical rest is paramount, but reassurance is also important because it diminishes patient fear and anxiety, which exert their toll in work on the heart. Elastic support in the form of pressure-graded panty hose is also important, especially in the latter half of pregnancy, as it limits many of the major hemodynamic fluctuations that accompany changes in maternal posture. Restriction of sodium intake to 2 g/day is recommended because it may limit the fluid retention and hydremia that normally are associated with pregnancy. Oral iron supplementation should be provided to prevent the so-called physiologic anemia of late pregnancy. Infections of any kind should be promptly and vigorously treated with antibiotics. All of these approaches to management tend to limit the demand placed on the heart and maintain the work of the heart within its functional capacity. This becomes increasingly important as pregnancy progresses since the elevated cardiac output in the last trimester is almost entirely maintained by an increase in heart rate [10]. Hence, limiting heart rate constitutes one of the most important aspects of care.

As previously stated, patients with significant mitral stenosis have an increased pulmonary blood volume during pregnancy [21], which makes them especially prone to develop pulmonary edema. The serial measurement of vital capacity is useful in detecting early signs of pulmonary congestion and is recommended, especially in the latter half of pregnancy.

For patients with rheumatic heart disease, the American Heart Association recommends rheumatic fever prophylaxis for life [22].

However, many authorities are modifying this approach, especially in older persons who have been free of recurrent disease for 10 years or more and who do not live in a geographic area in which there is a high incidence of the disease. However, the author recommends penicillin prophylaxis during pregnancy in the form of 1.2×10^6 U of benzathine penicillin intramuscularly every four weeks. At the time of labor and delivery, three intramuscular or intravenous injections of 1 g of ampicillin and 1.5 mg of gentamicin per kg (not to exceed 80 mg) is recommended as prophylaxis against subacute bacterial endocarditis. The first dose should be given during active labor; the second and third doses should be given eight hours apart in the early puerperium. This is the general regimen of subacute bacterial endocarditis prophylaxis recommended by the American Heart Association [22].

Realizing that there is controversy about the prophylactic use of digitalis in patients at risk of developing cardiac arrhythmias, I recommend its use in all pregnant patients with symptomatic mitral stenosis, particularly in those patients who show evidence of atrial irritability. Digitalis in therapeutic doses may effect a slowing of heart rate, but, more importantly, it may prevent a rapid ventricular response should the patient develop atrial fibrillation. The maternal mortality rate associated with atrial fibrillation in pregnancy approaches 15 percent [23].

During labor and for delivery, it is important to maintain patient comfort because pain elevates the heart rate. A segmental epidural anesthetic given early in labor is the procedure of choice. The advantages of this

technique are as follows: 1) it requires the least amount of anesthetic solution; 2) it can be given with the patient on her side (rotating from side
to side while the block takes effect); 3) it has the fewest cardiovascular
side effects (when epinephrine is omitted from the local anesthetic solution); 4) it interferes the least with uterine contractility; and 5) a perineal
dose can be given terminally, allowing the obstetrician to do a forceps
delivery, thereby avoiding maternal bearing down efforts in the second
stage of labor. In the critically ill patient with mitral stenosis, continuous
maternal electro–cardiographic monitoring during labor and the use of a
Swan-Ganz catheter are recommended.

In the past, maternal mortality from rheumatic heart disease was
thought to be highest around 28 to 32 weeks of gestation, when the cardiac
burden was thought to peak. However, recent data clearly show that the
time of maximum danger to these women is late in pregnancy and in the
puerperium [3,20]. Experience has shown that a successful outcome of
pregnancy is best achieved by strict medical management in the vast majority of instances; surgery (mitral valvotomy) is reserved for those few
patients who are unresponsive to conservative medical therapy [24,25].
Pregnancy, if survived, does not appear to shorten the expected life span
of the patient with mitral stenosis [26,27].

Rheumatic mitral stenosis is a progressive disease, and valvotomy
can only be considered as an interval and palliative procedure [28]. Therefore, if pregnancy is contemplated after surgery, it should not be unduly
delayed and is best undertaken when the patient is asymptomatic or mildly
symptomatic. It is important to emphasize the continued need for close
cardiologic supervision in these women during pregnancy. Two recent
studies showed a maternal mortality of 2 to 3 percent during pregnancy
after mitral valvotomy, [9,29]. As emphasized above, the time of maximum
risk is during late pregnancy and in the early puerperium, 14 of the 15
reported deaths occurred at this time.

MITRAL VALVE PROSTHESIS

The maternal mortality in women with valvular prostheses is surprisingly
low. In a literature review that appeared in 1971, only one maternal death
was encountered in 50 pregnancies. The fetal mortality, on the other hand,
was high, especially among the patients with mitral valve prostheses [30].
The poor fetal prognosis may be related to the use of oral anticoagulants
[31], but it may also be due to the relatively low fixed cardiac output at
rest and the subnormal rise with exercise that these patients experience,
[32,33].

The primary hemodynamic defect in patients with rigid mitral valve prostheses (ball or disk) is the same as in those with mitral stenosis: obstruction of blood flow during diastole from the left atrium to the left ventricle. The most dangerous hemodynamic changes associated with pregnancy are also similar, but with the additional risk of gestational and puerperal hyper-coagulability. Therapy is patterned after that recommended for patients with mitral stenosis with one major addition, i.e., anticoagulation. Based on the evidence in the literature, I do not recommend the use of oral anticoagulants in these women. Although there is little experience with the prolonged use of heparin, it offers the theoretic advantage of anticoagulation for the mother without risk to the fetus [34]. In the future, the use of porcine xenografts may allow women with mitral valve prostheses to negotiate pregnancy safely because these xenografts are less thrombogenic and in all likelihood will not require anticoagulant maintenance [35].

Patients with rigid prosthetic mitral valves, if first seen early in pregnancy, should be offered abortion as the safest therapeutic alternative. Should this not be acceptable, then strict medical management, as previously outlined in the section on mitral stenosis, should be instituted immediately.

Patients with aortic valve prostheses differ from those with mitral valve prostheses both hemodynamically and in pregnancy performance. They have a normal cardiac output at rest and a normal increase with both exercise [3,6,37] and pregnancy [38]. Thus, hemodynamically, pregnancy is not contraindicated. If a woman has experienced no problems with thromboembolism without anticoagulant maintenance, she may negotiate pregnancy safely [30]. However, careful medical supervision is required throughout, and full anticoagulation should be instituted in the early puerperium.

Congenital Cardiovascular Disease

The relative incidence of congenital heart disease has increased significantly during the past 30 years [2]. In part, this is due to the decline in the incidence of rheumatic fever, but it is also the result of cardiovascular surgery performed early in life, allowing these women to live to childbearing age. If the lesion has been completely repaired, pregnancy can ordinarily be undertaken without any increased risk. On the other hand, if the lesion is only partially corrected, then continued careful medical management is required.

In most forms of congenital heart disease, pregnancy is not hazardous to the mother. However, there are a few specific congenital cardiovascular defects in which pregnancy is exceedingly dangerous.

COARCTATION OF THE AORTA (COMPLICATED)

Evidence suggests that the risk of pregnancy in women with uncomplicated coarctation of the aorta is not as great as previously thought [39,40]. In fact, with uncomplicated coarctation of the aorta, pregnancy can be relatively safe for the mother, but there remains a substantial risk for the fetus [39]. Of the 14 maternal deaths reported in the literature, 8 occurred in patients with a significant associated cardiovascular defect, usually a bicuspid aortic valve [40]. Of the 14 maternal deaths, the majority were due to aortic rupture. Other causes of death included bacterial endocarditis, cerebral vascular accidents, and congestive heart failure.

The main hemodynamic defect in patients with coarctation of the aorta and a bicuspid aortic valve are obstruction to blood flow through the aorta and aortic regurgitation. The most dangerous cardiovascular changes accompanying pregnancy are the increased pulse pressure, increased cardiac output, changes in the wall of the aorta, and the potential of bacteremia at delivery. The most important aspect of management consists of strict limitation of all physical activity. The combination of lesions of obstruction to blood flow through the aorta and an incompetent aortic valve places a double burden on the left ventricle. The increased hemodynamic requirements of pregnancy (cardiac output and stroke volume) place additional demands on the left ventricle at rest and during exercise. In these women, even mild exercise causes a marked rise in upper extremity blood pressure and may prove dangerous. It is unclear what role is played by the histochemical changes in the media of the aorta during pregnancy, but potentially, this could be significant if one considers the mode of death in the majority of these patients [41,42]. Unfortunately, there is no test available to predict which patient has intrinsic disease of the ascending aorta and, therefore, who is at risk for aortic dissection and rupture.

The greatest maternal risk appears to be in the early peurperium, not during labor and vaginal delivery as previously thought. Five of the eight deaths reported by Goodwin occurred soon after delivery; none of them occurred during labor [40]. Close maternal observation is critical after delivery, and prophylaxis against subacute bacterial endocarditis is considered very important in these women, who are highly susceptible to bacterial seeding. During early labor, systemic analgesia should be used liberally to maintain patient comfort. In the active phase of labor, conduction anesthesia in the form of a segmental epidural anesthetic is recommended. A forceps delivery should be performed as soon as it is safe for both mother and fetus, to circumvent maternal bearing down efforts in the second stage.

There are sporadic reports of surgical correction of coarctation of the aorta during pregnancy [43,44]. However, the data support the concept that medical management is the most appropriate and logical approach and that surgery should be reserved for the nonpregnant woman when basal cardiovascular conditions prevail.

MARFAN'S SYNDROME

Experience with pregnancy in women with Marfan's syndrome is limited. However, from my experience and sporadic reports that have appeared in the literature, the overall hazards to the mother may be similar to those encountered for complicated coarctation of the aorta. My experience includes two sisters with Marfan's syndrome, both of whom suffered sudden aortic dissection, rupture, and death during pregnancy. A third patient dissected her aorta in early labor, delivered by an emergency cesarean section for fetal distress, and then underwent successful cardiovascular surgery in the early puerperium. A fourth patient negotiated two term pregnancies and vaginal deliveries without complication after refusing therapeutic abortion in each instance.

The disorder of connective tissue, most importantly the degeneration of the elastic lamellae in the media of the aorta, constitutes the most dangerous defect. The most dangerous cardiovascular changes accompanying pregnancy are the increased cardiac output, the increased pulse pressure, and, possibly the histologic changes in the wall of the aorta.

One cannot modify the histochemical changes that occur in the media of the aorta, but one can modify the stress placed on the aorta by the increment in cardiac output and pulse pressure. Medical therapy is basically patterned after that described for complicated coarctation of the aorta. Additionally, the use of propranolol is recommended. The reported value of this therapy suggests that a wide pulse pressure predisposes to aortic dissection in patients with Marfan's syndrome [45], and pregnancy potentially increases this risk. Although propranolol has potential undesirable side effects on uterine blood flow, on the fetus, and on uterine contractility [31], its use is nonetheless recommended.

During labor the patient should be kept on her side to avoid the significant changes in pulse pressure that accompany uterine contractions when supine. Patient comfort should be maintained with adequate systemic analgesia and epidural anesthesia. Delivery with the patient in the lateral (Sim's) position or supine with uterine displacement is recommended to avoid the large increment in pulse pressure accompanying delivery in the lithotomy position.

The outlook of pregnancy in women with the definitive diagnosis of Marfan's syndrome, evidence of subluxated ocular lenses, and aortic root disease [46] is bleak. Pregnancy should be avoided, and therapeutic abortion should be strongly recommended as early in gestation as possible. The maternal mortality may approach 50 percent.

PULMONARY HYPERTENSION

Pregnancy is strongly contraindicated in women with pulmonary hypertension, regardless of etiology. The maternal mortality in women with Eisenmenger's syndrome is over 30 percent [3,47]. In women with severe primary pulmonary hypertension, the maternal mortality rate is in excess of 50 percent [48,49]. When one looks at the outcome of pregnancy in women with congenital heart disease, the mere presence of pulmonary hypertension appears to identify those who are at risk of dying [50]. Even women with pulmonary hypertension who are asymptomatic before pregnancy are at risk of dying should they become pregnant.

Eisenmenger's syndrome shall be used as the representative lesion for this group of congenital cardiovascular diseases with pulmonary hypertension. The major hemodynamic defects of Eisenmenger's complex are pulmonary hypertension and a reversed or bidirectional shunt. The major pregnancy-related cardiovascular changes that are dangerous to these women include the increased cardiac output, increased blood volume, decreased systemic vascular resistance, potential hypotension from anesthesia, blood loss at delivery, and postpartum hypercoagulability.

In Eisenmenger's syndrome, pulmonary and systemic vascular resistances are essentially equal, and the shunt is balanced. A sudden rise in right-to-left shunting and cyanosis can occur in one of two ways. First, there can be a sudden rise in pulmonary vascular resistance. Second, there can be a sharp fall in systemic vascular resistance. The data collected from the literature would support the concept that these changes in vascular resistance most commonly occur late in pregnancy and particularly in the early puerperium, [47,49]. The cardiovascular changes most frequently responsible for death are hypovolemic shock at delivery and pulmonary intravascular thrombosis. During pregnancy congestive failure and sudden unexplained deaths (probably due to ventricular arrhythmias) have also been reported.

In patients with pulmonary hypertension, therapy is aimed at maintaining venous return. Pressure-graded elastic support for the legs is strongly recommended throughout pregnancy. Late in pregnancy and during parturition, avoidance of the supine position is imperative. Systemic analgesia is preferred during early labor, and pudendal block anesthesia is preferred for the delivery to circumvent the potential hypotension from conduction anesthesia. The patient should be allowed to labor on her side, and, if possible, delivery should be performed in the Sim's (lateral) position. Cross-matched blood should be available and should be given in case of excessive blood loss at delivery or at the earliest signs of vascular collapse. Elastic support for the legs should be maintained during labor and in the early puerperium to prevent venous pooling, particularly with early ambulation after delivery. Measures to lower pulmonary vascular resistance should be used at the earliest evidence of increasing cyanosis or increasing pulmonary vascular resistance. Oxygen inhalation can be useful in this regard, and occasionally the intravenous injection of tolazine hydrochloride may be necessary [48]. Antibiotic prophylaxis is important in patients who have pulmonary hypertension and associated cardiovascular disease to prevent subacute bacterial endocarditis. Anticoagulation therapy is recommended in the early puerperium in all patients with pulmonary hypertension because of the potential risk of intravascular pulmonary thrombosis [47]. Heparin therapy should be initiated within the first few hours after delivery.

Perhaps surgical delivery is indicated in women with Eisenmenger's syndrome. I am aware of two women who were delivered successfully by cesarean section under balanced general anesthesia and with Swan-Ganz hemodynamic monitoring.

PERIPARTUM CARDIOMYOPATHY

The etiology of peripartum cardiomyopathy, a relatively rare disease, is unknown. However, recent information reported by Melvin et al. [6] would suggest that, in at least some cases, a viral myocarditis might be responsible for the myocardiopathy. Clinically it may present as a wide spectrum of symptoms from transient mild myocardial failure to dysrrhythmia, thromboembolism, and death. Perhaps it is an extreme expression of the depressed left ventricular function commonly encountered in the early puerperium in normal women [51]. It is usually recognized within three months of delivery. It is more common in older and multiparous women and especially in those who have delivered twins or whose pregnancy was complicated by toxemia. It is also more common in women of low socioeconomic circumstances [52].

The primary hemodynamic defect is diffuse myocardial failure with pulmonary congestion. Therapy should consist of bed rest, diuresis, and digitalis. Because of the risk of thromboembolism, heparin anticoagulation should also be considered. In 50 percent of patients, the cardiomegaly persists, and in these women there is a significant risk of early death and of recurrence of the disease with subsequent pregnancies. The long-term prognosis is improved if the heart rapidly returns to normal size. However, future pregnancies are strongly contraindicated because of the high risk of recurrence.

Heart Disease and the Fetus

As in the mother, the outcome of pregnancy for the fetus is dependent not only on the specific cardiovascular lesions, but also on the functional capacity of the heart. Fetal mortality is not significantly elevated in mothers with asymptomatic or mildly symptomatic heart disease. It reaches 12 percent in mothers with class III heart disease and is as high as 31 percent in those with class IV heart disease [53]. However, it should be noted that 50 percent of the latter mortality is related to therapeutic abortion.

Recent data suggest that fetuses in mothers with cardiovascular disease may suffer from more subtle handicaps. There is an increased incidence of prematurity in women with asymptomatic and mildly symptomatic heart disease, and the mean birth weight of the infants delivered at term is lower than in a comparable control population [16,18]. Perhaps the intrauterine environment is less than ideal for the fetus, as it appears that even the mildly diseased maternal heart is incapable of meeting the increased demands of pregnancy. Serial hemodynamic studies during pregnancy in women with mild mitral stenosis showed the cardiac output at rest to be well below expected values throughout pregnancy, regardless of maternal position; during exercise the decrement was even greater [16]. In addition, patients with acquired mitral valvular disease had a wide AVO_2 (arteriovenous oxygen) difference in early pregnancy, both at rest and during exercise, compared with the relative hyperemic state found in normal women during the first half of pregnancy [54].

The data of Niswander et al. [18] support the contention that cardiac function is an important consideration in determining pregnancy outcome. These investigators, analyzing the cerebral palsy collaborative data, found that the stillbirth rate was more than twice as high in women with heart failure compared with those with heart disease but without failure, and was nearly four times as high as the rate for the total collaborative project. Similarly, the incidence of low birth weight ($\leq 2,500$ g) and of neonates with one-minute Apgar scores of ≤ 7 was highest in the heart failure group.

In women with congenital cardiovascular disease, it appears that the fetus suffers not only from its compromised intrauterine environment, but also from hereditary factors. If one parent has congenital heart disease, the incidence of congenital heart disease in the offspring is between 2 and 4 percent [55], a rate six times that of the general pupulation. If a sibling has congenital heart disease, the rates are similar. In 50 percent of cases, the same lesion recurs. If the mother has cyanotic heart disease, there is a high incidence of spontaneous abortion and prematurity. In contrast, the offspring of fathers with cyanotic heart disease are subject to no increased risk [56]. The fetal prognosis in women with cyanosis is directly dependent on the maternal hematocrit [57]. When the hematocrit is less than 48, the outcome of pregnancy is reasonably good. However, when the hematocrit of the mother is between 48 and 60, about 30 percent of pregnancies end in abortion, premature delivery, or infant death. If the hematocrit is greater than 60, less than 10 percent of pregnancies end with the birth of a living infant.

All these data emphasize the importance of early detection and correction of congenital heart disease. Similarly, when the functional severity of acquired maternal heart disease is improved by medical or surgical therapy, the prognosis for the fetus is improved.

Cardiovascular Drugs and the Fetus

Some of the potent cardiovascular drugs have potential harmful effects on the developing embryo and fetus. Analyzing the data concerning the use of these drugs is hazardous because it is frequently difficult to accurately determine whether one is seeing the result of the interaction of specific drugs with pregnancy or with the underlying cardiovascular disease or both.

ANTICOAGULANT DRUGS

Heparin, because of its large molecular size, does not cross the placenta and has never been shown to be harmful to the fetus when given in therapeutic doses to the mother at any time during pregnancy. Oral anticoagulants, on the other hand, not only have potential teratogenic effects when given in the first trimester, but also may cause a multitude of subtle physical deformities in the fetus from repetitive small hemorrhages when given during the second and third trimesters of pregnancy [58,59]. At least 12 cases of fatal hemorrhages in the fetus from the use of oral anticoagulants during pregnancy have been reported [60]. Most of the cases were associated with poor control of the anticoagulant therapy; however, control of oral anticoagulation can be difficult during pregnancy. In view of the data, in my opinion, the use of oral anticoagulants at any time during pregnancy is contraindicated.

ANTIARRHYTHMIC DRUGS

There are no reports of harmful effects to the fetus from the use of quinidine during pregnancy. Although quinidine shares many of the pharmacologic actions of quinine and is its *d*-isomer, it does not appear to have any significant oxytocic action. Therefore, quinidine appears safe to use during pregnancy. The choice of treatment for arrhythmias of recent onset is electroshock therapy. This has been used successfully during pregnancy in several instances [31] without producing any deleterious effects in the fetus.

Propranolol is a beta-adrenergic blocking agent that works directly on the heart through the beta receptors. Propranolol also has a direct quinidine-like action on the heart. In addition to its usefulness in the treatment of certain cardiac arrhythmias, it is effective in treating angina pectoris and hypertension. This drug should be used with caution during pregnancy because it has the potential of initiating premature labor through its beta-blocking action on the uterus [61]. The chronic increase in uterine tone induced by this drug could potentially lead to a small and infarcted placenta and a low-birth-weight infant, as suggested by some investigators [62]. The fact that this beta-adrenergic blocker enhances uterine contractions is demonstrated by the fact that it has been used successfully in the treatment of dysfunctional labor. Its reported effect on the neonate includes respiratory depression, hypoglycemia, and bradycardia, [62–64].

A new antiarrhythmic agent, disopyramide, will be reviewed briefly because of its reported oxytocin-like effect. This drug has electrophysiologic properties similar to quinidine and is effective in suppressing ventricular and supraventricular tachyarrhythmias. In a recent case report by Leonard et al. [65], this drug was used to treat cardiac arrhythmias due to mitral valve prolapse in a pregnant woman at 32 weeks of gestation; therapy resulted in the initiation of hypertonic uterine contractions. When the drug was stopped, the uterine contractions subsided. Because of the potential stimulating effect on the uterus of many of the antiarrhythemic agents, they must be used with caution during pregnancy and with careful monitoring of uterine activity and fetal response.

CARDIAC GLYCOSIDES

There is no report in the literature suggesting that the digitalis glycosides are teratogenic in animals or humans, nor is there any evidence that the digitalis compounds have any deleterious effect on the fetus later in pregnancy. A recent report, however, suggests that digitalis may have a myometrium-stimulating effect. It appears to influence the time of onset of labor and the duration of labor in women with heart disease [66]. It was found that spontaneous labor occurred more than a week earlier and lasted about half as long in cardiac patients taking digitalis compared with a control group of cardiac patients not taking digitalis. This interesting observation may have some merit because in the laboratory digitalis has been shown to increase uterine muscle tone in vitro [67]. Other indirect evidence of its potential effects on the uterus can be inferred from the following: the chemical structure of digitalis is similar to that of estrogen, and an estrogen surge has been shown to occur in some animals (possibly in humans as well) just before the initiation of labor [68].

Clinically, digitalis does not appear to have any significant myometrial stimulatory effect. Norris [67] attempted to induce labor at term by giving patients oral digitalis in digitalizing doses and 2× and 3× digitalizing doses. The study was double blinded with a placebo. He found no differences in the time of onset of labor, length of labor, or blood loss at delivery among any of the groups. Thus, cardiac glycosides do not appear to have any deleterious effects on the mother, fetus, or neonate. The indication for use should be the same as in the nonpregnant person, keeping in mind that higher doses may be required to maintain therapeutic levels.

DIURETICS (THIAZIDES)

Thiazide diuretics were used extensively in the past to treat edema of pregnancy and for prophylaxis against toxemia of pregnancy. The current understanding that dependent edema is a physiologic accompaniment of pregnancy and requires no therapy and the documentation that diuretics and sodium restriction do not prevent toxemia of pregnancy [69] have led to a marked and appropriate reduction in the use of these potentially harmful drugs. There is little doubt that the thiazide diuretics can reduce plasma volume during pregnancy, but there are no data to show whether this reduced volume is maintained by prolonged therapy.

The reported harmful effects to the fetus from the prolonged use of oral diuretics, especially late in pregnancy, include severe electrolyte imbalance, neonatal jaundice, thrombocytopenia, liver damage, and death [43,69,70]. These reports are infrequent and most commonly associated with large doses used for prolonged periods of time. The use of thiazide diuretics during pregnancy should, however, be limited to very specific clinical indications. The most common cardiovascular indication would be in the prevention or treatment of pulmonary edema. When using diuretic therapy, it is important to concurrently use potassium supplementation, especially if digitalis is also being used.

For a more extensive review of the effects of cardiovascular drugs on the mother, fetus, and neonate, the reader is referred to a recent review by Ueland et al. [31].

When managing a pregnant patient with cardiovascular disease, it is important to know the cardiovsacular changes that normally accompany pregnancy and parturition and how these interact with the particular lesion or lesions in question as well as how one can lessen maternal and fetal risks by introducing specific diagnostic and therapeutic measures. Table 9-1 summarizes my recommendations about whether pregnancy should be attempted in the presence of some of the more common and dangerous cardiovascular lesions.

Table 9–1

Recommendations Regarding Pregnancy

Cardiovascular Lesions	Usually Tolerated	Relatively Contraindicated	Absolutely Contraindicated
Mitral stenosis			
Asymptomatic to mild	+		
Moderate		+	
Severe			+
Atrial fibrillation			+
Post commissurotomy	+		
Prosthetic heart valves			
Aortic	+		
Mitral			+
Coarctation of aorta			
Simple	+		
Complicated			+
Marfan's syndrome			+
Eisenmenger's syndrome			+
Primary pulmonary hypertension			+
Mild		+	
Moderate to severe			+
Peripartal cardiomyopathy			+

References

1. Barnes, C.G. *Medical Disorders in Obstetrics Practice,* 3rd ed. Oxford: Blackwell, 1970.
2. Szekely, P., Snaith, L. *Heart Disease and Pregnancy.* Edinburgh: Churchill Livingstone, 1974.
3. Hibbard, L.T. Maternal mortality due to cardiac disease. *Clin. Obstet. Gynecol.* 18:27–36, 1975.
4. Clinch, J. Chorea gravidarum. *Hosp. Med.* 2:317–320, 1967.
5. Ueland, K., Metcalfe, J. Acute rheumatic fever in pregnancy. *Am. J. Obstet. Gynecol.* 95:586–587, 1966.
6. Melvin, K.R., Richardson, P.J., Olsen, E.G., et al. Peripartum cardiomyopathy due to myocarditis. *N. Engl. J. Med.* 307:731–734, 1982.
7. Jacoby, W., Jr. Pregnancy with tetralogy andd pentalogy of Fallot. *Am. J. Cardiol.* 14:866–873, 1964.
8. Nora, J.J., Nora, A.H. The evolution of specific genetic and environmental counseling in congenital heart diseases. *Circulation* 57:205–213, 1978.
9. Schenker, J.G., Polishuk, W.Z. Pregnancy following mitral valvotomy: a survey of 182 patients. *Obstet. Gynecol.* 32:214–220, 1968.
10. Ueland, K., Novy, M.J., Peterson, E.N., Metcalfe, J. Maternal cardiovascular dynamics: IV. The influence of gestational age on the maternal cardiovascular response to posture and exercise. *Am. J. Obstet. Gynecol.* 104:856–864, 1969.
11. Scott, D.B., Kerr, M.G. Inferior vena caval pressure in late pregnancy. *J. Obstet. Gynaecol. Br. Commonw.* 70:1044–1049, 1963.

12. Adams, J.Q. Cardiovascular physiology in normal pregnancy: studies with dye dilution technique. *Am. J. Obstet. Gynecol.* 67:741–759, 1954.
13. Pritchard, J.A. Changes in the blood volume during pregnancy and delivery. *Anesthesiology* 26:393–399, 1965.
14. Lund, C.J., Donovan, J.C. Blood volume during pregnancy. Significance of plasma and red cell volume. *Am. J. Obstet. Gynecol.* 98:393–403, 1967.
15. Hytten, F.E., Letich, I. *The physiology of human pregnancy*, 2nd ed. Oxford: Blackwell, 1971. p. 30–33.
16. Ueland, K., Akamatsu, T.J. Eng, M., Bonica, J.J., Hansen, J.M. Maternal cardiovascular dynamics. VI. Cesarean section under epidural anesthesia without epinephrine. *Am. J. Obstet. Gynecol.* 114:775–780, 1972.
17. Ueland, K., Hansen, J., Eng, M., Maternal cardiovascular dynamics. V. cesarean section under thiopental nitrous oxide and succinylcholine anesthesia. *Am. J. Obstet. Gynecol.* 108:615–622, 1970.
18. Niswander, K.R., Berendes, H., Deutschberger, J., et al. Fetal morbidity following potentialy anoxygenic obstetric conditions. V. Organic heart disease. *Am. J. Obstet. Gynecol.* 98:876–880, 1967.
19. Mortensen, J.D., Ellsworth, H.S. Pregnancy and cardiac surgery. *Circulation* 28:773, 1963.
20. Szekely, P., Turner, R., Snaith, L. Pregnancy and the changing patterns of rheumatic heart disease. *Br. Heart. J.* 35:1293–1303, 1973.
21. Gazioglu, K., Klatreider, N.L., Rosen, M., et al. Pulmonary function during pregnancy in normal women and in patients with cardiopulmonary disease. *Thorax* 25:445–450, 1970.
22. Kaplan, E.L., Bisno, A., Derrick, W., Prevention of rheumatic fever: AHA committee report. *Circulation* 55:223.226, 1977.
23. Szekely, P., Snaith, L. Atrial fibrillation and pregnancy. *Br. Med. J.* 1:1407–1410, 1961.
24. Gilchrist, A.R. Cardiological problems in young women: including those of pregnancy and puerperium. *Br. Med. J.* 1:209–216, 1963.
25. Szekely, P., Snaith, L. The place of cardiac surgery in the management of the pregnant woman with heart disease. *J. Obstet. Gynaecol. Br. Commonw.* 70:69–77, 1963.
26. Chesley, L.C. Rheumatic cardiac disease and pregnancy: long follow-up of women with severe cardiac impairment. *Obstet. Gynecol.* 29:560–570, 1967.
27. Miller, M.D., Metcalfe, J. Effect of pregnancy on the course of heart disease: re-evaluation of 106 cardiac patients three to five years after pregnancy. *Circulation* 13:481–488, 1956.
28. Ueland, K. Cardiac surgery and pregnancy. *Am. J. Obstet. Gynecol.* 92:148–162, 1965.
29. Wallace, W.A., Harken, D.E., Ellis, L.B. Pregnancy following closed mitral valvuloplasty: a long-term study with remarks concerning the necessity for careful cardiac management. *J. Am. Med. Assoc.* 217:297–304, 1971.
30. Buxbaum, A., Aygen, M.M., Shahin, W., et al. Pregnancy in patients with prosthetic heart valves. *Chest* 59:639–642, 1971.
31. Ueland, K., McAnulty, J.H., Ueland, F.R., Metcalfe, J. Cardiovascular diseases in pregnancy: special considerations in the use of cardiovascular drugs. *Clin. Obstet. Gynecol.* 24:809–823, 1981.

32. Hultgren, H., Hubis, H., Shumway, N. Cardiac function following mitral valve replacement. *Am. Heart J.* 75:302–312, 1968.
33. McHenry, M.M., Smaloff, E.A., Davey, T.B., et al. Hemodynamic results with full-flow orifice prosthetic valves. *Circulation* 35(Suppl.):24–33, 1967.
34. Spearing, G., Fraser, I., Turner, G., Dixon, G. Long-term self-administered subcutaneous heparin in pregnancy. *Br. Med. J.* 1:1457–1458, 1978.
35. Spray, T.L., Roberts, W.C. Structural changes in porcine xenografts used as substitute cardiac valves: gross and histologic observations in 51 glutaraldehyde-preserved Hancock valves in 41 patients. *Am. J. Cardiol.* 40:319–330, 1977.
36. Bristow, J.D., McCord, C.W., Starr, A., et al. Clinical and hemodynamic results of aortic valvular replacement with a ball-valve prosthesis. *Circulation* 29(Suppl. 1):36–46, 1964.
37. Ross, J., Jr., Morrow, A.G., Masson, D.T., et al. Left ventricular function following replacement of the aortic valve: hemodynamic response to muscular exercise. *Circulation* 33:507–516, 1966)
38. Ueland, K., Tatum, H.G., Metcalfe, J. Pregnancy and prosthetic heart valves: report of successful pregnancies in 2 patients with Starr-Edwards aortic valves. *Obstet. Gynecol.* 27:257–260, 1966.
39. Deal, K., Wooley, C.S. Coarctation of the aorta and pregnancy. *Ann. Intern. Med.* 78:706–710, 1973.
40. Goodwin, J.F. Pregnancy and coarctation of the aorta. *Clin. Obstet. Gynecol.* 4:645–664, 1961.
41. Cavanzo, F.J., Taylor, H.B. Effect of pregnancy on the human aorta and its relationship to dissecting aneurysms. *Am. J. Obstet. Gynecol.* 105:567–568, 1969.
42. Manalo-Estrella, P., Barker, A.E. Histopathologic findings in human aortic media associated with pregnancy: a study of 16 cases. *Arch. Pathol.* 83:336–341, 1967.
43. Mendelson, C.L. Cardiac disease in pregnancy: medical care cardiovascular surgery and obstetric management as related to maternal and fetal welfare. In C. E. Heaton, (ed.), *Obstetrics and Gynecology*. Philadelphia: F.A. Davis Co., 1960, p. 87.
44. Zitnik, R.S., Brandenburg, R.O., Sheldon, R., et al. Pregnancy and open-heart surgery. *Circulation* 39 (Suppl. 1):257–262, 1969.
45. Wheat, M.W., Jr., Harris, P.D., Malf, J.R., et al. Acute dissection aneurysms of the aorta: treatment and results in 64 patients. *J. Thorac. Cardiovasc. Surg.* 58:344–351, 1969.
46. Pyreitz, R.E., McKusick, VA. The marfan's syndrome: diagnosis and management. *N. Engl. J. Med.* 300:772–777, 1979.
47. Neilson, G., Galea, E.G., Blunt, A. Eisenmenger's syndrome and pregnancy. *Med. J. Aust.* 1:431–434, 1971.
48. Dresdale, D.T., Schultz, M., Michton, R.J. Primary pulmonary hypertension. I. Clinical and hemodynamic study. *Am. J. Med.* 11:686–705, 1951.
49. Jones, A.M., Howitt, G. Eisenmenger syndrome in pregnancy. *Br. Med. J.* 1:1627–1631, 1965.
50. Neilson, G., Galea, E.G., Blunt, A. Congenital heart disease and pregnancy. *Med. J. Aust.* 1:1086–1088,

51. Burg, J.R., Dodek, A., Kloster, F.E., et al. Alterations of systolic time intervals during pregnancy. *Circulation* 49:560–564, 1974.
52. Demakis, J.G., Rahimtoola, S.H. Peripartum cardiomyopathy. *Circulation* 44:964–968, 1971.
53. Burwell, C.S., Metcalfe, J. *Heart Disease and Pregnancy*. Boston: Little, Brown and Co., 1958.
54. Ueland, K., Novy, M.J., Metcalfe, J. Cardiorespiratory responses to pregnancy and exercise in normal women and patients with heart disease. *Am. J. Obstet. Gynecol.* 115:4–10, 1973.
55. Nora, J.J., Nora, A.H., Wexler, P. Hereditary and environmental aspects as they affect the fetus and newborn. *Clin. Obstet. Gynecol.* 24:851–861, 1981.
56. Neill, C.A., Swanson, S. Outcome of pregnancy in congenital heart disease (abstract). *Circulation* 24:1003–1004, 1961.
57. Cannell, D.E., Vernon, C.P. Congenital heart disease and pregnancy. *Am. J. Obstet. Gynecol.* 85:744–753, 1963.
58. Hirsch, J., Cade, J.F., Gallus, A.S. Anticoagulants in pregnancy. A review of indications and complications. *Am. Heart J.* 83:301–305, 1972.
59. Shaul, W.L., Hall, J.G. Multiple congenital anomalies associated with oral anticoagulants. *Am. J. Obstet. Gynecol.* 127:191–198, 1977.
60. Bloomfield, D.K. Fetal deaths and malformations associated with the use of coumadin derivatives in pregnancy. *Am. J. Obstet. Gynecol.* 107:883–888, 1970.
61. Barden, T.P., Stander, R.W. Myometrial and cardiovascular effects of an adrenergic blocking drug in human pregnancy. *Am. J. Obstet. Gynecol.* 101:91–99, 1968.
62. Sabom, M.B., Curry, C., Jr., Wise, DE. Propranolol therapy during pregnancy in a patient with idiopathic hypertrophic subaortic stenosis: is it safe? *South Med. J.* 71:328–329, 1978.
63. Gladstone, G.R., Hardof, A., Gersony, W.M. Propranolol administration during pregnancy: effects on the fetus. *J. Pediatr.* 86:962–964, 1975.
64. Habib, A., McCarthy, J.S. Effects on the neonate of propranolol administered during pregnancy. *J. Pediatr.* 91:808–811, 1977.
65. Leonard, R.F., Braun, R.E., Levy, A.M. Initiation of uterine contractions by disopyramide during pregnancy. *N. Engl. J. Med.* 299:84–85, 1978.
66. Weaver, J.B., Pearson, J.F. Influence of digitalis on time of onset and duration of labor in women with cardiac disease. *Br. Med. J.* 3:519–520, 1973.
67. Norris, P.R. The action of cardiac glycosides on the human uterus. *J. Obstet. Gynecol. Br. Commonw.* 1961.
68. Liggins, G.C. Parturition in the sheep and the human. *Basic Life Sci.* 4B:423–443, 1974.
69. Gray, M.J. Use and abuse of thiazides in pregnancy. *Clin. Obstet. Gynecol.* 11:568–578, 1968.
70. McAllister, C.J., Stull, C.G., Convey, N.G. Amniotic fluid levels of uric acid and creatinine in toxemia patients: possible relation to diuretic use. *Am. J. Obstet. Gynecol.* 115:560–563, 1973.

10

Management of Perinatal Infections

Charles J. Ingardia, M.D.

Toxoplasmosis

The protozoan parasite *Toxoplasma gondii* is an organism that is responsible for the congenital infection of approximately 3,000 infants per year in the United States. It is found in many species of birds and mammals throughout the world.

INCIDENCE

Infection with *T. gondii* is fairly common, with a prevalence up to 95 percent of persons tested in high-infestation areas. In this country, by age 30, up to 20 to 30 percent of persons will have antibodies to the organism. Because of the dearth of specific symptoms associated with the disease, diagnosis is often made only after serologic testing. It has been estimated that 4 to 6 of every 1,000 pregnancies will be characterized by a primary infection to the organism. Approximately 40 to 50 percent of these gravidas with primary infection will give birth to infants who are congenitally infected (2 to 3 per 1,000 live births). This corresponds to the prospective studies of Alford et al. [1] and Kimball et al. [2] in Alabama and New

York that placed the incidence from 1 per 750 to 1 per 1,350 live births, respectively. Much higher prevalence has been noted in Europe by Desmonts and Couvreur [3].

METHODS OF TRANSMISSION

T. gondii exists in three forms; the proliferative form (trophozoite), the tissue cyst (bradyzoite), and the oocyst. Toxoplasmosis is transmitted through direct or indirect contact with cat feces or poorly cooked meat. The incidence of sheep and swine infected with the parasite ranges from 5 to 15 percent. Beef is only rarely infected. The cat is the definitive host and itself gets infected from ingestion of rodents that carry the oocytes. With acute infection the cat sheds infectious oocysts for approximately 2 weeks and then ceases becoming infectious. The oocysts become infectious in 1 to 21 days after their excretion. The pregnant woman comes into contact with the feces directly or indirectly through infected soil or unwashed vegetables. The occysts may also be ingested by grazing animals or contact with contaminated soil. These animals then become infected after gastric juices liberate the organism in the cyst. Dissemination of the organism to all structures occurs then, with the eventual development of tissue cysts. The pregnant woman then can also be infected through the ingestion of tissue cysts from uncooked meat of infected animals. Heating

Figure 10–1
A. Toxoplasmosis trophozoites. B. Tissue cyst stage. C. Oocytes. *(From Fuchs, F., Kimball, A., Kean, B.H., The management of toxoplasmosis in pregnancy.* Clin. Perinat. *1:408–409, 1974.)*
SOURCE Fuchs, F., Clin. Perinat. 1:1974.

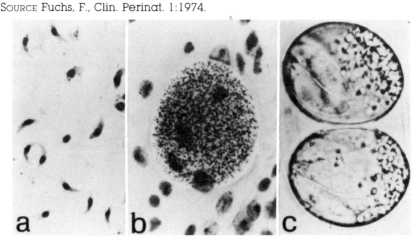

meat to 60°C or higher or freezing or drying it can destroy the organism. In this country, it is unclear which primary mode of infection is more important, infected cat feces or uncooked meat, but both may contribute to the prevalence of the disease (Figure 10–1).

MANIFESTATIONS

Maternal Toxoplasmosis in the adult is frequently asymptomatic (80 to 90 percent of cases). When signs and symptoms do occur they have been reported to include a mononucleosislike syndrome with malaise, mild fever, and cervical lymphadenopathy. In immunocompromised persons encephalitis, myocarditis, and pneumonitis may result.

Fetal Although a rare case of chronic maternal infection has been associated with congenital fetal infection, the infection of the fetoplacental unit comes from dissemination of trophozoite as a result of primary disease.

Several factors seem to influence the rate of transmission from mother to fetus. The risk of infection is lowest during the first trimester of pregnancy, with increased transmission in late gestation. If the mother is infected in the first trimester there is a 15 percent risk of fetal involvement. This increases to 40 to 50 percent in the second trimester and eventually up to 60 to 65 percent by term. Unfortunately, the severity of involvement is greatest earlier in gestation with a 60 percent risk of severe disease and a 9 percent risk of stillbirth when infection occurs in the first trimester. In the second and third trimester the majority of neonatal involvement is asymptomatic (45 and 92 percent, respectively). This increased severity in early fetal life may be the result of relative immaturity of fetal host immune mechanisms compared with those of a term fetus. The association of toxoplasmosis with premature labor has been reported, but the issue is not resolved.

Overall, about 75 percent of infants born live with congenital toxoplasma infection are asymptomatic at birth, with 10 percent displaying severe involvement and 15 percent having mild symptomatic disease.

In the symptomatic neonate the complete triad of hydrocephalus, chorioretinitis, and intracranial calcification may be present, but is uncommon. Other associated signs are hepatosplenomegaly, jaundice, and thrombocytopenia along with central nervous system disease or chorioretinitis. In symptomatic neonates, the most common manifestation is ocular. The characteristic lesion is focal necrotizing retinitis (Figure 10-2). Associated ocular lesions include anterior uveitis, microopthalmia, optic atrophy, and cataracts. Ocular disease is often seen in association with central nervous system involvement. This central nervous system involvement includes the typical intracranial calcifications, but also hydrocephalus, microcephaly, mental retardation, and epilepsy.

Figure 10–2
Chorioretinitis.

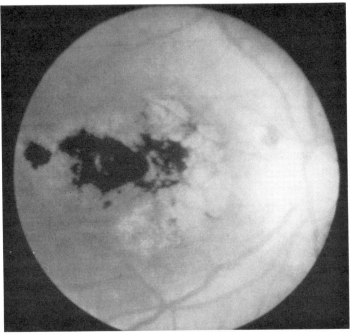

The asymptomatic neonate is apparently not without serious future morbidity. In a recent series of Wilson and Remington [4], up to 85 percent of infants who were followed developed serious sequelae, including chorioretinitis (75 percent), severe neurologic disability (8 percent), and retarded mental development (15 percent).

DIAGNOSIS

The diagnosis of toxoplasmosis can be made with isolation of the organism in suspected tissues or presence of immune response (i.e., antibody production) to the organism. At the present time the diagnosis of toxoplasmosis for the most part rests in serologic examination.

After primary infection, antibody of primarily IgM is produced. The onset of IgM production is within one week of infection, with a peak at one month and then a decline to generally undetectable levels by three to four months. The antibody of IgG also begins production within one to two weeks, with peak levels at one to two months; IgG antibody may be present for many years after primary infection.

Several serologic tests are available. The Sabin Feldman dye test is a very sensitive and reliable test for the detection of toxoplasma antibody. More widely available is an indirect fluorescent antibody assay (IFA). Hemagglutination and complement fixation tests are also available.

The diagnosis of acute toxoplasmosis is made if seroconversion is noted from negative to positive antibody status or with a fourfold rise noted between initial and convalescent serum taken three to four weeks apart. Primary infection can be susbstantiated as well by an increase in the IFA IgM fraction of greater than 1 to 80. A negative IFA IgM (less than 1 to 10) indicates a primary infection of at least three weeks before sampling.

It is imperative that significant titers be substantiated by a reference laboratory before management decisions are made. The presence of rheumatoid factor or a positive antinuclear antibody will give a falsely elevated IFA IgM, and tests for rheumatoid factor and antinuclear antibody should be ordered when a positive IFA IgM result is obtained.

MANAGEMENT

Maternal The presence of significant titers, particularly with a large IgM fraction, indicates recent infection, and gravidas so diagnosed should be questioned about timing in gestation of possible associated symptoms (fever, lymphopathy, and so on). Despite serologic analysis and historical data it is at times impossible to determine with certainty the timing of infection in gestation. The risks at each trimester and the severity of illness need to be discussed with parents. Induced abortion may be the choice early in pregnancy, but only one-half of primary infections occur before 20 weeks of gestational age, therefore, other options need to be discussed.

The use of spiramycin in France, reported by Desmonts and Couveur [5], and pyrimethamine and sulfadiazine in Germany, reported by Kraubig [6], has been associated with a 50 percent reduction of expected fetal infection. Spiramycin is not available in the United States, and pyrimethamine is considered potentially teratogenic in the first trimester. Sulfadiazine should be eliminated near term because of its association with neonatal hyperbilirubinemia. It is apparent that these drugs act in reducing the risk of infection, but will not reverse damage done by the organism before treatment. The length of course of therapy is also in debate, and at least a 28 to 40-day course is advised. When using pyrimethamine it is necesary to give folinic acid to prevent bone marrow toxicity, which is occasionally seen with the drug. Complete blood cell counts and platelet counts should be performed biweekly. The dosages are: pyrimethamine, 25 mg per day for 28 days, plus sulfadiazine, 1 g four times a day; folinic acid, 5 mg two to three times per week.The option of treatment should be discussed with parents along with the aforementioned potential risks of medication to mother and fetus.

NEONATAL

The diagnosis of toxoplasmos is in the neonate can be made with evidence of the stigmata of disease (i.e., hydrocephalus, cerebral calcifications, and so on as well as serologic confirmation. The presence of IFA IgM in neonatal blood is particularly significant, since no passive transfer of IgM from the mother occurs. Its presence in high titers confirms congenital infection. The IFA IgG test or Sabin Feldman dye test will be positive in all infants whose mothers have detectable IgG antibodies because it crosses the placenta. The decline in IgG antibodies seen in uninfected neonates can occasionally be seen in an infected neonate as well until about 1 to 2 years of life, when the infected infant continues to have detectable antibody and the noninfected infant does not. Isolation of toxoplasmas from tissues (i.e., placenta) is also possible as a means to confirm the diagnosis.

PREVENTION

Since 80 to 90 percent of women with toxoplasma infection are asymptomatic, most infections in gravidas will not be detected unless routine serologic examination is performed. In an idealistic setting the toxoplasma screen in performed at the initial prenatal visit; if negative, it is performed again at 20 weeks and again near term to detect primary infection in pregnancy. If positive, the nature of the immunoglobulin, i.e., IgM or IgG, is assayed at a reference laboratory to determine whether this is a primary or chronic smoldering infection. The issue of cost effectivenss of the program of routine screening for all gravidas is not resolved; until it is, physicians must decide on an individual basis who to screen (i.e., cat owners). An alternative and far less costly approach is to assume that all gravidas and those contemplating pregnancy should be assumed to be susceptible to toxoplasmosis and preventative recommendation should be followed. They include the following: (1) cooking meats to 66°C (150°F); (2) avoiding handling raw meats and doing so with gloves if necessary; (3) if raw meat is handled, washing hands thoroughly; (4)washing fruits and vegetables thoroughly; (5) avoiding cleaning cat litter boxes or cleaning with gloves; (6) disinfecting cat litter boxes every 24 hours with near boiling water for 5 minutes; (7) wearing gloves while gardening and washing thoroughly afterwards. These measures should be discussed with all pregnant patients by their concerned obstetricians. These simple precautions may make a major inpact in the reduction of this disease.

Cytomegalovirus Infection

Structure

The cytomegalovirus, (CMV) is a DNA virus of the herpesvirus family. The virus was isolated in 1956, but its characteristic intranuclear inclusion bodies and large cells were recognized as early as 1915. The virus consists of a deoxyribonucleic acid core enclosed by icosahedral capsid. The complex is surrounded by one or more oval membranes. The virus is labile and very susceptible to freezing, low pH (less than 5.0), and exposure to ultraviolet light for 5 minutes.

Frequency

It has been demonstrated that CMV can be isolated in 2 or 3 percent of pregnant women at term, and neonatal CMV infection is present up to 1 to 2 percent. Virus shedding has been detected from the urine, cervix, and nasopharynx. Virus isolation from the cervix and urine displays some gestational influences, with increased frequency of positive cultures with advancing gestational age.

Maternal Disease

After acquisition of the virus via respiratory or venereal routes or infected blood products, a primary infection ensues. In over 90 percent of persons the infection is asymptomatic. Very rarely, an infectious mononucleosis-like syndrome may be present. Unlike toxoplasmosis, the diagnosis is made through culturing of the cells from infected sites. After primary infection, the infected person undergoes persistent excretion of the virus for a number of years. This persistent excretion may be due to reinfection with different CMV serotypes (six serotypes in all) or, like herpes simplex virus, remain in a latent phase in tissues only to be reactivated at various times. In pregnancy, asymptomatic sources of infection include the cervix (5 to 15 percent), urinary tract 5 to 1 percent), breast milk (25 percent), and nasopharynx (2 percent), as reported by Reynolds et al. [7].

Fetal and Neonatal Disease

About 0.5 to 2 percent of infants are born with detectable CMV virus. An additional 3 to 5 percent of infants may acquire the infection from delivery through the infected cervix or from ingestion of infected breast

137

milk. Neonatal CMV infection outbreaks have occasionally been reported in nurseries due to close contacts with infectious sources.

The great majority of infants infected with CMV are asymptomatic at birth (90 to 95 percent), as reported by Knox [8]. CMV can be associated with extensive tissue destruction of all organs or can isolate or affect a single organ system. Hepatosplenomegaly is the most common abnormality seen when the infant is symptomatic. Hyperbilirubinemia, which occurs in 50 percent of symptomatic neonates, may be present in initially high levels or may become elevated over several days. Petechia, purpura, and thrombocytopenia may also be present. The petechia may be transient or may be one of the only signs of the disease. Microcephaly or hydrocephaly can occasionally be seen, most often in conjunction with periventricular calcifications. Chorioretinitis has also been reported (Figure 10–3).

The followup of infected neonates shows a tendency for chronic morbidity, usually in the form of seizures, optic atropy, diplegia, and sensorineural deafness. In fact, up to 17 percent of infants born with CMV develop progressive hearing loss in childhood. In addition, lower IQ and behavioral problems have been noted more frequently in these children, as reported by Hanshaw et al. [9].

Figure 10–3

Generalized purpura and hepato splenomegaly. *(From Hanshaw, J.B., Dudgeon, J. A. Viral Diseases of the Fetus and Newborn Philadelphia: W.B. Saunders, 1978, p. 117.)*

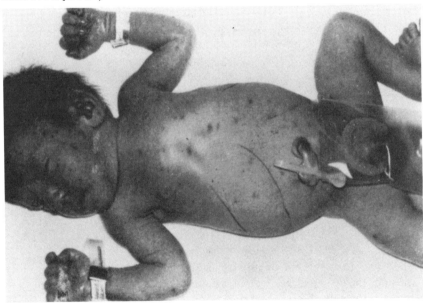

DIAGNOSIS

The definitive diagnosis of CMV infection is the isolation of the virus. If the virus is isolated within two weeks of birth it can be assumed that it is a congenital infection and not acquired in parturition or in the neonatal period. The virus can be cultured from urine, throat, eyes, and rectum, although urine cultures are the most frequent source. Inclusion-bearing cells in spun-down urine samples may also indicate infection, although a negative cytology does not rule out congenital CMV.

Serologic examination can be of help in the diagnosis of CMV, but is less sensitive with more technical difficulties than virus isolation. It must be kept in mind tha several strains of CMV virus exists; therefore the presence of CMV antibody does not necessarily afford protection in subsequent pregnancies. CMV virus has also a variable antigenic composition that may account for the fact that only 80 to 90 percent of infants with positive virus isolation eventually respond with antibody formation. There may be some cross-reactivity with other herpeslike virus antibodies as well (i.e., varicella virus). CMV antibody can be detected through complement fixation, hemagglutination, neutralization, and fluorescent antibody tests. The fluorescent antibody tests allows for qualitative analysis, i.e., IgG or IgM, which may help distinguish passive maternal antibody transfer or congenital CMV infection. Most serotypes share common complement fixation antigens; and although it will not distinguish among serotypes, this is a sensitive assay to detect CMV antibody.

MANAGEMENT

No satisfactory treatment is available at the present time for the infant with CMV infection. The use of antiviral agents, arabinofuranosyladenosine (Ara-A) or arabinofuranosylcytosine (Ara-C), have been associated with only a temporary suppression of CMV infection when the drugs were utilized. At the present time isolation of the child from uninfected or pregnant persons is advisable.

The development of an attenuated virus vaccine is being studied, although it is unclear whether there is a potential for oncogenesis or chronic virus shedding after vaccination.

Hepatitis B Infection

STRUCTURE

The hepatitis B virus (HBV) is a 42-nm DNA virus that has several distinct antigens. These antigens include a surface antigen (HbsAg) that has five

Figure 10–4

a, Surface antigen (spherical form). b, Surface antigen (tubular form). c, Dane particle (core and surface antigen). *(From Drew, W.L. Viral Infections: A Clinical Approach Philadelphia: F. A. Davis, 1976, p. 190.)*

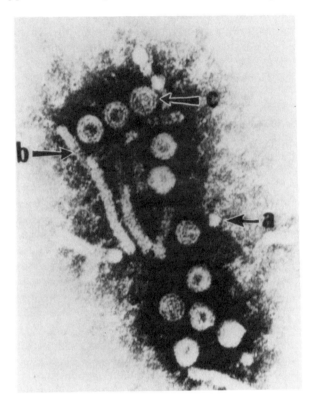

antigenic determinants, a, d, y, w, and r,and a core antigen (HbcAg). HbeAg (e antigen) may also be present in serum of actively infected persons, although its source is unclear. These antigens and their characteristic antibodies can be utilized as helpful markers of the disease process (Figure 10–4).

EPIDEMIOLOGY

The presence of HbsAg indicates active infection. There are marked geographic differences in the prevalence of HBV carrier states. Chronic carriers of HbsAg occur in 1 to 2 percent of the population in the United States, whereas up to 15 percent of Asian populations have been so classified. Transmission of the HBV viruses is through contact with infected blood, saliva, secretions, and seminal fluid. Perinatal infection of neonates with HbsAg can occur through transplacental tranfer from viremia either through an acute infection or chronic carrier state. It is also possible that neonatal infection is conferred through vaginal delivery and contact with infected secretions or blood. Breast milk has also been implicated as a source of infection, although the role this plays in neonatal acquisition is unclear. The risk of acquiring the virus is greater with overt maternal illness than with the chronic antigenemia state, as reported by Stevens et al. [10].

The risk of antenatal acquisition is greatest near term, with over 70 percent of infected mothers transmitting the infection to their fetuses compared with 10 percent of first-trimester patients, as reported by Schweitzer [11]. Okada et al. [12] reported that the presence of HbeAg in the mother was almost, always associated with neonatal infection.

MATERNAL INFECTION

The incubation for HBV is variable, but is usually 60 to 180 days. The patient may have fever, nausea, headache, and upper abdominal pain. With the fever, or within several days if it is subsiding, jaundice appears that may persist up to a month. The urine darkens with the appearance of jaundice. Hepatosplenomegaly is usually evident. After this appearance of jaundice there is slow recovery, but in 10 percent of cases state of chronic infection exists. There is no evidence that the course of HBV infection is altered by the pregnancy, although earlier reports of increased mortality associated with hepatitis have been noted. Although transplacental infection can be detected, no teratogenic damage has been reported.

LABORATORY

An elevation of serum glutamic-oxaloacetic transaminase, serum glutamic-pyruvic transaminase, lactic dehydrogenase, deoxyribonucleic acid polymerase and bilirubin occurs. The serum glutamic-pyruvic transaminase level is raised for about 50 days after exposure to the virus and may last for 30 to 60 days. These abnormal liver function studies may be helpful in diagnosis, but serologic evaluation to detect the presence of specific antigens and their corresponding antibodies is more specific. The serologic response in relation to clinical disease of the patients affected with HBV is displayed in Figure 10–5. It must be remembered that in about 1 percent of patients the HbsAg maybe absent by the time jaundice or other manifestations of clinical disease are present. The presence of HbeAg indicates

Figure 10–5

Hepatitis B antigenemic and antibody response after exposure.

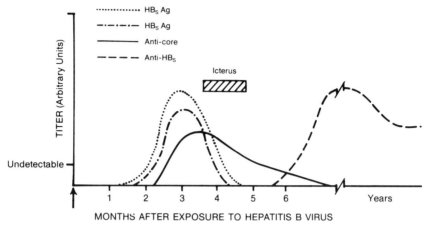

MONTHS AFTER EXPOSURE TO HEPATITIS B VIRUS

increased infectivity of the gravida, both to contacts and the fetus. With the disappearance of HbeAg the risk of infection is greatly reduced. The HbeAg usually clears in 6 to 8 weeks after the onset of symptoms. A carrier is defined as a person with persistent HbsAg and no detectable HbsAb response after several months with the disease.

MANAGEMENT OF THE GRAVIDA WITH OVERT HBV INFECTION

A general management scheme for all patients with HBV infection should be followed, including increased rest, adequate foods, and normal diet (low-protein diet if the patient shows signs of encephalopathy). The patient should be considered infectious when HbeAg or HbsAg is present without corresponding antibody. Since blood and saliva secretions are infectious sources, precautions should be taken when handling the patient's blood either for laboratory work or through inadvertent contact during surgery. Towels, razors, washcloths, and drinking and eating utensils should be separated from general family use. Sexual intercourse should be refrained from during active infection. Immune globulin prophylaxis should be provided to close contacts.

MANAGEMENT OF THE GRAVIDA EXPOSED TO HBV

The gravida exposed to HBV because of known contact with sources should have immune globulin in the hopes of modifying the disease. The

HBIg (hepatitis B immune globulin) should be given as soon as possible after exposure or within 7 days in a dose of 0.05 to 0.07 ml/kg. Repeat the dose in 25 days.

NEONATAL INFECTION WITH HBV

The neonate with HBV is most frequently asymptomatic. Occasionally, they may become icteric by three to four months of age or show evidence of elevated liver function in test studies. No specific therapy in infected persons is indicated, except precautionary measures to protect contacts. Sever et al. [13] recommend the utilization of hyperimmune HBIg in these infants to help modify the course of hepititis.

MANAGEMENT OF THE NEONATE EXPOSED TO HBV

The presence of HbsAge or HbeAg in maternal blood indicates the greatest risk of vertical transmission as mentioned above, and this may be in the form of contact with maternal secretions or blood in neonatal acquisition for breast milk or close maternal contact. These infants are at risk, and prophylaxis with HBIg is indicated. The dosage for neonates is 0.5 ml/kg. This regimen is repeated at monthly intervals with doses of 0.16 ml/kg for six months. Kohler et al. [14] report that this prophylaxis program helps to prevent or delay the onset of HBV infection.

HEPATITIS B VACCINE

The protection from fragments of HbsAg for hepatitis B vaccine has been recently introduced. It will no doubt aid in reducing the incidence of HBV infection. Its safety during the course of pregnancy is not established.

Herpes Simplex Virus

Herpes simplex virus (HSV) has been recognized as a cause of perinatal infections since the 1930s, but the interest in this disease awaited further elucidations in the 1960s and 1970s, when the full spectrum of the disease was recognized, and its relationship with maternal genital infection was studied by Nahmias et al. [15]. Although the incidence of genital herpes has risen in recent years, the incidence of neonatal infection is estimated to be 120 cases per year in the United States, as reported by Boehm et al. [16].

143

VIRUS

The viruses of the herpes families are compromised of double-stranded deoxyribonucleic acid. There is separation of the virus into two types, type 1 (HSV-1) and HSV-2, as reported by Amstey [17], because of biochemical, clinical, and biological characteristics of each type. HSV-1 generally involves the lips and mouth, whereas HSV-2 involves genital areas. However, up to 10 to 20 percent of genital infections can be caused by HSV-1 virus, and HSV-2 infection can cause stomatitis. Intrinsic to the nature of the virus is a tendency for latency in neural tissue, where reactivation can be triggered by emotional or hormonal changes.

DIAGNOSIS

Clinical   The appearance of multiple vulvar, cervical, or perineal ulcerations is characteristic of genital infections. A primary infection with HSV is usually characterized by multiple lesions, lymphadenapathy, viremia, and occasional constitutional symptoms. Significant virus shedding in primary disease lasts longer (three to six weeks) than from recurrent or reactivation of the disease (one to two weeks). The discomfort often associated with these lesions occasionally requires analgesia. Occasionally dysuria, fever, and backache can be observed. The lesions ulcerate, scab, and then heal over, all within a matter of one to two weeks.

Serology   Infection with HSV engenders both a cellular and immunologic response. The antibody produced is relatively specific for each serotype (type 1 or type 2), but-cross reactivity exists between them, and the presence of antibody does not prevent the occasional reactivation of the virus or offer prognosis for neonatal outcome. Since it is difficult without neutralization testing to distinguish between type 1 and type 2 antibody, serologic examination is not helpful in the diagnosis and prognosis for this disease.

Epidemiology   The virus is transmitted by infected secretions of infected sexual partners. The risk of acquisition of HSV after exposure to a partner with lesions is about 75 to 80 percent. The incubation period generally varies, but is about 7 to 14 days. It has been estimated that up to 5 percent of women and 15 percent of men remain as asymptomatic carriers of the disease, and 10 to 15 percent of patients will experience a recurrence of the disease.

The frequency of HSV-2 antibody has been established up to 10 to 15 percent of the population. Viral culturing studies indicate an incidence of 0.65 percent in asymptomatic pregnant patients, as reported by Bolognese et al. [18]. Nahmias et al. [19] reported a lower rate of asymptomatic patients at term (1 in 250 to 1 in 1,000).

144

Although transplacental transmission from maternal viremia is possible, it is rare. In almost all cases, fetal or neonatal infection is from vertical transmission at delivery from genital involvement. Factors associated with added neonatal risk are ruptured membranes for greater than four to six hours, direct fetal monitoring, and overt lesions. The risk to the fetus after delivery through infected genital areas has been reported by Nahmias, et al. to be 40 percent, although a much lower frequency is possible. The rate of neonatal infection may range from 1 in 7,500 to 1 in 30,000. Nosocomial infection from infected nursery personnel or other neonates has been reported by Linnemann et al. [20].

HSV Infection And Pregnancy   In the review by Nahmias et al. [15], symptomatic HSV infection was associated with higher pregnancy risk both in the form of spontaneous abortion (20 to 50 percent) and prematurity, although the etiology of this problem is unclear. Whether these problems may be related to an ascending chorioamniotis or some other indirect effect from HSV infection is not known.

HSV infection in the first trimester has on rare occasion been seen in association with a series of congenital anomalies that include cerebral or hepatic calfications, bony abnormalities of the hand, and patent ductus arteriosus.

After neonatal viral acquisition, an incubation of 7 to 10 days ensues, with the neonate displaying few symptoms. After the incubation period, the infants may have nonspecific symptoms such as fever, poor feeding, icterus, or seizures. The spectrum of disease of perinatal HSV can vary from isolated lesions of the skin, eyes, or oral cavity (15 percent) to disseminated infection (70 percent) of all major organs and the central nervous system. Lesions of the skin are only present in half of the cases. Nahmias et al. [15] report that the presence of passive antibodies does not protect the neonate from disease. The result of disseminated neonatal infection can be devastating, with a mortality rate of 50 percent and a 60 percent risk of serious neurologic sequelae in survivors.

DIAGNOSIS

The diagnosis of HSV infection can be made with the use of various techniques. HSV is a readily cultured virus that can produce cytopathic changes within 24 to 48 hours after inoculation. Various media can be used, including chicken embryo cells, rabbit kidney cells and amnion cells. Specimens need to be transported in ice to the culturing laboratory.

Various methods of indirect viral detection can be utilized, but are less sensitive. These include election microscopy, fluorescent antibody tests, pap smears, and biopsy. Because these histopathologic techniques need cellular material, it renders the validity less reliable. In studies by

Boehm et al. [16], where culturing techniques were used in conjuction with cytologic analysis, it can be seen that cytologic analysis has no role in predicting infection.

Humoral response can be utilized, and there are several methods for measuring antibody, including indirect fluorescent antibody assays, complement fixation tests, indirect hemagglutination, inhibition tests, and neutralization tests. None of these tests is helpful early in the diagnosis of neonatal infection because of the normal delay in immunologic response. Since these infections are of neonatal, not fetal origin, IgM evaluation is of no aid. Hemagglutination tests can distinguish between HSV-2 and HSV-1, but significant cross-reactivity exists. It appears that serologic evaluation has no role to play in the management of perinatal HSV infection.

INTERPARTUM MANAGEMENT

The management of the gravida with a history of HSV infection (or with a partner with HSV infection) should include frequent visual inspection of the perineal and cervical areas. If a documented herpetic lesion occurs early in pregnancy, its onset and disappearance should be recorded, and a confirmatory viral culture should be done. The basis of management in pregnancy should rest on viral isolation. In all gravidas with a positive history, cervical and viral cultures should be obtained at 37 to 38 weeks. A negative culture and evidence of no new lesions at parturition allows vaginal delivery with safety, as reported by Boehm et al. [16]. A positive culture within two weeks of labor or the presence of new lesions warrants cesarean section, if membranes have been ruptured for less than four hours. Although no guarantee can be made that the fetus of a culture-positive mother will not be infected if membranes have been ruptured over four hours, one can argue that even in these circumstances vaginal delivery may pose an added risk. If vaginal delivery is planned, internal fetal monitoring, with its risk of leading to herpetic scalp lesions, should be abandoned.

NOSOCOMIAL ACQUSITION

The extent of nosocomial HSV infection is unknown. Postnatal neonatal acquisition from infected mothers and personnel with cold sores, hand lesions, and so on, could be possible. In these circumstances it appears prudent to cover lesions, if possible, and to limit exposure to persons with lesions until the lesions are crusted over. HSV is quickly destroyed by soap and water, and handwashing should be employed. The infected neonate should be isolated to prevent contamination of other neonates.

References

1. Alford, C.A., Stagno, S., Reynolds, D.W. Congenital toxoplasmosis clinical, laboratory, and therapeutic considerations with special reference to subclinical disease. *Bull. N.Y. Acad. Med.* 50:160, 1974.
2. Kimball, A.C., Kean, G.H., Fuchs, F. Congenital toxoplasmosis: a prospective study of 4,048 obstetric patients. *Am. J. Obstet. Gynecol.* 111:211, 1971.
3. Desmonts, G., Couvreru, J. Toxoplasmosis: a study of epidemiology and serological asp-cts of perinatal infection. In Krugman, S., Gershon, A. A. (eds.), *Infections of the Fetus and the Newbown Infant,* vol. 3. New York: Alan R. Liss, 1976, p. 115.
4. Wilson, C.B., Remington, J.S. What can be done to prevent congenital toxoplasmosis. *Am. J. Obstet. Gynecol.* 148:357–363, 1980.
5. Desmonts, G., Couveur, J. Congenital toxoplasmosis: a prospective study of the offspring of 542 women who acquired toxoplasmosis during pregnancy. In Thalhammer, O., Baumgarten, K., Pollak, A. (eds.), Syllabus from *Perinatal Medicine Sixth European Congress: Vienna, 1976,* pp. 51–50.
6. Kraubig, H. 2vr prophylaxe der kumatelr toxoplasmose. *Arch. Gynaekol.* 202: 92, 1965.
7. Reynolds, D.W., Stagno, S. Hosty, T.S., et al. Maternal cytomegalovirus excretion and perinatal infection. *N. Engl. J. Med.* 289:1, 1973.
8. Knox, G. Specific viral infections: cytomegalovirus. In Depp, R., Eschenbach, D., Sciarra, J. (eds.), *Obstetrics and Gynecology,* vol. 3. Philadelphia: Harper & Row, 1971, p. 45.
9. Hanshaw, J.B., Scheiner, A.P., Mosley, A.W., et al. School failure and deafness after "silent" congenital cytomegalovirus infection. *N. Engl. J. Med.* 295:468, 1976.
10. Stevens, C.E., Beasley, R.P. Tsui, J., et al. Vertical transmission of hepatitis B antigen in Taiwan. *N. Engl. J. Med.* 292:771, 1975.
11. Schweitzer, I.L. Vertical transmission of the hepatitis B surface antigen. *Am. J. Med. Sci.* 270:287, 1975.
12. Okada, K., Kamiyama, I., Inomath, M., et al. "e" antigen and enti-d in the serum of asymptomatic carrier mothers as indicators of positive and negative transmission of hepatitis B virus to their infants. *N. Engl. J. Med.* 294:746, 1976.
13. In Sever, J.L., Larsen, J.W., Grossman, J.H. (eds.), Hepatitis B. *Handbook of Perinatal Infections,* Chapter 5. Boston: Little, Brown and Co., 1979, pp. 37–43.
14. Kohler, P.F., Dubois, R.S., Merrill, D.A., et al. Prevention of chronic neonate hapatitis B virus infection with antibody to hepatitis B surface antigen. *N. Engl. J. Med.* 219:1378, 1974.
15. Nahmias, A.J., Josey, W., Naib, Z.M. Perinatal risk associated with maternal genital herpes simplex infection. *Am. J. Obstet. Gynecol.* 110:825, 1971.
16. Boehm, F., Estes, W., Wright, P., et al. Management of genital herpes simplex virus infection occurring during pregnancy. *Am. J. Obstet. Gynecol.* 141:735, 1981.
17. Amstey, M.S. Current concept of herpes virus infection in the women. *Am. J. Obstet. Gynecol.* 117:717, 1973.

18. Bolognese, R.J., Corson, S., Fuccillo, D., et al. Herpesvirus hominis type II infections in asymptomatic pregnant women. *Obstet. Gynecol.* 48:507, 1976.
19. Nahmias, A.J., Josey, W.E., Naib, Z.M. Significance of herpes simplex virus infection during pregnancy. *Clin. Obstet. Gynecol.* 15:929, 1972.
20. Linnemann, C.C., Jr., Buchman, T.G., Light, I.J., et al. Transmission of herpes simplex virus type I in a nursery in the newborn—identification of viral isolates by DNA fingerprinting. *Lancet* 1:964, 1978.

11

Psychosocial Effects of Long-Term Antepartal Hospitalization

Dona J. Snyder, R.N., Ph.D.*

In the last few decades we have witnessed dramatic advances in the care of childbearing women and at the same time the development of an interesting and perplexing paradox.

On the one hand, health care professionals of all types and the public as well now place great emphasis on enhancing the normality of the child-bearing experience for all women. Childbearing is seen as an integral part of a life cycle for parents and children, and the ultimate goal of health care is to support and enhance parent-child relationships right from the moment of conception. Such things as full participation of all family members and parent-infant bonding have become essential concerns. This viewpoint is supported by a large body of literature from many disciplines, such as the works of Bowlby [1,2], Rubin [3,4], and Klaus and Kennel [5], as well as by a vast amount of lay, consumer-oriented literature.

On the other hand, in contrast to this idealized view of maternity care, there has arisen a marked increase in the ability of health care professionals to utilize sophisticated technologic interventions to improve the physiologic outcomes of high-risk pregnancies. These interventions

* The author would like to acknowledge her two coresearchers, Mary Joan Wheaton, B.S.N., R.N., and Sylvia Freeman, B.S.N., R.N., for their valuable contributions to this research.

frequently require removing the mother from the "normal" mainstream of childbearing and may often interfere with, or make virtually impossible, the "ideal" childbearing experiences so highly prized by everyone. Concern over the effects of such interventions on the normal course of childbearing is also reflected in both lay and professional literature [6].

One frequent aspect of such high-risk interventions is maternal hospitalization for extended periods during the latter months of pregnancy. Much of the literature supports the advantages of such hospitalization in terms of the physiologic outcome of pregnancy [7,8]. Yet, many health care professionals caring for these mothers have begun expressing a sense of "dis-ease" about the practice. Very often they find the mothers to be difficult to care for, demanding, emotional, and not totally complaint. They are identified as posing real problems in terms of both medical and nursing management.

A search of the recent literature, however, revealed little, if any, research attempting to define or explain the broad parameters of the experience of antepartal hospitalization for high-risk pregnancy. There are many studies that approach the problem in strictly physiologic terms and propose and evaluate particular treatment modalities, such as medications, bed rest, and so on [9,10]. Yet, nowhere could any work be found that viewed childbearing in a broader framework and attempted to look at the whole constellation of factors, not just the physiologic, that are attendant on antepartal hospitalization in the latter stages of pregnancy.

The purpose of this study, then, was to begin the task of defining the psychosocial parameters of long-term antepartal hospitalization for high-risk pregnancy. The specific research question was, "What are the expectant mother's perceptions of and responses to long-term hospitalization during the antepartal period for management of a high-risk condition?" It is anticipated that this particular study will be the first step in a series of studies aimed at increasing our understanding of this complex phenomenon.

Conceptual Framework

The conceptual framework upon which this research is based views the childbearing experience in terms of a holistic model consisting of interactions between five major systems—physiologic pregnancy, the mother's self system, the peer and family system, the societal system, and the cultural system [11]. In addition to the interactions of these systems, the idea of "trajectory" is also an essential part of the model. A trajectory is defined as a person's preconceived idea of how an experience will progress and is based on past experiences, knowledge related to the experience, and observations of others going through similar experiences. The accuracy and realism of such a trajectory may vary, but, regardless of such variations, it is a major factor in determining how a person will cope with the particular experience as it occurs. Together, then, these systems and the defined trajectory interact in a unique way to determine how each individual woman will experience and respond to childbearing and antepartal hospitalization.

Methodology

Because so little previous work has been done in this area, a grounded theory methodology was selected [12–14]. This is inductive phenomenological approach that moves from data to theory and begins with no preconceived ideas about the phenomenon being studied. The researcher moves back and forth between data collection and data analysis as a "theory" gradually emerges. Data collection relies primarily on observation of the phenomenon as it occurs, and data analysis involves the identification of categories of observed behavior. This is an ongoing process, and the study reported here is only a beginning. A theory of psychosocial responses to antepartal hospitalization has not yet been generated, but the data reported here do give us some interesting clues as to what such a theory might contain.

The research sample consisted of seven antepartal women who were hospitalized for a high-risk condition at some time during the last half of their pregnancy. Hospitalization occurred in the maternity unit of a major medical center that admits both antepartal and postpartal patients. Admitting diagnoses included one or more of the following: premature labor, placenta previa, subchorionic hematoma, incompetent cervix, vaginal bleeding, and triplet gestation. The women ranged in age from 18 to 30 years (mean, 25.5 years), and gestation at admission ranged from 25.5 to 35 weeks (mean, 29.5 weeks). The mean length of hospitalization was 6.75 weeks, with a range of 3 to 11.5 weeks. All subjects were married, and all but one were white.

After explanation of the study purpose and the signing of an informed consent, in accord with the requirements of the Institutional Review Board for the Protection of Human Subjects, each woman was interviewed on a weekly basis by either the major researcher or a research assistant. The same interviewer conducted all sessions with a given subject. The interviews were nondirective, i.e., no set interview schedule was used. We talked about what the mother wanted to discuss. No particular topics were suggested, but we did encourage the subjects to elaborate on a topic once it was introduced. The subject's permission was obtained for us to take notes during the interview, and these notes were then converted into a process recording format immediately after the session. We included as much "verbatim" material in our recordings as possible, and we made notes about the environment, the subject's nonverbal behavior, and significant events that occurred in the previous week, such as amniocentesis and ultrasound. A total of 26 interviews were conducted, varying in length from 1 to 2.5 hours.

Data Analysis

The recordings of each interview were analyzed independently by the major researcher and two coresearchers. Each analyzed behaviors in terms of two major areas. First to be identified were those behaviors that seemed to indicate stressors being experienced by the hospitalized mother. Stressors were defined as those experiences or concerns described by the subject as being disturbing or worrisome. These independent analyses were compared and compiled, and similar stressors were then grouped into five major categories. These categories were not necessarily mutually exclusive, and no attempt was made to rate or rank them as to intensity or to consider their interaction. Such an analysis will depend on future research.

Next to be identified were those behaviors that seemed to represent coping mechanisms being used by the mother. Coping mechanisms were defined as ways that the subject tried to deal with stressors and stressful situations in the attempt to make them more manageable. The identified coping behaviors were then also grouped into five major categories. No effort was made to evaluate the efficacy of these coping behaviors or how "healthy" they were.

In the remainder of this paper I describe the data in terms of these identified categories of stressors and coping mechanisms. Again, it is important to remember that, at this time, these are descriptive only and that no conclusion as to level of stress, efficacy of coping, and so on should be extrapolated from these data.

Stressors

HIGH-RISK CONDITION

The first category of stressors comprised those directly related to the particular high-risk condition or incident. Five different groups of behaviors fell into this category.

First, the indefinite trajectory of the high-risk condition itself concerned the mothers. Pregnancy was no longer going the way they thought it would, and they could not project what would be happening to them. They did not know how this pregnancy would end. Most expressed the feeling that this would go on forever, and this feeling seemed to be underscored when physicians and nurses frequently put off their projected delivery dates. A feeling of frustration that nothing was happening was expressed, and the mothers felt helpless because they did not not know what was going on inside their bodies. Anxiety over waiting for test outcomes that might mark progress was very high, and disappointment if desired progress was not confirmed was great. For those mothers who had a previous pregnancy with a bad outcome, the tendency to describe the current pregnancy in similar negative terms was apparent.

The constancy of the situation was also cited. A frequent comment was, "It never goes away." Mothers sat all day tuned in to contractions or fetal movements. One stated, "I can't forget about this whole thing even for a little while. The baby is moving around and is always there to remind me." Constant questions by nurses or physicians relative to contractions, movement, or other symptoms only served to focus the mothers more intently on their plight.

Most women in the latter stages of pregnancy do tend to express concern about an undesirable outcome to their experience. Fantasies of sick babies, maternal death or injury, and monsters are common [15–17]. Yet, for these hospitalized high-risk mothers this fantasy had roots in present reality. Each had legitimate concerns about the questionable outcome of this pregnancy. The possibility of a complicated delivery and separation from their sick infant was not far-fetched, and they seemed to think about it a great deal. The often-voiced reassurance, "Don't worry," was an impossibility for them. They could not help but worry about themeselves and their infants.

Many of the treatment modalities prescribed for the high-risk condition were certainly perceived as stress producing. Admissions were often abrupt and accompanied by such frightening symptoms as bleeding and strong contractions. Mothers described these experiences in great detail. Ritodrine therapy was particularly identified as being especially frightening. Complaints included the side effects of heart palpitations, extreme nervousness, and, as one woman described it, "feeling like I was going to jump out of my skin." Two mothers decided to discontinue ritodrine therapy on their own accord, regardless of the consequences, because it was so distressing. Other treatments like bed rest, nothing by mouth for a week, and nonstress tests were singled out as being distasteful.

Finally, it became apparent that the mothers began to experience a real loss of self in the high-risk condition. They perceived that most of the concern and interest, in the part of both health care professionals and family members, centered on the infant, not on themselves. They perceived their own needs and wishes as secondary. One mother expressed this clearly when when said, "I'm a person too, not just something that happens to be wrapped around a baby!" This sense of loss of self was also related to a feeling of not being understood. "No one knows what this feels like," was a common complaint. It was further exacerbated by "guilt trips" stimulated by health care professionals when the mother had negative feelings about her treatment and her pregnancy. Such statements as "of course you want to do this for your baby" did not help. Often these mothers were not entirely sure that they agreed with this.

HOSPITALIZATION

The second category of stressors was related to hospitalization itself. Confinement to the hospital with accompanying separation from their usual social environment was perceived as stress producing by all of the mothers. The term "prison" was used very frequently, and mothers often described themselves as prisoners. One remarked, "Charles Manson had a better cell than I do." All described a tremendous sense of boredom with days marked by television programs, which only served to increase their sense of separation from the world. Many found it difficult to understand why hospitalization was necessary since they were receiving little if any active therapy and they did not see themsevles as sick. They also expressed a sense of guilt about the dependency caused by such confinement.

Hosptial routines, policies, and regulations proved stressful as well. Sleep deprivation was a frequent complaint. They described being awakened for medications and fetal heart tone checks as well as by noises of various kinds and by other patients. The effect of stress caused by such sleep deprivation on the high-risk pregnancy itself is a question that has never been addressed. Lack of privacy was also a real concern. Both physicians and nurses were described as "barging in at embarrassing times without knocking." Doctor's visits during bath time or when the mother was on the bedpan were especially embarrassing. The lack of privacy to discuss personal things with husbands or other family members also was frequently cited. Husbands and wives had little privacy to talk to each other or exchange carresses. Lack of control over simple body needs, such as selecting foods, using bedpans, or taking bedbaths was also a source of consternation. The enforced dependence of hospitalization was very hard to tolerate for these women who did not really perceive themselves as ill. Visiting hours were viewed as restrictive and further enhanced the sense of social isolation mentioned earlier. The hustle, bustle, and noise of hospital units were also singled out, especiallly that of the labor and delivery unit. Furthermore, the mothers were upset by frequent transfers between units in the maternity department depending on their condition.

All of the mothers identified other patients, primarily roommates, as a real problem. They cited things such as lack of privacy, especially during visiting hours, having to share such things as television and telephone, and general incompatability. If the roomate had a normal baby the mothers complained of being disturbed at night for feedings and about visiting restrictions when the baby was in the room. In addition, they felt that the presence of normal baby only served to emphasize their own plight. If the roommate also had a high-risk problem things were not necessarily better. One woman, whose roommate had a stillbirth said, "I thought I had everything pretty well under control, I convinced myself that everything was going to be okay. Then when this happened last night it all came back! I got so scared again!" Two mothers were transferred to private rooms when the stress of roommates became too great.

Cost of hospitalization was also identified as a stressor. Even though most of the mothers were covered by either insurance or perinatal funds, they were aware of the tremendous cost of their treatment, and fears and guilt about this surfaced. One mother was especially stressed when she returned to her room and found a huge hospital bill lying on her table. She saw all of their family resources being depleted by this bill, and she felt guilty and frightened.

FAMILY RELATIONSHIPS

The third group of stressors comprised those concerned with family relationships. Four of the seven women were very concerned about the stress placed on their husbands. Husbands were described as very fatigued by freqent trips to the hospital, often over long distances, along with their other work and family responsibilities. Several asked their husbands not to visit so often because all they did was fall asleep in the chair when they came. Husbands, on their part, were very worried about not being able to be available or present during a crisis or the delivery. One woman related that her husband was even afraid to take a shower or go to the grocery store for fear of missing a call from the hospital. In general, husbands seemed to feel peripheral to the whole experience and isolated, and their wives worried about this. Two mothers described increased tension between themselves and their husbands, and one was worried that her husband was "playing around." Two felt that they had let their husbands down because they would not be able to participate in the delivery as planned.

Concern over children and their care was identified as stress producing. Also, the mothers felt guilty about the extra responsibilities that their hospitalization was placing on other family members such as mothers, mothers-in-law, and sisters. Yet, it was interesting that several voiced concern that things were going too well at home without them. They seemed to feel that their family members really did not need them, and

155

they were concerned about losing their own role in the family. Anxiety over going home and resuming the roles of wife and mother was described. Several worried that they would not know how to act when they got home.

LOSS OF NORMAL EXPERIENCES OF LIFE AND OF CHILDBEARING

The fourth group of stressors comprised those related to the loss of normal life experiences. Most mothers complained about the loss of normal activities of daily living. Such little things as not being able to get a suntan were grieved over. One woman wistfully said, "I've had the same $12 in my purse for 6 weeks." Things that would ordinarily seem trivial often became very important and were mourned.

The loss of normal experiences related to childbearing were particularly felt. Childbearing has been identified by our society as an event of great social significance, and many rituals and perquisites surround it. These mothers expressed a real feeling of loss of these perquisites of pregnancy. Several, said, "This has taken all the fun out of pregnancy!" Such things as baby showers, being waited on by family members, and showing off maternity clothes were denied to these women and missed by them. Among these normal experiences are the rituals of preparing for the baby. Nesting, as this is usually called, has been identified as an important activity or task of pregnancy [18]. It is generally seen as one of the ways that the expectant mother begins to separate herself from her fetus and to prepare for taking on the role of mother to him as an infant. These mothers, however had lost the opportunity to nest. Other family members performed some of the activities, such as purchasing baby clothes, but this was not a substitute for the process.

Finally, it was apparent that most of the mothers were grieving over the *loss of their normal trajectory for pregnancy*. One described her previous pregnancy as a "beautiful experience" and had tears in her eyes as she compared it to the present high-risk pregnancy. Several expressed a sense of betrayal by the current circumstances and were very disturbed that their trajectory had not come true.

RELATIONSHIPS WITH HEALTH CARE PROFESSIONALS

The final group of stressors comprised those stemming from relationships with health care professionals. Most of us consider ourselves as healers, so it was disturbing to learn that we also served as sources of stress for these hospitalized mothers.

First, the numbers of health care personnel with whom each mother

156

was interacting was mentioned frequently. One mother counted seventeen different health care personnel entering her room in one eight-hour shift. They found the number of physicians who were responsible for their care to be very confusing. Often a group of two to four attending physicians saw each patient as well as several residents and, of course, medical students. One mother said, "They keep changing. I really don't know which one is mine!" (with the emphasis on "mine"). She then described her relationship with her obstetrician from the referring hospital in very wistful terms, saying, "I really knew her. I felt I could really talk to her." Another stated, "I don't really know who my doctor is. That bothers me. Who is deciding what to do?" Several wondered why they had to be examined by so many different doctors and were amazed that no one seemed to know what the other doctors had found. They recognized the need for medical students to learn, but they were disturbed by frequent exams and questions by students they really did not know.

The number of nurses with whom they had to relate on a daily basis was also a source of stress. Several women expressed a desire for a "nurse of my own," saying that it was difficult to convey one's wishes, needs, and preferences to a different nurse every day. They were also upset that they often could not tell the nurses from the aides or licenced practical nurses because all wore scrub clothes. One described being very embarrassed after she discussed a personal problem at great length with someone she thought was a nurse, only to find out that she was a nurse aide. Several also confided that there were some nurses with whom they really did not get along as well as with others, and they felt they should have the option of requesting not to be cared for by these nurses. Sometimes this request was honored and sometimes it was not, primarily due to staffing patterns and patient census.

A related concern was worry over coordination of care, both medical and nursing. Mothers often described getting confusing and contradictory messages from both physicians and nurses. For example, one person would say, "We'll probably section you at 36 weeks," to be followed by someone else commenting, "It looks like we'll be able to get you to 37 or 38 weeks." These kinds of contradictions, although not momentous to us and certainly understandable in light of the patient's changing condition, were perceived by these women as obvious signs that their care was fragmented and that no one was really in charge with an organized plan of care.

Finally, and perhaps most distressing for us to hear, was the definte perception that we, as health care professionals, really did not understand what they were going through. They frequently used words like, "You really don't know what this feels like," and, "You don't know what it's like to sit here every day and just watch TV." This feeling was addressed to nurses and physicians of both sexes. Some mothers did seem to feel that women physicians and nurses were a little more likely to understand.

The frequent use of the phrase "don't worry" by all health care professionals only seemed to heighten this feeling of not being understood. Several said that it is impossible not to worry and felt that we as health care people should know that.

Coping Mechanisms

Our data also showed that these hospitalized mothers did exhibit various types of coping behaviors in their attempt to deal with the stressors engendered by their high-risk condition and confinement to the hospital. Six categories of such coping mechanisms were identified. All of the subjects in this research sample used several or even all of them during their hospital stay, and health care personnel recognized and supported the mechanisms in varied degrees.

DENIAL

Some form of denial was utilized by all of the subjects in dealing with their situation. They often denied the presence or severity of their particular high-risk situation. This was evidenced by behaviors such as not wanting to learn about what might happen to them. Several adamantly refused the trips to the Neonantal Intensive Care Unit or Labor and Delivery Suite that nurses feel are so necessary in preparing a patient for her delivery. Others really did not want to participate in their delivery experience. They were quite willing to turn it over to the doctors and nurses and said, "Just put me out. I don't want to know."

The reality of the baby and the possibility of its survival after delivery were also denied. One woman said, "I keep dreaming that the baby has been delivered but I never see what sex it is or what it looks like." Talking about what the baby would be like and naming the baby were usually avoided. The mother of triplets had several name books on her table for weeks but did not begin to look at them until the last minute. Furthermore, trying to engage these women in speculations about mothering activities generally proved fruitless.

Indeed, as we perused the data, it semed that these mothers were shifting the focus of their attention from their fetuses to themselves and their particular high-risk condition. In comparing this with the heightened concern of the normal third-trimester mother with the realities of her baby and her imminent assumption of the maternal role, questions arise as to how this high-risk experience affects eventual postpartal adaptation. Further study of the effects of this experience on maternal-fetal attachment and completion of the tasks of pregnancy is certainly warranted.

RATIONALIZATION

Some form of rationalization was also a common coping mechanism. For instance, several women clearly identified themselves as being healthy while it was only their pregnancy that was ill. There seemed to be an attempt to separate self from pregnancy, perhaps in an attempt to decrease the perceived threat of the high-risk condition to self. Others rationalized that they probably would have needed the high-risk treatment anyway. One commented, "I probably would have needed a section anyway so this isn't so bad." (There was no medical justification for this statement.) Another justified her confinement by saying, "The baby is better off here near the high-risk nursey, so I guess I'm glad I'm here." Several were really convinced that they would progress just as well at home and attempted to shift the blame for their hospitalizations and attendant costs and family disruptions to their physicians. One mother commented, "I'm only here because he [the physician] wants me here."

CONTROL

Some very interesting, and at times maddening to hospital personnel, coping behaviors used by these mothers were the ways they attempted to exert control over their lives and their daily activities. For instance, in the matter of control of their immediate environment most of the mothers took over as much of their room as possible, spreading out belongings to stake out their claims. Several attemtped to keep out other roommates or to specify clearly what kind of patient might be admitted to the other bed. Control of relationships was expressed through attempts to say who could care for them, who could visit, and even who could call on the telephone. They also tried to control their own treatment plans by setting limits on the options available to physicians and nurses. One mother said, 'I won't stay here after 36 weeks. I don't care what the doctor says!" Two women actively pursued the cessation of their ritodrine therapy in spite of physician and nurse opposition. Several commented that they really could go home if they wanted to, i.e., they were in control. Control of self care activities was also important. They liked to take showers, and so on, when they wanted to, and such a simple thing as being able to control the opening of their own pill packets and the taking of their own medications was coveted. All of these controlling activities seemed to help these women in their expressed need to "keep myself together."

ACCOMPLISHMENT

Another interesting coping mechanism was seen in the various ways that these women tried to convince themselves that they were really accomplishing something in the face of long, tedious days of seemingly little or no progress.

Many expressed great pride at the length of time that they had maintained this pregnancy. This was viewed as a real accomplishment. Several were amazed at how long they had lasted in their confinement. "I never thought I would get this far," was a frequent comment, and they seemed to view their "good behavior" and compliance with a real sense of pride. Some marked ongoing days and significant events on a calendar and then used this as a basis for seeing what they had achieved.

Pride in their own good mothering was also expressed. This often took the form of bragging about past successes in pregnancy and mothering. Past pregnancies were described in detail, and long accounts of how they managed their children, homes, and even pets were common. They also expressed pride in their willingness to accept hospitalization and other distressing treatments for this pregnancy. They liked it when this feeling was reinforced by significant health care personnel. They also achieved a sense of pride in noting what they were sacrificing for their husbands and families.

Some seemed to find great comfort in achieving goals in tangible activities. They set definite goals for themselves in projects such as handwork and reading. When these goals were successfully achieved they reported it with great pride. Products of such handwork were exhibited to everyone that came to visit and seemed to mean much more than just a way to pass the time.

TRAJECTORY DEFINITION

A fifth group of coping behaviors was related to the mother's definition of her trajectory for this pregnancy. As was stated earlier, the way one perceives the trajectory of a particular experience is closely related to the way one copes with that experience. When the original trajectory is disrupted, a new one must be constructed to take the disrupting variables into account. Thus, these mothers had to revamp their particular trajectories in light of their high-risk conditions.

Five of the seven clearly attempted to set a particular end for their experience by saying, in many ways, "This is when I think it will end." Some were very adamant about it and marked the endings very clearly on the calendar. These endings often were not very realistic, and the mothers were shattered when their new trajectories were dashed.

Identifying the condition of the fetus at various points was another interesting trajectory-setting behavior. They decided at what point the baby would be likely to survive delivery by comparing themselves with their own past pregnancies or to other women, such as mothers and sisters, at similar gestations. Such old wives' tales as, "Seven-month babies do better than eight-month babies," were used to reassure them in a trajectory that showed signs of possible premature delivery. Looking at babies in the newborn and special care nurseries was also a tactic. They tried to find babies of gestation comparable to their own fetus to determine whether their own baby would survive. Again, their perceptions of their own baby at various gestations were not always realistic, but it was difficult to dislodge these perceptions.

They frequently sought the confirmation of physicians and nurses for their perceived trajectories. One woman welcomed vaginal exams to confirm that she was really on target. Ultra-sound and amniocentesis results were of vital concern, and the hours spent waiting for them were long and painful. If the woman had a history of a "bad pregnancy," then her current trajectory tended to be defined in negative terms and the need for medical confirmation of progress became even more vital. One woman with a past history of premature delivery due to an incompetent cervix could only view her current pregnancy (which was going well after a circlage procedure) in negative terms, and she was constantly seeking medical confirmation that her trajectory was wrong.

SOCIAL SUPPORT SYSTEMS

Finally, and to no one's surprise, the use of social support systems as coping mechanisms was very apparent. Contact with home was crucial. Several women spent much time making things for home, as if this formed some kind of a bond for them. When passes were allowed they were generally appreciated, although some did say that it was very difficult being "a visitor in your own house." Some husbands were very fearful of precipitous deliveries while they had their wives away from the hospital, but they generally overcame these fears and took their wives home. One mother did not tell her husband about the onset of mild contractions while she was on a pass because she did not think he could cope with that.

Maintaining contact with significant others was also important. Visiting hours were anticipated eagerly. As all who care for these patients would know, they were constantly on the phone. The intrusion of roommates on such contacts was not appreciated. Visits by their children were eagerly anticipated, and any rejection behaviors on the part of the children were described as very disturbing. One mother related her toddler's rejection with great emotion and then reported with great relief the next week that the child had greeted her with enthusiasm.

Occasionally certain health care personnel (physicians or nurses) were singled out as support persons, and the mothers really looked forward to their visits. Certain physicians and nurses might be called by first names and always were described as being friends as well as professionals. These persons were identified as "my" doctor or nurse even if the health care professionals did not see themselves as such.

Summary and Conclusions

To summarize, two broad conclusions seem to emerge from this initial study of hospitalized high-risk mothers: first, that antepartal hospitalization for high-risk pregnancy is definitely a stress-producing experience; and second, that stressors arise from a wide variety of sources, both physiologic and psychosocial. This research undertook only the task of identifying and describing various stressors. Little is known about the interactions of such stressors with the process of childbearing and their subsequent effect on outcomes, either physiologic or psychosocial, nor have the long-term effects of such stressful experiences on future mothering behaviors and mother-child relationships been adequately investigated.

Further, our data indicate that high-risk mothers do cope with their confinement and their high-risk condition in a variety of ways. Once again, these coping mechanisms were only identified and described. This research did not attempt to rate them or to evaluate their efficacy. Also, it did not attempt to answer the very pertinent question of how we as health care professionals might assist the mothers in developing and utilizing healthy and efficient coping mechanisms.

Indeed, this study generates a great many more questions than it answers, and we believe that that is its significance. If we hope to provide quality care for this important and growing group of childbearing women, we as health care professionals must begin to generate sound research data upon which to base our professional actions and decisions. And, we must commit ourselves to a holistic approach to childbearing, one which takes into account the myriad of variables interacting to make up this complex and essential experience.

References

1. Bowlby, J. The nature of the child's tie to his mother. *Int. J. Psychoanal.* 39:350–373, 1958.
2. Bowlby, J. *Attachment and Loss,* vol. 1. New York: Basic Books, Inc., 1969.
3. Rubin, R. Basic maternal behavior. *Nurs. Outlook* 9:683–686 1961.
4. Rubin, R. Maternal touch. *Nurs. Outlook* 11:828–831, 1963.
5. Klaus, M.H., Kennell, J.H. *Parent-Infant Bonding,* 2nd ed. St. Louis: C. V. Mosby, 1982.

6. Brody, H., Thompson, V.R. The maximum strategy in modern obstetrics. *J. Fam. Pract.* 6:977–986, 1981.

7. Boehm, F, Haire, M. One-way maternal transport: an evolving concept. *Am. J. Obstet. Gynecol.* 134:484–492, 1979.

8. Harris, T., Isaman, J., Giles, H. Improved neonatal survival through maternal transport. *Obstet. Gynecol.* 52:294–300, 1978.

9. Herron, M.A., Katz, M., Creasy, R.K. Evaluation of a preterm birth prevention program: a preliminary report. *Obstet. Gynecol.* 59:452–456, 1982.

10. Merkatz, I.R., Peter, J.B., Borden, T.P. Ritrodrine hydrochloride: a betamimetic agent for use in preterm labor. II. Evidence of efficacy. *Obstet. Gynecol.* 56:7–12, 1980.

11. Snyder, D.J. The high-risk mother viewed in relation to a holistic model of the childbearing experience. *J. Obstet. Gynecol. Neonat. Nurs.* 8:164–170, 1979.

12. Glaser, B., Straus, A. *The Discovery of Grounded Theory: Strategies for Qualitative Research.* Chicago: Aldine, 1967.

13. Sims, L. The grounded theory approach in nursing research. *Nurs. Res.* 30:356–359, 1981.

14. Stern, P.N. Grounded theory methodology; its uses and processes. *Image* 12:18–23, 1980.

15. Deutsch, H. *The Psychology of Women,* vol. 2. New York: Grune and Stratton, 1945.

16. Leifer, M. *Psychological Effects of Motherhood.* New York: Praeger Publishers, 1980.

17. Oakley, A. *Becoming a Mother.* New York: Schocken Books, 1980.

12

Spiritual and Emotional Issues When Pregnancy Fails

Ann C. Schoup, M. Div.

Although this chapter will emphasize the needs of parents whose babies are in critical or terminal situations, it is important to be aware that all parents whose pregnancy has complications go through similar emotional and spiritual experiences. Among the common spiritual questions of these parents are the following: Why me? What did I or we do wrong? Why is God punishing me? Why doesn't God answer my prayer? I've always lived a respectable life, why is God so cruel? If my baby dies what will happen to him? To her? Is there a heaven? What is it like? There are so many people who don't want their babies and have healthy babies, why is it so easy for them and so hard for me?

Rarely is this time of questioning and grief appropriate to engage in God talk or theology. It is a time for caring and for trying to understand. Young couples who are going through the trauma of infant illness or death are frightened, confused, shocked, overwhelmed, angry, guilt-ridden, and inclined to feel that no one understands what they are going through. Most people who are the care givers have not personally experienced what it is like to have a baby die or a newborn in an intensive care unit. Our concerns must not only be to provide the best possible medical care for the mother and the sick baby, but also to be sensitive to the general needs (physical, spiritual, and emotional) of the parents and to be responsive to external issues that influence their reactions and relationship to the newborn child, the institutional care givers, and other significant persons in their lives. Too often we categorize and stereotype rather than listen. We get caught up in procedure, systems, and time schedules and lose sight of the human beings who are the reason for everything we do.

Although the emotional trauma of critical and terminal illness is beyond verbal description, we can improve our sensitivity if we invite those who have first-hand experience to talk with us about their needs and feelings. Many are quite open in their conversations. It is also important to know what it is like for a couple after they have been away from the hospital for several months or even years. Occasionally I call a couple and ask, "As you look back, what was the experience like?"

I want to share two of those conversations, typical of many others, as a way of helping us see something of what parents see and feel. The first is with a father whose child died in the Special Care Nursery when he was six months old. The father remembers:

The first thing we both said was, "why me?" We were in a state of shock and awe of the technology and staff for weeks. During that time we never really saw our baby. We saw only the tubes, the machines, all the technological equipment, and all those marvelously trained people. We never really understood what they were saying, but we were sure they would make our baby well. We had a lot of hope. The hardest thing, then, and up to the end was that we could never really do anything for our baby ourselves. We were encouraged to touch, to hold, to change diapers, but none of that made up for the sense of helplessness we had. The staff were doing all the really important things for our baby.

After several weeks we found it increasingly difficult to be hopeful and felt a sense of despair. That was also the period of time that we lost our awe of the medical team and felt sure there was more they could be doing if they really cared. We became very critical of everyone and everything. That seemed to go on for many weeks, but eventually we came to realize that we had to make the best of a bad situation and somehow keep on living. We both had other things we had to do.

That's also about the time we regained new respect for the staff, but it was different this time. We didn't have them on a pedestal any more, but grew to appreciate staff members as human beings, for their dedication, the quality of care they gave our baby day after day even though there didn't seem to be any hope of taking the baby home. They never stopped caring about us or our baby even when we were not very responsive.

Through it all our faith in God was strengthened with the help of our pastor. He helped us keep hope when everything looked hopeless. You have to have hope to keep on going. Through his help we are a lot closer to God than we were before. Our family is a lot closer, too. I have to say we're a stronger family for what we went through.

A mother whose daughter was in and out of the intensive care unit for three and a half months before her death has a similar, yet very different story to share:

It means so much that they were willing to tell us over and over what they were doing, why they were doing things. We couldn't seem to remember from one minute to the next, nor could we really concentrate. Nothing ever looked very encouraging, and we had ourselves so programmed for disaster that we didn't know how to respond when we got a bit of good news from time to time.

After I had the baby home for awhile I had to take her to the doctor for a checkup. I will never forget the doctor that day because he asked me how I was doing. I could hardly believe it. He really cared about how I was doing and not just about the baby.

Later when the baby was in the hospital and we were approaching the end my husband and I practically lived there. Often I could sense significant changes before they were noted by doctors and nurses. I was very angry one evening when I overheard a young doctor say, after I'd expressed concern about a problem he wasn't attending to, "These parents think they know everything because they have been in the hospital for a few weeks." It turned out that there really was a problem and I was right to insist on having my baby's doctor called. A mother gets to know a lot about her baby.

One of the things I noticed is that medical people don't want to listen to a nonprofessional. They talk down to us as though taking care of our child was a favor they are granting us. They are being paid, and if someone is doing a favor it is the parents who do the institution and its staff a favor by choosing to use their services. Another thing I noticed is that if parents are calm and quiet their concerns are often minimized. If a woman is hysterical she's passed off as just another hysterical mother.

When I was with my baby I really appreciated the times someone brought me a cup of coffee or came and talked with me about her. Some people always wanted to distract me. I resented that. I wasn't going to have years with my baby. I didn't feel I could afford to spend my precious time chit chatting about other things.

When my baby died we all just hugged each other. I'm so glad people didn't talk then. The hugs and just being together were so much more meaningful than empty words.

I've kept a diary all along. As I've looked back I realize I was really crazy for months. I beat and yelled at our dog for nothing. I felt I was losing my mind. I'd walk away from people in the middle of a conversation. I couldn't sleep. When I did I had a nightmare every time about the hospital. During the day I'd have flashbacks when I would see all the tubes, the scars, the pain our baby had been through.

I felt absolutely useless. When the baby was home there had been care I had to give every two hours. When she was in the hospital I was there constantly. Suddenly there was absolutely nothing. I was envious of all children, especially of handicapped children. If only my baby could be alive and handicapped instead of dead. At one point we put the house up for sale to get away from all the memories. No one bought it so we're still there.

I never cried except by myself. I had to be strong for everyone. I had been the cause of everyone else's hurt and pain. I couldn't add to their problems by being weak in addition. So I did and continue to do my crying in private.

As these stories indicate, the responses and needs of parents when a newborn is critically ill or dies differ. Even so, all seem to find that reorganization of life and acceptance is related to finding a person or persons who will permit them to grieve, to share their story until the pain and agony can be put aside and one is free to live and laugh again.

To provide support to grieving couples we have organized a self-help group. The Caring Connection. Membership is open to parents from anywhere, and there are no dues because we want to be available to any parent who is in need of the support of someone who has had a similar experience.

The way health care professionals relate to parents at the time of a newborn's death makes a great difference in how they feel about themselves and how they work through their grief.

Among the issues frequently seen to be important by parents are the following:

1) Provision for and respect for spiritual needs. In a time of trauma even persons who have not been close to their faith system are frequently comforted by relationship to appropriate religious leaders and provision for rituals and liturgies. It is often a time when healing can take place within the faith system if there has been prior disinterest or alienation. For parents who come from Christian traditions baptism is very important. When there is not an immediate crisis parents usually prefer to be consulted in case there is a particular priest or pastor they wish to invite for the sacramental service. Baptism is a sacrament in which God's blessings are invoked upon the child, but also a time when parents are making a statement about their relationship to God. If at all possible both parents, or at least one parent, and other significant adults who may be in the area need to be included. Certainly they should be consulted to be sure it is a sacrament that is desired and has meaning to the parents. Increasingly we live in a pluralistic society. We cannot assume that all families come from Christian traditions. Baptism of infants from Jewish, Hindu, Muslim, or other non-Christian traditions is not appropriate. To be more effective and more holistic in our care in a pluralistic society, we need to know about other family support systems. What are typical responses to trauma for persons from other cultures and traditions? What do various faith traditions teach or feel about autopsy? What are the preferred forms and necessary rituals for burial? Are there differences in the official position of the faith system and the practices and needs of members of a particular group?

2) It is extremely important for the parents to name, to see, and to hold their baby at the time of death. Mothers and fathers are rarely aware that naming, seeing, and holding are normal and therapeutic responses. Frequently they need the encouragement of their physician to find the courage to respond to the suggestion of the nurse and chaplain. Mothers who choose not to see and hold their babies are often haunted by regrets later in life. Even when there are anomalies the parents who see and hold appear to do better in grief resolution than those who do not. What is imagined is usually far worse than the reality. When parents see and hold their baby they need to be given private space and time. In our hospital the chaplain joins the couple briefly for a prayer of dedication and commitment. Often during a time of prayer the bereaved father finds himself free to cry. Repeatedly bereaved mothers have said that when their husbands cried they knew they cared as much as they did.

3) When parents have not seen their child before death, they need to be prepared clearly, but sensitively, for what they will see. Clinical words and descriptions frequently sound brutal to nonclinical persons. Search for everyday word pictures that describe what will be seen. Recently a young medical resident reminded me that a mental translation is very difficult. I sympathize, yet the couple are usually so in awe of medical personnel that they cannot say they do not understand or that the choice of words is offensive. Difficult as it is, the responsibility for sensitive and clear communication resides with the professional.

4) Parents need to be given permission to cry or not cry and to claim their feelings of anger, fear, confusion, and guilt. They need to hear from medical persons that their emotions are appropriate, that you, too, have feelings of sadness, anger, and helplessness. Cry with parents if that is an emotion you feel at the time. They will not see you as unprofessional, but rather as a person to whom they and their infant are more than a number or dollar sign. It is natural that some deaths will affect you as the care giver more deeply than others.

5) Mementos that will assist the parents with future reality orientation are greatly cherished. Sometimes couples do not think so at the time of hospital discharge, yet even when they go home without them they generally return to pick them up. Among the items appreciated are: baptismal certificate, water used for baptism, hospital identification band, picture, measuring tape, baby's comb, footprints, lock of hair, and baby blanket or shirt.

6) Both parents are hurting, but each will express grief in a different way. Do not focus on one and ignore the other.

7) Parents whose child dies long for their physician to be present with them for a time, to give them a hug, to look them in the eyes, to stay quietly with them for a few minutes. Usually touch and presence are far more important than words. What do you say? Something like, "I don't really know what to say; nothing I can think of feels very comforting at

this time." Use the baby's name. Among the commonly used statements that parents find very irritating are these: you're young, you can have another baby; your baby wouldn't have been normal so it's probably for the best; you'll get over it in time; thank goodness you never took it home; fortunately you never really knew your baby; it was God's will; it just wasn't meant to be, so you'll have to accept it; just be grateful you have . . .

8) Parents who experience the death of a newborn rarely have any idea what the next steps are. After some initial time for grieving has been provided, someone on the team needs to give infomation about the next steps, clarifying issues related to autopsies and final disposition. I prefer to be called as soon as we know that an infant is in trouble. It gives me an opportunity to begin building a relationship before decisions need to be made.

In our hospital, when the physician desires an autopsy it is his or her responsibility to raise the question and clarify the process. Many couples do not understand what an autopsy entails.

Many of the decisions revolve around the question of how to dispose of the remains. That decision-making process must allow time for the couple to have adequate conversation with each other, significant family members, and religious leaders from their faith tradition. Since nurses and physicians are often asked what to do, I want to review the disposition alternatives in a general way. In our hospital the chaplain assists the couple through this process of decision making and signing of forms.

Most hospitals have some method of disposing of the infant's body at no cost to the couple. Frequently couples are unaware of other alternatives and make this choice too hastily. They do not realize that avoiding direct confrontation with the pain of loss at this time may cause increased pain later and merely delay the grief process.

Many funeral directors provide all or most of their funeral services at no cost. Couples need to know that when they ask for information about charges they are not being beggars, but simply seeking a service that is commonly provided in these unusual circumstances. Parents should see the casket that will be used. Also, they should know how the baby will be transported to the cemetery.

Cemetery costs vary considerably. Burial in an infant's area of a cemetery is usually quite reasonable.

Another common alternative is burial in the grave of a relative. In that case permission needs to be given by the nearest living relative whose grave will be used. The couple will be charged the opening and closing fees. Later in life when the couple make decisions about their own burial plots they can have the baby transferred if they so desire.

Frequently religious groups have financial assistance available for young couples who have no resources to meet cemetery costs. In general their pastor, priest, or religious leader can counsel them best in this area.

Social service personnel and hospital chaplains are also sources of information.

There is no need to be in a hurry about the burial itself. The primary time factor is that the funeral director who will be providing his services needs to file for a burial permit. Clarify this issue with informed personnel in your state. Generally, husbands and grandparents do not need to proceed with a burial before the mother is discharged from the hospital. Although well-meaning relatives, funeral directors, or parish pastors often wish to protect the mother from the pain of planning the funeral or from the funeral itself, it is extremely important for the mother to be a participant in making the plans and attending the funeral. This is another point where the physician's encouragement, along with that of the patient's nurse and chaplain, is very important.

Some options in relation to burial and accompanying rituals are: a) service with immediate family, close friends, parents of the infant, religious leader, and funeral director; b) service with parents of the infant, religious leader, and funeral director; c) burial by religious leader and funeral director; d) burial by parents and funeral director; e) burial by funeral director; f) burial by a funeral director with a memorial service in the couple's place of worship at a later time; g) funeral with wake and approach as for an adult; this involves different financial arrangements and will vary from funeral director to funeral director. Burial is important because it provides a ritual of closure, a place for parents to return when they need a time and place for remembering, and as something specific parents can do for the baby that has died.

Someone needs to prepare the couple for some of the problems that may be ahead. It is wise to discuss a number of issues while the mother is still hospitalized. The couple sould be alerted to the wide array of emotions that they may experience as they move through the grief cycle. They may hurt longer than they anticipate. Their loss may place stress on their personal relationships, emotionally as well as sexually. They may feel frustration and anger toward family members, relatives, and friends who seem to be unconcerned or say things that hurt rather than ease. There is the possibility of pain at holidays, invitations to showers, birth announcements, going to a grocery store and seeing an infant in a grocery cart, phantom crying, nightmares, carrying around of dolls, and feelings of going crazy. It is important to include siblings in the funeral when there are other children and to recognize needs of grandparents and other family members.

There are undoubtedly insights yet to be understood in the area of perinatal loss. Persons who have not had first-hand experience but are committed to holistic health care will feel challenged to continue to grow in their understanding, to give care, and also to pay great attention to emotional and spiritual issues.

13

Selected Legal Aspects of Perinatal Care

Nancy J. Brent, R.N., M.S., J.D.

This chapter is intended to provide the reader with a brief overview of the subject matter presented. It is not intended to be a source of specific legal advice in specific situations or a substitute for legal advice. The reader is encouraged to seek competent legal advice when it is required.

With the many advances in medical science and technology, it is an understatement to say that the practice of perinatal medicine is not what it used to be 10 or 15 years ago. The advances that have been made have allowed infants who years ago could not have survived to, at the very least, have fighting chance at life. As positive as that end result is, the survival of these infants raises new legal and ethical issues that must be faced by health care providers. For example, if the infant has a serious birth defect, what will the quality of that infant's life be? Can—and should—treatment be withheld? What if the family clearly indicates that they cannot afford the medical care necessary to keep that child alive? These and other questions are not easy ones, and, of course, no one answer exists for all of the complex situations that the health care professional faces on a daily basis. Yet, a brief look at some of the general legal issues involved in perinatal medicine is necessary to begin to provide some framework for the health professional to grapple with as he attempts to resolve, at least in his own mind, the complex legal and ethical dilemmas in perinatal medicine today.

This chapter is limited to three general areas of discussion. The first section covers defective newborns and some of the implications for medical and nursing practice. Terminally ill infants are discussed on the second portion of this article, with particular emphasis on the decision to resuscitate or not resuscitate. Last, the Uniform Anatomical Gift Act is discussed in relation to the transplantation of dead infant's body organs.

There are many proponents of the view that the decision concerning whether to treat or not to treat a newbown with a severe congenital anomaly should rest with the physician and the parents of the newborn [1–3]. In addition, this approach to the decision-making process concerning treatment issues has been formally supported by the American Medical Association's Judicial Council, which held that "the decision whether to exert maximal efforts to sustain life (of seriously deformed newborns) should be the choice of the parents" [4]. Recently, however, concerns about such issues as whether the parents were being given adequate and complete information to make the decision (informed consent), whether the rights of the family members involved and the rights of the deformed infant were being equitably balanced, and what was to be done when a conflict arose between the doctor and the parents has resulted in the legal system's increasing involvement in this decision-making process.

The legal system's increasing involvement in the area of whether treatment should be withheld or given to defective newborns has not been as much in the form of direct novel intervention in litigated cases involving treatment decisions [5] as it has been in the application of existing statutes and case law intended for other circumstances to these treatment decisions. Precedents in the areas of family law, constitutional law, criminal law [6], and civil law have gained new import in delineating the possible avenues and ramifications for decision making with respect to defective newborns. A brief look at each of these areas and its application to treatment decisions may prove useful in aiding the health professional's awareness of the potential legal issues involved in that decision-making process.

Family law principles involve the balance of the parents' and the defective newborn's rights with the duties and statutory powers of the state to protect the welfare of its citizens. Inherent in this balancing are the general legal principles that parents have a strong, but rebuttable, right to make decisions concerning their children, and that the state can attempt to intervene under the *parens patriae* doctrine when it is clear that the welfare of one of its citizens, including a defective newborn, cannot be protected by that person himself. Clearly, then, there is a potential conflict between these two legal principles; it often raises its head when the parents make a decision concerning medical treatment, and the state, exercising its duty to protect one of its citizens under its neglect and abuse statutes, does not agree with that decision and takes action on behalf of the infant.

A third legal principle involved in this balancing includes, of course, the rights, wishes, and interests of the child involved in the controversy. These rights, wishes, and interests are, at best, difficult to define because the child often cannot define or articulate them due to his age, the infirmity involved, or both. In addition, society and the law are skeptical of the child's ability to know what is best for him, except in certain circumstances. In some states, for example, the parent or guardian of a minor must give consent for medical treatment unless the child is pregnant, married, or otherwise emancipated [7]. In addition, certain states allow the minor to give consent for treatment for venereal disease, drug abuse, and alcoholism if the minor is 12 years of age or older [8]. Also, many Mental Health Codes have codified the rights of minors to consent to treatment and to release of their mental health records [9]. As a result, this legal principle is dealt with by having adults make decisions for a child's rights, wishes, and interests.

When these principles are acted out in relation to treatment decisions concerning defective newborns, it is clear that, at the very least, the principles become more complex and are in conflict with each other. To begin with, the parents, when faced with the birth of a defective newborn, are understandably traumatized, distraught, and confused. As a result, their ability to make informed, reasoned decisions concerning the treatment to be given to their defective newborn—or the treatment to be withheld— can be affected by such issues as the costs of caring for the defective newborn, the impact of the defective newborn on siblings, and the guilt, anger, and loss of self-esteem felt by the parents. These issues, although real and significant, are rarely delved into by the courts when treatment issues are litigated [10]. As a result, the decisions to treat or not to treat often simply acknowledge the right of the parents to make such decisions without any analysis by the legal system as to the potential conflicts these issues might raise with the interests, wishes, and rights of the defective infant.

As a result of these potential conflicts, the legal mechanism of appointing a guardian for the defective infant is being utilized with increasing frequency, both in litigated and nonlitigated cases. This mechanism is particularly useful when the parents appear to be unable to make a decision, when the two parents disagree, when the parents are not concerned about the defective newborn's well-being, when their interests are in conflict with those of the child, and when the parents and the physician disagree about withholding or instituting treatment.

Although certainly a plus in aiding the resolution of conflict(s) concerning treatment decisions for defective newborns, the appointment of a guardian is not always the answer in this controversy. The guardian may solve the problem of providing "protection" for the defective infant's rights wishes, and interests, but his presence does not help the decision maker, for example, the court, decide which factor or factors should be given the most weight in deciding whose position—the defective newborn's, the parents', the state's, the doctor's or the guardian's—should be given final approval. To help with this process, several approaches have been proposed.

One approach, the best interest of the infant approach, focuses on doing what furthers the best interests of the defective newborn. Clearly, this approach underlines the defective newborn's interest in life [11], and is a logical exercise of the state's parens patriae power. Three factors have been suggested as valuable in coming to a decision utilizing this approach: treatment is available that would clearly benefit the defective newborn; all treatment is probably futile; and the probable benefits to the defective newborn from a variety of treatment choices are not clear [12]. If it is clear that treatment can benefit the child, then it should be instituted. If, however, all treatment available will not benefit the defective newborn, and the physicians, parents, and other actors in the decision-making process are in agreement, then treatment should be withheld, with the understanding that comfort measures, including feeding, physical contact with the child, and medications, can be provided until death occurs. The third option, when the benefits and treatments available to the defective newborn are unclear, is more difficult. The President's Commission for the Study of Ethical Problems in Medicine and Biomedical and Behavioral Research suggests that developing guidelines for those defective newborns who will receive life-sustaning treatment and for those who will not is one way to deal with this aspect of determining what is in the best interest of the defective newborn, especially if these guidelines would lead to more objective decision making [13].

The latter factor suggested—that of developing objective criteria for determining which defective children will receive treatment and which will not—overlaps with a second overall approach in determining treatment issues for defective newborns, that of the quality of life approach [14]. This approach considers what type of life the defective infant would live if treatment were given. The basic premise underlying this approach is if the quality of life would be poor, then death is the preferred option. The determination of the quality of life takes into account the quality as it would be experienced by the defective newborn in terms of pain and suffering, the necessity for surgical and medical intervention(s), and the ability to carry out and experience those tasks and feelings associated with being a full-fledged member of the human race. This approach has its obvious drawbacks. Indeed, some of the cases decided concerning the withdrawal of treatment for incompetent adults or minors utilizing this argument have not met with total acceptance by the courts [15–17].

One other approach, the ordinary/extraordinary treatment approach [18], has not been particularly useful in resolving the conflicts concerning a decision to treat or not to treat a defective newborn. What is ordinary or extraordinary treatment depends on the factual circumstances of each particular situation; as a result, few, if any, guidelines can be gleaned from it.

Clearly, family law principles as applied to treatment decisions for defective newborns do not present a complete picture concerning all of the legal issues involved in these decisions, for the focus is mainly on the competing intrafamily interests in determining how to resolve a particular situation and the state's intervention into those interests. Criminal law, on the other hand, is not concerned with competing family interests, but rather with the utilization of applicable state and federal statutes to protect its citizens.

One such statute that may be utilized when attempting to determine treatment decisions concerning defective newborns is a state's child abuse or neglect statutes. The Federal Child Abuse Prevention and Treatment Act [19] may be amended to include provisions for ensuring that defective newborns receive appropriate care (H.R. 1904 and S. 1003). The Senate Bill reportedly contains provisions for loss of federal financial assistance if an institution does not comply with proposed regulations suggested by the Department of Health and Human Services. Although these statutes vary from state to state in the interest of protecting the neglected or abused child, the state can, when necessary, take custody of the child, provide foster home placement, appoint a guardian for the child, terminate (temporarily or permanently) parental rights, and impose fines, imprisonment, or both on the offenders. Withholding or refusing medical treatment for a child is often one of the conditions under which the statute(s) applies. Thus, when a family has decided that treatment for their defective newborn should not be instituted, or when the family and the physician so decide, a call to the designated reporting agency by a "concerned person" could begin the investigation and proceedings of child abuse or neglect against the family, the physician, the hospital, or all three.

Despite the jurisdiction of the state to intervene in such situations, the court's task is no easier when in this situation than it is when it intervenes on the basis of family law principles, for the various interests and approaches discussed thus far must be taken into consideration in deciding whether any of the various penalties will be enforced against the alleged offenders as well as whether medical treatment will be instituted for the defective newbown.

Other criminal statutes that might be utilized when defective newborns are not provided treatment are those that involve the commission of an act, or the failure to carry out a legal duty, that results in injury or death. Thus, the applicability of such charges as murder, voluntary manslaughter, and involuntary manslaughter are possible, depending on how the respective statutes are worded. It is important to note that to date there have been no criminal prosecutions of either parents or physicans for withholding treatment that resulted in the death of a defective newborn [20,21]. Whether this will continue to be the case in the future remains to be seen.

Principles of constitutional law have also been applied to the treatment decisions of defective newborns. Three principles utilized most often are those of equal protection, due process, and the right to privacy [22]. Perhaps the one that has received the most national attention, however, is that of equal protection. In response to the Infant Doe case [23], in which an infant with Down's syndrome and a deformed esophagus that prevented him from taking food died after his parents refused to consent to surgery to repair the defect, the Reagan administration began to reinforce and underscore its position of nondiscrimination concerning handicapped persons. Citing Section 504 of the Rehabilitation Act of 1973 [24], the Office for Civil Rights reminded federally funded health care providers that federal monies would be lost if discrimination against handicapped persons—especially defective newborns—occurred while providing medical care: "No otherwise qualified handicapped individual . . . shall, solely by reason of his handicap, be excluded from the participation in, be denied the benefits of, or be subjected to discrimination under any program or activity receiving Federal financial assistance . . ." The Office of Civil Rights, in its May 18, 1982 notice, also specifically referred to infants with Down's syndrome as being covered by Section 504 of the Rehabilitation Act. To ensure that no discrimination against handicapped (defective) newborns was occurring, a Health and Human Services regulation was enacted requiring federally funded hospitals to post notices stating that treatment and routine care cannot be withheld from defective newborns and provided a "hot-line" to call if treatment was withheld. When a call was received, the Office of Civil Rights would intervene immediately to protect the defective newborn.

The American Academy of Pediatrics filed suit against the Secretary of Health and Human Services [25] alleging, among other things, that the Department did not follow its own procedures for rule making, and that the intrusion into the family-physician relationship was a violation of those parties' constitutional rights. The United States District Court for the District of Columbia agreed and held that the regulation was "arbitrary and capricious." The Court also indicated that public comment was necessary before such a grave intrusion into medical and human decisions is taken by the government. The Department of Health and Human Services appealed the decision and lost that round as well. However, shortly after the decision was handed down, a "new regulation" was proposed by the Department which solicits public comment, retains the "hot-line," and adds the phrase "futile therapies which merely temporarily prolong the process of dying of an infant born terminally ill . . ." are not required [26]. This debate is not over yet, and only time will tell whether any compromise is reached between the divided factions of this difficult issue. Another attempt by the Government to ensure that defective newborns will receive treatment is the proposed amendments to the Child Abuse Prevention and Treatment Act. Two bills (H.R. 1904 and S. 1003) would allow the Health and Human Services Department to study and recommend procedures for treating seriously ill newborns in health care facilities receiving federal monies. Congress will be debating these bills in the future [19].

A final area of law that could be applied to treatment issues, is, of course, that of civil liability. Where injury or death occurs as a result of acts or omissions on the part of the health professional, that health professional could be named in a suit for professional negligence (malpractice) on the premise that a legal duty was owed to the defective newborn, and that that duty was breached. In addition, the "new" actions of wrongful birth, wrongful life, and wrongful death may have increasing applicability to the treatment decisions of defective newborns.

What, if anything, can be gleaned from this brief overview of the legal issues involved in treatment issues for defective newborns? At the very least, the issues are confusing, at times contradictory, and somewhat frightening. Even so, certain guidelines do emerge. To begin with, both the hospital and the physician have a duty to ensure that, whatever the treatment decision, the decision be an informed one [27]. If there is any concern that this is not the case, then judicial guidance should be sought. If, on the other hand, the decision is made by one who is fully informed and legally entitled to make the decision, then the hospital and physician should abide by that decision. The decision-making process and the ultimate decision should, of course, be well-documented in the patient's chart.

In addition, it is important that the institution have well-defined policies and procedures concerning consent, including who should obtain it and how it is to be documented on the patient's chart. Clearly defined policies and procedures should also be developed concerning the internal decision-making process itself. The development of an "ethics committee" or similar body that would review difficult cases or the utilization of a medical consultation to confirm what appears to be a fatal condition have been suggested by the President's Commission for the Study of Ethical Problems in Medicine and Biomedical Behavioral Research [28] as two ways to deal with the difficult decisions in these cases. The Commission also recommends that where review is not possible before the decision is made, retrospective reviews would at least guard against future "bad" decisions being made [29]. Whatever the established internal procedures, if they do not function to ensure a decision that is at least somewhat comfortable for all involved, then judicial intervention should be obtained.

Last, but not least, it is important for those health professionals working with defective newborns to be given an opportunity to share and work through their own feelings, thoughts, and concerns about treatment issues. In doing so, they will hopefully be able to deal with the stress associated with treatment decisions for defective newborns.

Stress concerning treatment decisions is also felt by those working with terminally ill infants, for often a decision must be made concerning whether resuscitation measures should be instituted for a terminally ill infant. Many, if not all, of the same legal issues that have just been discussed covering treatment issues for the defective newborn have applicability for the terminally ill infant. Clearly, substituted consent, fully informed consent to withhold or institute resuscitation measures, all of the respective parties' interests, rights, and concerns, and potential liabilities for health professionals are duplicated here. However, the decision to resuscitate or not resuscitate—the latter being known infamously as DNR—has a better developed "legal history," if you will, than do the treatment decisions of defective newborns. In 1974, The American Heart Association and The National Academy of Sciences, in its "Standards for Cardiopulmonary Resuscitation and Emergency Cardiac Care" statement, indicated that "Cardiopulmonary Resuscitation is not indicated in certain situations, such as in cases of terminal, irreversible illness where death is not unexpected." [30].

After that statement was published, many hospitals began developing policies and procedures concerning resuscitation. Difficulties did not arise, for the most part, for competent, adult patients who refused resuscitation. The better policies indicated that the decision must be documented, and a written order not to resuscitate be placed in the patient's chart. If a verbal order was given—and it could only be given in certain, limited circumstances—two persons had to hear the order, document the order, and sign their names as witnesses, and the physician had to countersign that verbal order within a certain time frame. If the establishment procedure was not followed, then the order not to resuscitate could not be carried out.

Difficulties did arise, and continue to arise, for incompetent adults or minors who could not make the decision for themselves. Cases such as *In re Shirley Dinnerstein* [31], in which a hopelessly ill, 67-year-old woman with Alzheimer's disease, whose family, guardian, and physician all agreed that a DNR order was appropriate and wanted to know if such an order was legal, are somewhat helpful. In that case, the Court held that when an illness is terminal, such an order is appropriate and should be made by the medical profession [32]. The Court further held that judicial intervention should occur only when the physician "fails to exercise that degree of skill and care of the average qualified practitioner" when making such decisions [33].

As clear cut as that decision may sound, however, decisions from other states have not been so clear, especially in relation to minors. This uncertainty creates understandable difficulties for physicians, nurses, and the institution and often results in decisions to resuscitate all minors "just to be safe" or not resuscitating certain terminally ill infants, but not documenting the decision and not writing a DNR order.

A better approach to the problem of resuscitation with terminally ill children is to develop clear policies concerning the internal decision-making that will have to take place. Provisions should be included for consultation with the minor's family and guardian (if one is present), the physician, and other appropriate health team members, such as the nursing staff. As was indicated earlier, if agreed to, the order should be in writing and should be periodically reviewed for renewal or cancellation. Obviously, consultation with the institution's legal department is essential to determine whether any cases, statutes, or opinions of the State's Attorney General might provide guidance in developing those policies. Of course, provision should include the importance of obtaining judicial guidance when agreement is not forthcoming, or when it is clear than an informed consent or refusal is not possible.

The last topic to be discussed is that of transplantation of dead infant's body organs and the Uniform Anatomical Gift Act [34]. The Act, adopted in some form in all of the fifty states and the District of Columbia, spells out the procedures for donating body parts once death has occurred. The Act also defines death, for the purposes of the Act, as "irreversible cessation of total brain function, according to usual and customary standards of medical practice [35]. This is an important definition to remember, for although the definition of death in a particular state may not be brain death for the purposes of determining when death occurs in other situations, it is the standard for determining when death occurs for transplantation purposes.

The Act's consent provisions for transplantation purposes are clear. In the case of a dead infant, either parent, a guardian of the person of the deceased infant at the time of his or her death, or any person authorized or under obligation to dispose of the body, in that order [36], can give all or any part of the infant's body to donees specified in the Act. It is important to note that the time of death of the donor is to be determined by a physician who does not participate in the procedures for removing or transplanting that part [37].

With the importance of responding quickly in transplant situations once death has occurred, the Act is a ready guideline for hospitals, physicians, nurses, and other health professionals who are involved in some way in this decision. Hospital policies should reflect the Act's substantive parts. Familiarity with the Act and relevant hospital policies is essential to provide protection for the dead infant and his family and, at the same time, provide an orderly transition of the body part or parts to a donee in need.

I hope that this brief overview of some of the legal aspects of perinatal medicine has been enlightening, interesting, and informative. If none of those hoped-for results occurred, I hoped that, at the very least, an appreciation of the complex legal issues involved in providing care to patients and their families has been developed. The old adage that ignorance is bliss simply cannot apply here. By becoming more knowledgeable about the legal issues involved in this speciality area, you can protect your rights and the rights of your patients and their families and, at the same time, utilize that knowledge to improve the quality of the care you provide rather than be stymied by it.

References

1. Duff, R.S., Campbell, A. G. M. Moral and ethical dilemmas in the special care nursery. *N. Engl. J. Med.* 289:890, (1973).
2. Stahlman, M.T. Ethical dilemmas in perinatal medicine. *J. Pediatr.* 94:615, 1979.
3. Rickham, R.P., The ethics of surgery on newborn infants. *Clin. Pediatr.* 8:251, 1969.
4. Judicial Council of the American Medical Association. *Current Opinions.* Chicago, Ill: American Medical Association, 1982, p. 9.
5. Longino, P.H. *Withholding Treatment from Defective Newborns: Who Decides, and on What Criteria?* 31:Univ. Kan. L. Rev. 377, 381 (1983).
6. Baumgardner, K. L. *Defective Newborns: Inconsistent Application of Legal Principles Emphasized by the Infant Doe Case,* 14 Tex. Tech. L. Review 569, 570 (1983).
7. Illinois Revisesd Statutes Chapter 111 §4501(1961) and 111–½ §4651(1969).
8. Illinois Revised Statutes Chapter 111 §4504 (1980).
9. Illinois Mental Health and Developmental Disabilities Code and Confidentiality Act, Illinois Revised Statutes, Chapter 91–½ §1–100 *et seq.* (1969) and Chapter 91–½ §801 *et. seq.* (1969).
10. Longino, *supra* note 3, at 389.
11. *Id.,* at 394.
12. President's Commission for the Study of Ethical Problems in Medicine and Biomedical and Behavioral Research. Seriously Ill Newborns, in *Deciding to Forego Life-Sustaining Treatment.* Washington, D.C.: U.S. Government Printing Office, 1983, p. 217.
13. *Id.,* at 221.

14. Longino, *supra* note 3, at 395.
15. In re Quinlan, 355 A. 2d 647 (1976).
16. Maine Medical Center v. Houle, Main Super. Ct. Civ. Action No. 74:149 (1974).
17. Superintendent of Belchertown v. Saikewicz, 370 N.E. 2d 417 (1977).
18. Longino, *supra* note 3, at 397.
19. Public Law 93–247, 88 Statutes 4 (1973).
20. *Id.*, at 406.
21. Cosby, M.G. *The Legacy of Infant Doe*, 34 BAYLOR L. REV. 699, 710 (1982).
22. Baumgardner, *supra* note 4, at 582–588.
23. In Re Guardianship of Infant Doe, No. 1-782A157 (Ind. April 14, 1982).
24. 29. U.S.C. 794, Section 504.
25. American Academy of Pediatrics v. Heckler, no. 83-0774, United States District Court for the District of Columbia, April 14, 1983.
26. 48 FED. REG. 30, 846, July 5, 1983.
27. Longino, *supra* note 3, at 390.
28. President's Commission, *supra* note 8, at 227.
29. *Id.*, at 228.
30. National Conference Steering Committee. Standards for cardiopulmonary resuscitation (CPR) and emergency cardiac care (ECC). *J. Am. Med. Assoc.* 837 and 864, 1974.
31. 380 N.E. 2nd 134 (Mass. App. Ct. 1978).
32. *Id.*
33. *Id.*, at 139.
34. *Uniform Anatomical Gift Act,* Illinois Revised Statutes, Chapter 110–½ §302(b), 1969.
35. *Id.*
36. *Id.*, §303(b).
37. *Id.*, §308(b).

14

Neonatology Practice: A New Challenge

Girdhar L. Ahuja, M.D.

In the last two decades many advancements have been made not only in the care of sick newborns, but also in understanding pathophysiologic changes in the fetus and newborn. Today the use of the ultrasound for determining fetal gestational age, arterial catheterization for blood gases, continuous distending airway pressure, and the use of mechanical ventilators are routine in perinatal care. Tomorrow, we are looking forward to routine use of combined transcutaneous oxygen and carbon dioxide monitoring, prevention of premature labor, and prenatal diagnosis of fetal deformities and genetic disorders.

In the last 10 years we have also witnessed the reorganization of perinatal care, which is still in the developmental stage in some states [1]. Developmental and educational reorganization in Wisconsin has produced a significant reduction in perinatal morbidity and neonatal mortality in that state [2]. Baum has noted that the majority of infants are born in private institutions [3]. Recently perinatal care has been subdivided into level I (primary care), level II (secondary or intermediate care), and level III (tertiary care) centers. A level III nursery is usually established in a university hospital. I question whether it is the only route available.

In this chapter I discuss the organization of perinatal care in a family-centered hospital not affiliated with a medical school and without a graduate training program in obstetrics or pediatrics. Organization and data will be presented that suggest that the care provided is as good as that at most university centers and, in some ways, better. Problems that have been encountered will also be reviewed.

Selection of the Hospital

Combined planning by the medical staff (obstetrics, pediatrics, and family practice) and the administration resulted in a contract with the hospital that allowed me to assume the duties of a part-time director of nurseries and educator of perinatal medicine to the nursing staff, the medical staff, and paramedical personnel involved in the care of all newborns. A short perinatal course for expectant parents was alrady in existence. Educational needs are subgrouped as follows: administration, nursing and paramedical staff, medical staff, and parents.

ADMINISTRATIVE EDUCATION

Weekly conferences were held by the director with an administrator, the nursing supervisor covering the prenatal and postnatal family center and the nurseries, and the head nurse of the special care nursery. In our institution the admitting nursery is staffed by the nurses of the special care nursery, and they provide maximum observation and care to every newborn infant. Besides the purchase of equipment, the patient/nurse ratios during all shifts and holidays and future needs are regularly reviewed.

NURSING AND PARAMEDICAL STAFF EDUCATION

Nurses are the central core of all patient care, particularly newborns who not only are small, but also whose needs are different. Realizing individual nurses' needs, attitudes, and experience, education was provided by bedside teaching, practical procedures, and formal lectures. In my point of view, bedside teaching is extremely important. Two meetings per week have been arranged; one during a day shift and the other for an evening shift. Night shift personnel chose either of two sessions. Invariably all subjects are covered with both groups; however, nurses chose the subject material. It covers physiologic changes at birth, assessment of gestation, symptoms and signs of various disorders, and the nurse's role in the patient management. Paramedical staff, i.e., respiratory therapy and obstetric personnel, are encouraged to attend. Some of topics discussed are asphyxia, resuscitation, apnea, temperature regulation, jaundice, caloric and fluid requirements, and physical and emotional needs of the sick newborn. The family practice house staff on rotation are encouraged to attend the same sessions as well. Techniques, precautions, and the advantages and disadvantages of many practical procedures are discussed, including use of the Hope bag, nasogastric feeding, transpyloric feeding, starting of intravenous fluids, radial artery blood sampling, use of oxygen, and endotrachael intubation. Each nurse is individually supervised and certified by the director when proficient in doing procedures like intravenous infusion, radial artery blood sampling, and arterial catheter blood sampling. Formal lectures with audiovisual aids are combined with medical staff education.

MEDICAL STAFF EDUCATION

I organized the lectures for education of the medical staff on a weekly basis for all personnel of the institution, which includes not only medical and nursing staff, but also respiratory therapy, dietary, pharmacy, and pastoral personnel. The topics discussed are quite varied and include asphyxia at birth, respiratory distress syndrome, infections of the newborn, nutritional needs, prevention of iatrogenic problems, stress and strain of high-risk infant care, role of parents, care of the siblings and family, coping with death, and availability of supportive agencies. These conferences are well attended. Our speakers are predominantly physicians in practice, with occasional guest speakers from the referral centers in the city. Our conferences have been approved by the Indiana Chapter of American Academy of Family Physicians, hour for hour for continuing medical education.

EDUCATION OF PARENTS

The education of parents is an integral part of the care provided at Saint Francis Hospital Center. After the admission of the infant, the parents are constantly given updated information by a team of care providers: a physician, a nurse, a social worker, and, if needed, a minister or chaplain. The importance of touching, calling infants by their first name, and "enfacing" are stressed. Visits by grandparents and close relatives who may be involved in the care of the infant after discharge as well as by siblings (via the window) are routine at our institution. For the last three years, sibling visits have been encouraged for normal newborns as well. Parents are trained in caring for their infants, changing of diapers, and changing posture or position; they are also trained in use of hope bag, tube feeds, and use of oxygen whenever circumstances warrant. Training parents for intragastric tube feeds, changing gastrostomy tube, and changing of dressings is not unusual.

Three sets of parents have been trained to take care of central hyperalimentation at home. We individualize each infant's needs and allow the parents to participate in his care. We have sent growing premature infants home weighing four pounds or less when the parents have been properly educated. This type of education required the teamwork of a physician, nursing staff, and paramedical staff as well as lots of patience and time.

Organization of the Nursery

Along with the teaching program, the special care nursery was initially organized to accomodate four sick infants with adequate facilities for oxygen, vacuum suction, electrical outlets, cardiorespiratory monitoring, and oxygen analyzers. This capacity is now increased to eight in the last two years. There is no capability to monitor central arterial pressure at present; however, a DINAMAP = 847 neonatal monitor is used to measure blood pressure indirectly. For the last four years, two types of pressure ventilators have been used to provide constant positive airway pressure, intermittent mandatory ventilation, and controlled ventilation with or without end expiratory pressure. Previously trained and certified nursing staff draw a sample either by arterial catheter or a radial artery puncture for blood gas analysis routinely during all shifts. There is an initial standing order sheet for each new admission which authorizes the nurses to order oxygen to relieve cyanosis, blood gases, chest x rays, and blood glucose tests as considered clinically necessary if there is difficulty in contacting the physician of the infant. It is our standing policy that attending physicians must see their patients within four hours of admission, or earlier if the condition warrants. As outlined above, there is a continuing education program for both physicians and the nursing staff. (Off duty nurses are paid overtime to attend teaching conferences.) The nurses are also trained to read x rays for the position of endotracheal tubes and arterial catheters and also to identify a pneumomediastinum and pneumothorax. Because of the availability of an anesthetist on duty, there has not been the need for the nurses to intubate any neonates, although there is at present an ongoing program for teaching endotracheal intubation.

Results

Through 1972 and 1974, the number of deliveries at Saint Francis Hospital Center has been rather stable at about 1,600 per year. The exact data regarding the morbidity and mortality of high-risk infants are unknown because sick infants were transported to one of the two referral centers. As a routine practice, deaths at the level III nursery were not included

185

Figure 14–1
Incidence of high-risk infants against live births.
ST. FRANCIS HOSPITAL CENTER
1975-1981

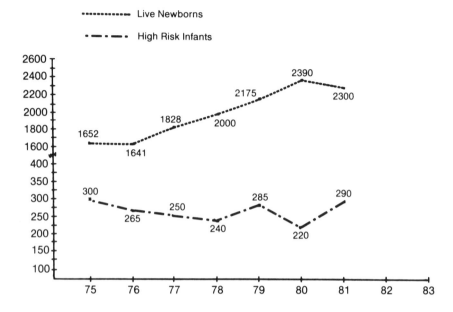

in neonatal and perinatal deaths of the primary hospital. Since January 1975, the number of deliveries has generally increased at Saint Francis (Figure 14–1). All 1981 data have been averaged on the basis of the first 11 months. A list of high-risk neonatal categories was made as a guideline for admission to the special care nursery with approval of the obstetric, pediatric, and family practice medical staff. Any infant found to have a problem during the 4 to 6 hour period of observation in the admitting nursery or any infant in the family centered postnatal unit who develops a problem is admitted to the special care nursery. In the last six years, the number of infants admitted to the special care nursery has slowly fallen because of improved prenatal care, fetal monitoring, and intrapartum care. The infants born by a repeat elective cesarean section or born to a mother with a medical condition are no longer automatic admissions to the special care nursery facility. Even asymptomatic babies born by emergency cesarean section or with a history of prolonged rupture of membranes are transferred to the regular nursery after an initial period of observation that can be extended up to eight hours on hourly charge basis. Thus, in spite of the progressive increase in the number of births (1,650 in 1975 to 2,390 in 1980) at Saint Francis, admissions to the special

Figure 14–2

Statistics on admissions to the Special Care Nursery at Saint Francis Hospital Center in 1978.

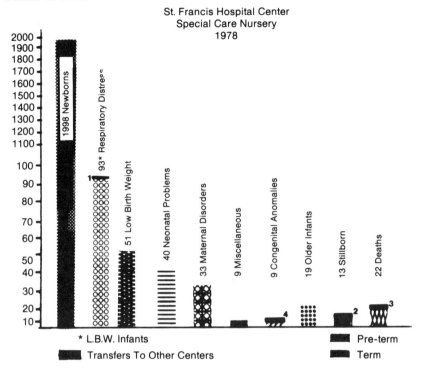

St. Francis Hospital Center
Special Care Nursery
1978

* L.B.W. Infants   Pre-term

Transfers To Other Centers   Term

care nursery have fallen from 300 in 1975 to 220 in 1980 (Figure 14–1). Figure 14–2 shows the number of births, categories of infants admitted to the special care nursery, number of infants transferred, and number of deaths during 1978. Figure 14–3 shows the admission distribution in various subgroup categories from 1975 through 1981.

Because of the acquisition and use of ventilators and the addition of two pediatric surgeons to the staff, the number of very sick infants transferred to other institutions has progressively fallen (Figure 14–4). The major indication for a transfer now is congenital heart disease, since we cannot do cardiac catheterization or surgery, although we have added two-dimensional neonatal echocardiography as one of our diagnostic tools.

The essence of the care provided has been the teamwork between physicans involved in perinatal care, continuing education of both doctors and nurses, and communication among all people involved including laboratory technicians, respiratory therapists, radiologists, social service personnel, parents, and pastoral personnel. Our combined efforts have resulted in a low perinatal mortality rate (number of deaths per 1,000 de-

Figure 14–3

Statistics on admissions to the Special Care Nursery at Saint Francis Hospital Center from 1975 through 1981.

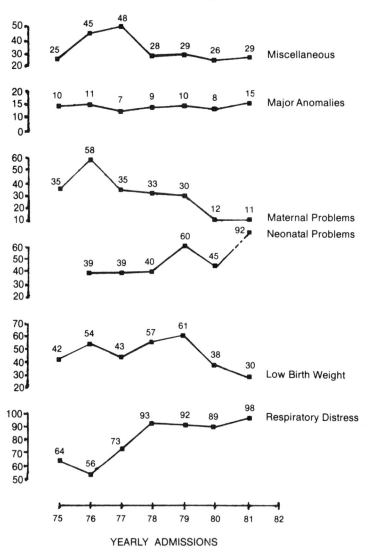

St. Francis Hospital Center
Special Care Nursery

188

Figure 14–4

Mortality rate per 1,000 births and transfers.

ST. FRANCIS HOSPITAL CENTER
1975-1981

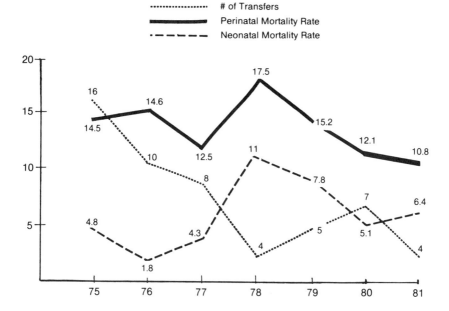

liveries, i.e., stillborns and neonatal deaths), which has remained between 10.8 and 17.5 (Figure 14–4) and has slowly fallen over the last four years. The neonatal mortality rate (number of deaths per 1,000 live-born infants up to 28 days of age) has remained low as well. Since we began to use ventilators, 1978 through 1981, neonatal mortality, including neonates with major congenital anomalies, has gradually declined from 11 to 6.4 deaths per 1,000 births (Figure 14–4). These data include the infants who were born at Saint Francis, but were tranferred to two other referral centers where they eventually died. The 1978 data reveal a higher rate than previous years because they include six babies of less than 700 g who were born with heart rates, of less than 40 beats per minute and were counted as live births. One infant is also included as a newborn death, although he died of bronchopulmonary dysplasia at the age of 2.5 months, but never left the special care nursery. A perinatal mortality committee has been established which examines perinatal deaths to determine whether the care given to the mother, fetus, and neonate could have been improved.

Organization of the Practice

Our goals to provide good quality care are as follows: 1) care for high-risk infants, 2) education and training (as discussed above), 3) follow-up care of high-risk infants, 4) follow-up care of normal newborns, especially siblings (pediatric practice), 5) consultations for nurseries and pediatrics, 6) self-education, 7) meeting obligations to various medical staff committees and meetings.

Because of my obligations as the part-time director of nurseries and an educator at Saint Francis Hospital Center, it was decided to locate my office at the adjacent Medical Arts Building. At present, I have patient care commitments mainly at Saint Francis and Community Hospital. Methodist Hospital has a large pediatric graduate training program and a tertiary perinatal care center, where I took my fellowship in neonatology for two years and continue my affiliation by conducting weekly teaching rounds in the special care nursery.

Simultaneous to organizing my office practice and part-time directorship at Saint Francis, I have contracted to be a teacher at Saint Vincent Hospital and an instructor for the pediatric nurse associate training program at Methodist Hospital.

In the office, my main objective has been to follow high-risk infants' families, including the siblings. Obviously, caring for normal newborn infants and siblings is an essential part of the economics of the practice, but pediatric practice has to be greatly restricted because of my time involvement with high-risk babies. Office hours are set from 12:00 noon to 5:00 p.m., four days a week, as the mornings fulfill the rest of my obligations. However, the patient follow-ups and consultations are seen by appointment only, with the understanding that the appointment may be cancelled if an acute emergency arises in either the nursery or the delivery room. All telephone calls from the parents are returned by me personally at the end of office hours or later from my home. The office nursing staff usually provide emotional support to comfort some of the anxious parents. All parents receive a booklet upon the infant's dismissal from the hospital providing guidance for routine infant problems, automotive safety recommendations, immunizations, and outline of growth and development records. On each visit the parents are given an outline of recommendations in writing. This has been very successful in enhancing parental compliance.

High-risk infant follow-up includes evaluation of physical growth, neurologic and ophthalmic evaluation, audiology screening, and developmental evaluation at six-month intervals. Whenever necessary, speech evaluation is performed between 16 months and two years. Other necessary referrals are made as the need arises.

Personal continuing education is a regular and built-in process since I prepare at least two didactic presentations a month for the Saint Francis conferences and once-weekly teaching rounds with the pediatric house staff at Methodist Hospital special care nursery. Regular attendance or weekly pediatric grand rounds and conferences on topics in perinatal medicine and section meetings at various hospitals provide the stimulus to learn. I manage to attend three to four newborn or perinatal medicine national or regional symposia each year.

Problems

Saint Francis Hospital Center is a modest size institution with a rising delivery rate from 1,600 per year in 1974 to nearly 2,400 per year during 1980 and 1981, of which about 12 percent are admitted to the special care nursery. This presents a great challenge as well as a difficult task in providing immediate care for the sick neonate in the delivery room. Obviously, continuing education of the nursing and medical staff has played a very significant role in providing this care around the clock. With increasing coordination and cooperation between obstetric and nursery staff, both specialists (obstetrician and neonatologist or pediatrician) are present for high-risk deliveries. Prior personal communication with the neonatologist or pediatrician markedly increases the chances of familiarization with prospective parents before delivery. The need to provide this care puts constraints on the personal and social life of the neonatologist and limits the amount of time available for continuing education and for vacation. (I strongly believe that it is the responsibility of referral centers to co-ordinate time-off arrangements and provide coverage in all level II care nurseries in a regional reorganization of perinatal care.) With strict discipline and determination to accept the demanding tasks, these problems can be overcome. Obviously other members of the pediatric and obstetric staff have to cooperate and share the care of high-risk infants.

Insurance coverage remains a large problem. In our community about 25 to 30 percent of couples do not have third-party coverage, and half of the remaining parents have only partial coverage. To compound the problem, disproportionately higher percentages of high-risk infants are born to young mothers (couples), single mothers, and those of lower economic group, who frequently have little or no third-party coverage. Continued follow-up pediatric care should improve the chances for payment in some cases. The hospital must provide remuneration to the neonatologist to direct and guide the nursery and for continuing education to the nursing and medical staff. The physician can then supplement his income by fee-for-service payment for direct patient care.

It is unfortunate that if the infant dies, the parents are often forgotten. Previous constant parental support and time spent educating the parents about the disease and problems of high-risk neonates increases the confidence of the parents in the physician. The practice of referring to infants by their first names by all people involved in their care helps bring warmth and closeness and helps later when counseling grieving parents. In cases where the baby dies, I and the nurses who provided most of the infants' care meet with the parents at three weeks and three months after the death.

Conclusion

Since the nurseries at Saint Francis Hospital Center were upgraded in 1974, the care of newborns has vastly improved. In spite of an increase in total births by about 50 percent over the past six years, fewer babies were admitted to the special care nursery, and few babies were transported to level III nurseries. Both neonatal and perinatal mortality has remained low. Nearly all mothers are now being monitored (external and internal fetal monitor) during labor. Above all, quality care is being provided by a team consisting of the nursing staff, paramedical personnel, family physicians, and specialists, both obstetrics and pediatric, without disrupting the usual health care system, that is, a family unit, a community hospital, and the private physician.

References

1. Salisbury, A. J. Progress in "regionalization" of perinatal care. *Clin. Perinatol.* 3:267–270, 1976.
2. Schneider, J. M. In *Regionalization of Perinatal Care: Report of the Sixty Sixth Ross Conference on Pediatric Research.* Columbus, Ohio: Ross Laboratories, August, 1974.
3. Baum, R. S. The large private hospital and neonatal intensive care. *Clin. Perinatol.* 3:304–314, 1976.

15

Arterial Oxygen Monitoring: Using the Searle Umbilical Artery Catheter-Tip Electrode in Neonates

Manohar Rathi, M.D., Vasundhara Kakodkar, M.D., and Michael J. Tidd, M.D.

The need for monitoring arterial oxygen tension (PaO$_2$) in premature and other high-risk neonates has been recognized for at least as long as the complications of oxygen therapy. Intermittent sampling was the only option available until it was recognized that it might be technically feasible to produce compact, continuously operating electrochemical oxygen sensors based on the Clark cell [1] or related devices small enough for intraarterial placement in neonates. A number of devices based on monopolar or bipolar Clark cells [2] or silver-lead-oxygen fuel cells [3,4] were produced on a prototype basis, but in most cases the formidable technologic problems involved in miniaturization and manufacturing led to unsatisfactory performance in clinical use.

However, by 1975 a miniaturized bipolar polarographic oxygen electrode (oxygen probe) suitable for large-scale production had been developed and was introduced [5] into clinical practice in Europe [6,7]. Substantial experience has now been accumulated with this device, and it has recently become available in the United States [8] and Canada [9]. Over approximately the same period, transcutaneous oxygen monitoring was also developed and introduced. Enough information is now available about each technique to make comparative evaluation of their relative advantages and their respective limitations. In this chapter we review these and provide some practical guidance to the use of catheter-tip electrodes based on over two years of experience with them in a neonatal intensive care unit.

Some of the data were obtained by the authors during a clinical investigation of 5-Fr oxygen probes that is to be reported in detail elsewhere. Briefly, 47 neonates (median birthweight, 2.3 kg; range, 1.1 to 4.6 kg) requiring umbilical artery catheters (UACs) in the course of ordinary clinical treatment were managed with Searle oxygen probes instead. The probes were inserted at a median age of 4.3 hours (range, 0.42 to 111.63 hours). PaO_2 readings from the probes were compared periodically with PaO_2 readings by conventional blood gas analyzer obtained on samples withdrawn from the sampling lumen of the probe. The probe was recalibrated at intervals as indicated by the accuracy required for satisfactory clinical management in each set of circumstances, using the blood gas analyzer as the standard. Glucose-electrolyte solutions were administered via the sampling lumen. Infusion fluids were heparinized in only two infants. Cumulative probe survival was calculated by using the life table technique of Potter [10]. In addition to these data collected during the first 12 months of our experience with the probe, we have drawn on subsequent experience obtained with both 4- and 5-Fr probes and with heparinized infusion fluids.

Principles of Operation

Both transcutaneous and umbilical artery catheter oxygen electrodes are based on the electrochemical reduction of oxygen at the surface of a silver, gold, or platinum cathode that acts as a catalyst. Each of these metals has specific electrochemical properties that are importantly different in certain clinical circumstances, although oxygen is reduced at the surface of each. If a fixed polarizing voltage, typically a few hundred millivolts, is applied continuously between an anode (usually a silver/silver chloride reference electrode) and the cathode, and the access of oxygen to the electrode is simultaneously limited by means of an overlying oxygen-permeable membrane, it is possible to arrange conditions such that all oxygen reaching the cathode is electrochemically reduced according to the overall equation, $2H_2O + O_2 + 4\bar{e} \text{ --- } 4OH^-$. An electrolyte layer beneath the membrane on the face of the electrode permits the liberated electrons to flow as a current that is proportional to the rate of diffusion of oxygen to the cathode. Thus, under appropriate conditions, the current is proportional to the oxygen tension at the outer surface of the oxygen-permeable membrane, which is in contact either with skin (transcutaneous) or flowing blood (intravascular).

If the current output of such a catheter-tip device held at constant

194

Figure 15-1

Schematic representation of relationship between polarizing voltage and current flow for a typical Searle oxygen probe equilibrated with oxygen-nitrogen and oxygen-nitrous oxide gas mixtures. The percentage of oxygen is indicated above each plateau. There is a small current at zero oxygen concentration. *(Based on data from the following: Hahn, C.E.W., Brooks, W.N., Albery, W.J., Rolfe, P. O_2 and N_2O analysis with a single intravascular catheter electrode.* Anaesthesia *34:263–266, 1979. Brooks, W.N., Hahn, C.E.W., Foex, P. On-line PO_2 and PN_2O analysis with an in-vivo catheter electrode.* Br. J. Anaesth. *52:715–721, 1980.)*

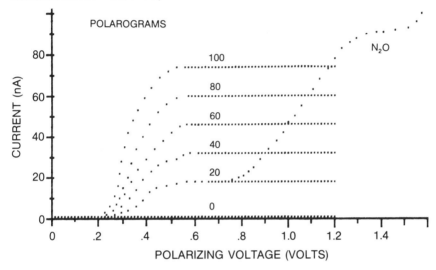

oxygen tension is plotted against a varying polarizing voltage the resulting current-voltage curve (polarogram) shows that the current flow is substantially independent of the polarizing voltage over a range of several hundred millivolts. Within this range the current output can be made to be virtually linearly proportional to pO_2 [5,11]. Figure 15-1 is a schematic representation of the relationship between polarizing voltage and current flow for a typical Searle probe at 37°C in stirred saline equilibrated with oxygen-nitrogen gas mixtures at the concentrations of oxygen shown. Above about 0.6 V there is a clear plateau for each concentration, the level of which is related to concentration, but which is independent of voltage.

The polarizing voltage applied to the Searle electrode (described later) is 750 mV. This voltage is sufficient to cause some electrochemical reduction of nitrous oxide, if present according to the equation, $N_2O + H_2O + 2\bar{e} \text{ --- } N_2 + 2OH^-$. The curve labeled N_2O in Figure 15-1 indicates the approximate current-voltage relationship for a mixture of 20 percent O_2 and 80 percent N_2O. There is an increasing additional current due to

195

N_2O reduction above about 0.7 V. The formation of nitrogen bubbles under the sensor membrane [11] interfering with oxygen diffusion, the production of spurious electrical signals from nitrous oxide reduction, and the additional possibility of interference from the electrochemical reduction of brominated anesthetic agents, particularly halothane [12–14], at the silver cathode makes the use of such devices inadvisable during anesthesia and for some time after until the anesthetic agents have been eliminated.

Bipolar electrodes with platinum or gold cathodes, which are electrochemically indifferent to N_2O, are nevertheless also liable to such interference, because silver from the anode (Ag-AgCl reference electrode) may be electroplated onto the electrochemically active surface of the cathode [11].

Description of the Device

The elements of the Searle neonatal oxygen monitoring system* consist of an umbilical artery catheter electrode attached by means of a screened connecting cable to a battery-powered monitor, which, after calibration, displays the PaO_2 on an analog scale. The monitor also contains adjustable high and low alarms, a low battery alarm, and calibration controls.

If the monitor is to be used with a strip chart recorder, it is necessary to connect it to a recorder interface unit, which maintains the electrical isolation of the monitor from ground to protect the patient from electrical shock hazards from ground leakage currents.

The construction of the tip of the oxygen probe is illustrated in detail in Figure 15–2. The sampling port and sampling lumen are connected to a Luer connector to permit sampling and are quite separate from the lumen carrying the electrical conductors.

Insertion

The insertion of the catheter electrode into an umbilical artery follows standard aseptic insertion techniques. Some users have found it helpful to stiffen the catheter by precooling, but we have not found this to be necessary. Both 4- and 5-Fr catheters are available, and selection is based largely on the weight of the infant, the smaller size being recommended for infants of 1 kg or less.

Certain additional precautions are advisable to maximize the chance of subsequent satisfactory function. As mentioned above, the anode and cathode at the tip of the catheter are covered with a delicate polymer

*Orange Medical Instruments, Costa Mesa, California.

Figure 15–2

Details of construction of the Searle oxygen probe. (A) Longitudinal section through tip of catheter and oxygen sensor. (B) Cross section of shaft of catheter showing bilumen construction with cathode (small) and anode (large) conductors in one lumen. The other lumen is used for sampling and infusion. (C) Cross section of a conventional UAC for comparison showing larger internal diameter. *(Modified in part from Parker, D., Soutter, L. P. In vivo monitoring of blood PO_2 in newborn infants. In Payne, J.P. (ed.), Current Status of Oxygen Measurements in Biology and Medicine, London: Butterworth, 1975, pp. 269–283.)*

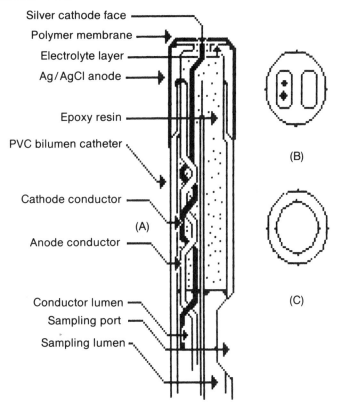

membrane that is easily damaged by injudicious handling with metal instruments. Membrane function may also be seriously disturbed by the undetected accumulation of a layer of dried blood or Wharton's jelly over it during multiple insertion attempts. Such a layer may act as a nidus for subsequent thrombus formation, with adverse consequences for both the infant and the probe function. Gentle cleaning with heparinized saline is suggested if there is any suspicion of foreign material on the probe.

Activation, Stabilization, and Initial Calibration

After insertion, water diffuses through the polymer covering the sensor and establishes a conducting electrolyte layer at the face of the anode and cathode. This process is a gradual one during which the sensitivity of the device increases (not necessarily smoothly) to a maximum over a variable period, which in our experience may be as short as 10 to 20 minutes, but which rarely exceeds an hour. Although this process of stabilization can be followed easily in the laboratory, where ambient oxygen tension can be held constant, it is not necessarily so easy to judge when stability has been achieved in vivo. With experience a judgement can usually be made that a probe is approaching or has reached stability.

A provisional calibration should then be carried out by performing a conventional blood gas analysis on a sample withdrawn from the sampling lumen and comparing the result with the monitor reading at the time of sampling. In the event of a significant discrepancy the current monitor reading should be adjusted to a new (corrected) value, which is obtained by multiplying the current (uncorrected) value by the ratio (blood gas analyzer PaO_2/monitor PaO_2 reading at the time of sampling) and adjusting the uncorrected monitor reading to the correct value immediately. Check calibrations after suitable intervals (15 to 30 minutes) should be performed until there is consistent agreement between PaO_2 by blood gas analyzer and the corresponding monitor PaO_2 reading for the sampling. For routine trend monitoring purposes agreement to within 10 percent to 1.33 kPa (10 mmHg) is satisfactory.

Recalibration

Periodic comparisons of monitor PaO_2 readings with the results of arterial blood gas analysis should be made. We made such comparisons at a median interval of about three hours. The median interval between calibrations was just over 9 hours. As would be expected, small discrepancies between monitor and analyzer readings (< 1.33 kPa) led to recalibration in only a small proportion (8.4 percent) of cases, whereas differences of 1.33 kPa or more usually led to an appropriate calibration adjustment.

The accuracy of a given calibration or recalibration is related both to the accuracy with which the monitor can be read (accuracy is adversely affected when the reading is varying rapidly) and to the accuracy with which the monitor reading reflects the PaO_2 at the time the sample is withdrawn. Changes in oxygen tension at the outer surface of the sensor membrane are not reflected instantaneously at the cathode because of the diffusion resistance of the membrane. Thus, the instantaneous reading of the monitor is related in a complex way to recent PaO_2 changes. The monitor reading lags behind the PaO_2, and it has been found empirically by Wilkinson et al. [8] that the correlation between monitor and blood gas analyzer results is improved significantly if the monitor reading used in the calibration calculation is obtained 45 seconds after the blood sample is withdrawn, rather than at the time of withdrawal. There is little to be gained from the adoption of such a procedure when the PaO_2 is stable, but it appears worthwhile when calibration is being attempted when the PaO_2 is very variable.

Relationship Between Monitor and Blood Gas Analyzer Readings

The results of comparisons between monitor and blood gas analyzer PaO_2 for a subset of 453 paired observations where the monitor had been calibrated in accordance with the recommended directions for routine clinical monitoring are illustrated in Figure 15–3. The monitor was regarded as remaining satisfactorily calibrated if the reading was within 10 percent of the corresponding blood gas analyzer result and at least 60 minutes had elapsed since insertion. The paired observations were plotted on the scattergram. The majority (66 percent) of the readings fell within the 10 percent range lines, indicating that there was a relatively good chance that the monitor would require only occasional adjustment.

The extent to which monitor and analyzer readings were concordant was obscured by the use of a "clinical" calibration standard, which accepted as satisfactory agreement between monitor and analyzer to within about 10 percent. We therefore examined a larger subset of 542 paired observations to calculate the extent to which the calibration factor (defined as the ratio of monitor/analyzer readings) would have subsequently deviated from perfect calibration at the following calibration check had the calibration been exact (calibration factor of 1) on each prior occasion. The data base was larger than that for Figure 15–3, since changes in valid calibration factors outside the 0.9 to 1.1 range were accepted. The frequency distribution of the calculated calibration factors is shown in Figure 15–4. Clinically acceptable calibration is indicated by calibration factors of 0.9 to 1.1, and 58 percent of values were in this range. Widening the range to 0.8 to 1.2 covered 85 percent of values. These figures may overestimate the divergence since inspection of the data strongly suggested that not infrequently an erroneous "calibration" was followed by a correction on the next calibration. This gave rise to wide swings in the correction factor on each such occasion. The occurrence of pairs of large deviations strongly suggests that the true underlying change in probe calibration had been small and that at least some of these paired deviations may have been artifacts.

199

Figure 15–3

Relationship of arterial oxygen tension measured by blood gas analyzer and as estimated by oxygen probe for 453 paired observations (see text for details). The least squares fit linear regression line is flanked by + 10 percent and − 10 percent range lines. Each point is an open square, and heavy overprinting of data points has occurred due to clustering near and between the range lines.

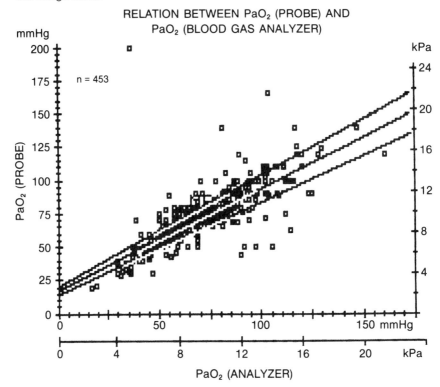

RELATION BETWEEN PaO$_2$ (PROBE) AND PaO$_2$ (BLOOD GAS ANALYZER)

PaO$_2$ (ANALYZER)

Catheter Positioning

There are indications that high placement of conventional umbilical artery catheters may result in a lower incidence of certain vascular complications in the lower limbs [15,16]. To the best of our knowledge there are no published data on the effect of sensor-tip position on the incidence of vascular complications. Our policy has been to place the probe tip at T6 to T8; in the largest published series [17], the probe tip was placed at L2 early in the investigation and later revised to L4. In our series of 47 infants the device was removed because of circulatory impairment in three cases (6.4 percent), which was similar to the 6.7 percent (18/268) incidence of removal for comparable reasons in the series of Pollitzer et al. [17]. How-

Figure 15–4

Frequency distribution histogram for 542 calibration factors (blood gas analyzer reading/monitor reading). Perfect calibration is indicated by a value of 1.00. The data indicate the extent to which calibration would have deviated from ideal between calibrations if the probe had been recalibrated at each calibration check. The data are in part calculated since in practice not all checks led to a recalibration.

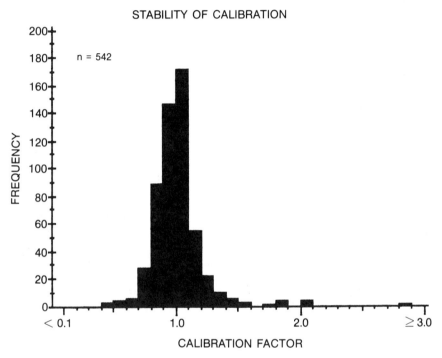

ever, the patient populations differed in material respects, particularly birth weight, and this apparent lack of major effect of positioning should be interpreted with caution.

Sampling Lumen Management

The effective use of a catheter-tip PaO_2 electrode is dependent not only on the satisfactory technical performance of the sensor itself, but also on the ability to check the sensor calibration periodically. Thus the maintenance of the patency of the sampling lumen is critical. Because of the presence of the second lumen carrying the conductors to the sensor, the sampling lumen diameter is considerably smaller than that of a comparably sized conventional umbilical artery catheter (Figure 15–2). This slows the

201

Figure 15–5

Cumulative overall probe failure rate by time showing contributions from sensor failure (i.e., sensor-specific) and catheter-associated (i.e., not sensor-specific) causes. The failure rate at time zero includes probes that failed ever to function satisfactorily and that were therefore usually removed shortly thereafter. Standard errors of the estimates of the cumulative overall failure rates are indicated.

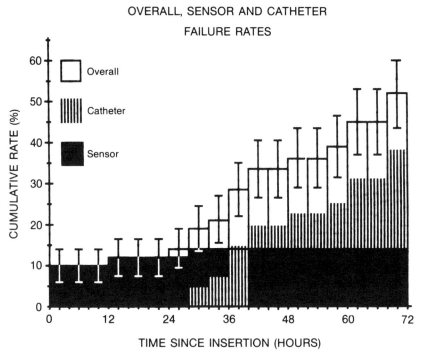

OVERALL, SENSOR AND CATHETER

FAILURE RATES

rate at which blood can be withdrawn during sampling, prolonging the procedure. For this reason the use of a heparinized saline flush to keep the lumen clear of blood as far as possible during insertion is recommended to minimize the risk of formation of a nidus of thrombus, which may subsequently propagate and lead to blockage during later sampling. Based on our experience with both heparinized and unheparinized sampling lumen fluid infusions, we feel that the use of heparinized sampling lumen infusions is generally desirable (see below).

The overall cumulative probe failure rates by time, together with the contributions from sensor failure and failure attributed to loss of catheter function or complications of catheter use, are illustrated in Figure 15–5. In our experience, sampling lumen occlusion was undoubtedly the most frequent cause of system failure and usually occurred while the sensor was operating satisfactorily. Pollitzer et al. [17] observed a sampling lumen occlusion rate of 10 percent after a mean of 55 hours of use. In our hands the catheter-associated failure rate was 22 percent after the same interval. Sampling lumen occlusion accounted for most of this. The infusion of heparinized fluids (2 U/ml at 2 ml/hour or more) through the sampling lumen was routine in their series, whereas we employed heparinized fluids in only two cases. It seems very likely that this marked difference in occlusion rates was due to their use of heparin. Rajani et al. [18] have found that constant infusion of heparin (1 U/ml) at a rate of between 100 and 200 U of heparin per kg per day in infants weighing 1 kg or more produced an increase in conventional UAC functional half-life from about two days to seven days.

In spite of our initial reluctance we now use heparin in the sampling fluid infusion as a routine in most infants, recognizing that there may be a small risk of accidental heparinization. In practice this does not seem to represent a problem, since neither Rajani et al. [18] nor Pollitzer et al. [17] found evidence of complications attributable to heparinization at these levels. This has also been our recent experience since we changed our policy to one of routine use of heparinized (1 U/ml) infusions. On balance the benefit of heparinizing the infusion fluid in keeping the lumen open and the system functional outweighs the risks involved.

Functional Lifetime in Relation to Clinical Need

It is evident both from our experience and from the extensive series reported by others [17,19] that a small proportion of probes fail ever to function in vivo. Defects in manufacturing and unrecognized damage during insertion [20] are responsible for some of these. However, Pollitzer et al. [17] found that nearly half of the probes that were nonfunctional in vivo functioned satisfactorily in vitro when tested later. The explanation for this is not clear.

Once the oxygen monitoring system has been inserted, activated, and stabilized satisfactorily, the cumulative probability of it becoming nonoperational because of sensor failure in the period up to 72 hours from insertion is quite small—about 6 percent in our hands, excluding initial failures (Figure 15–5, solid histogram). We found no system failures or withdrawals due to problems attributable to the catheter (e.g., circulatory impairment, sampling lumen occlusion, and so on) until 28 to 32 hours after insertion (Figure 15-5). Catheter-related problems (principally lumen blockage) then occurred with a probability of about 1 percent per hour, so that by 72 hours about 37 percent of probes had been removed for such reasons (Figure 15–5, hatched histogram). These problems comprised 14 cases of lumen occlusion and 2 cases of circulatory impairment.

The risk of having to remove a catheter for catheter-related problems is, of course, not unique to catheter-electrodes, and catheter removals would have been expected had conventional UACs been used. Rajani et al. [18] found that about 37 percent of conventional UACs with unheparinized infusion fluids in their series had failed by about 42 hours. Strict comparisons between our experience and that of Rajani et al. [18] are difficult to make because of differences in study population parameters, catheters, and so on. Nevertheless, it is clear that, although the sampling lumen of the probe is considerably smaller in diameter (and thus perhaps more liable to occlusion) than the conventional catheters used by Rajani et al. [18], the rate of loss of function due to occlusion is certainly not excessive in comparison with their unheparinized controls.

The overall functional half-life of the oxygen electrode catheter was about 70 hours (Figure 15–5, open histogram). This figure, taken on its own, gives an exaggerated impression of the impact of system failure on clinical mangement. The time of greatest need for continuous PaO_2 measurement was usually in the early phase of acute illness. Probe system failure in the first 24 hours after stabilization was uncommon in our hands (about 6 percent), and, apart from an occasional sensor failure, most of the failures after 24 hours were due to recognized complications of catheterization per se rather than to problems uniquely attributable to oxygen probes. Our view is that even when used with unheparinized infusion fluids, problems with lumen patency in these catheters are broadly similar in frequency and nature to those seen with conventional UACs.

The option of insertion of a substitute catheter was also available if loss of sampling lumen patency occurred. In the case of sensor failure, intermittent PaO_2 analyses rather than replacement of the catheter was also sometimes practical. In our series, loss of system function occurred at a time judged sufficiently serious to necessitate insertion of a substitute probe in five (11 percent) cases.

Complications

The complications that may occur with the oxygen probe are generally similar to those that occur with conventional UACs. These have been well described elsewhere [15,16,21]. Pollitzer et al. [17] examined the frequency of complications in their series of infants with severe respiratory illnesses. The incidence of arterial thrombosis and of other complications of catheterization was similar to that reported for conventional UACs.

Use During Transportation of Neonates

Recent studies have indicated that, with the exception of transportation in fully equipped mobile neonatal intensive care units, it is usual for arterial oxygen tension to move to unacceptably high or low levels, even in experienced hands [22]. We have had some experience with the use of this monitoring system during transportation of sick neonates in an urban environment. The monitoring system, being lightweight, compact, and battery powered, can be used without a chart recorder to follow PaO_2 during transportation. Radio transmissions from the transporting vehicle may cause some interference to the monitor readings, but these are readily recognized and output normalizes rapidly.

Except when highly specialized transporting vehicles are used, it is not usually possible to perform sensor recalibrations during transit. Provided that the sensor is adequately stabilized and calibrated before the commencement of transportation, this does not present a serious problem. However, to be reasonably certain that a sensor is stabilized, about 60 minutes should be allowed after insertion, and check calibrations should be performed before departure. To reduce the possibility of delays in departure implicit in these requirements, it may be helpful to ensure that referring hospitals are in a position to insert oxygen probes, if indicated, before the arrival of the transport team. It may also be possible to commence activation in vitro by immersion of the sensor tip aseptically in sterile warm physiologic saline (solutions not containing electrolytes deactivate the sensor and should not be used for this purpose) before the arrival of the transport team.

It should be noted here that attempts to precalibrate the electrode by immersing it in solutions of known PaO_2 before insertion have been made [20]. These have been reported as moderately successful, but are not recommended. The main difficulties with such attempts are that the probe is dependent on the consumption of oxygen, albeit in tiny amounts, for normal operation. Thus, a reliable output is conditional upon a continuing flow of fluid past the sensor. Without this, the electrical output falls, producing a falsely low signal. Another important factor is that the electrical output of the probe is temperature dependent (about $+3$ percent per degree Celsius), and even a small unrecognized difference in temperature between the calibration solution and the infant would lead to clinically significant discrepancies.

In our experimental work with this device during transportation of sick neonates we allowed an average of only about 14 minutes (range, 7 to 20 minutes) between insertion and calibration. It became clear subsequently that insufficient time had been allowed for stabilization and that this accounted for the indicated PaO_2s being about 2.66 kPa higher than the corresponding measurements by blood gas analyzer on arrival in the receiving unit.

Provided that the pretransportation calibration precautions mentioned earlier are taken, the indications from our experience are that the probe may prove to be of value in controlling oxygen administration during transport. The experimental use of conventional transcutaneous monitoring

205

equipment during transport has also been reported, with encouraging results [23], and it seems probable that the probe will be similarly useful since the need for monitoring in these circumstances is no less than in the neonatal intensive care units.

Comparative Characteristics of Oxygen Catheter-Electrodes and Transcutaneous Oxygen Electrodes

There is no doubt that continuous monitoring of trends in arterial oxygen tension has become an indispensible tool in the management of severe cardiorespiratory disorders in neonates. The consequences of hypoxemia on the central nervous system and on closure of the ductus and of hyperoxygenation on pulmonary and ocular tissues are well recognized. Intermittent arterial sampling, whether by arterial puncture, arterialized capillary sampling, or umbilical artery catheter, can be highly misleading, especially in the absence of information on the rate of change of PaO_2. A continuous indicator of PaO_2 is usually required. Transcutaneous and intravascular electrodes both provide continuity of measurement, although the need for periodic resiting and recalibration of heated transcutaneous electrodes results in some disturbance to the infant and loss of monitoring time in the order of 15 minutes per resiting. This can amount to a significant proportion of monitoring time in the very premature infant, where resiting every two hours may be necessary. The procedure also consumes staff time, and in our experience the oxygen probe system is less demanding in this respect. The transcutaneous method has the undoubted advantage of noninvasiveness, but in some seriously ill infants arterial access through a UAC may be mandatory. The invasive device provides all of the advantages of a conventional UAC, and if one is to be inserted little is lost and much can be gained by inserting an oxygen probe. By this means full arterial blood gas measurements may be obtained whenever required in addition to continuous arterial oxygen tension readouts. Although some transcutaneous systems also provide estimates of PtcCo (transcutaneous carbon dioxide levels) they do not yet provide sufficient accuracy or precision to obviate the need for intermittent direct arterial sampling for calibration checks, pH determinations, and assessment of full acid-base status.

It is useful to bear in mind that invasive and transcutaneous electrodes do not measure the same parameters of oxygenation. Transcutaneous electrodes measure a combination of central circulatory oxygenation and adequacy of tissue perfusion in the skin. The latter is dependent upon blood pressure [7], cardiac output, and the level of circulating catecholamines. Early indications of circulatory failure may be available by comparing PaO_2 and $PtCO_2$ readings. $PtCO_2$ readings will be low in the event of peripheral hypoperfusion.

Although the response time of a transcutaneous electrode in vitro is more rapid in general than that of the probe, the damping effect of skin resistance on oxygen diffusion in vivo lengthens this considerably. Clinically, the probe responds a little more rapidly than macrocathode and microcathode transcutaneous sensors [24], but the difference is not large enough to be of any real importance.

The risks of the intravascular electrode are essentially those of conventional UACs. It appears that where continuous PaO_2 and intermittent $PaCO_2$ and pH measurements are necessary, or that continuous access to the arterial system is required, then the balance of advantages is in favor of the probe, particularly during the early management of infants with severe respiratory disorders [17]. In infants primarily requiring only monitoring of oxygenation once the acute phase of illness is over, or where infants are less seriously ill, transcutaneous monitoring appears preferable.

References

1. Clark, L.C., Jr. Monitor and control of blood and tissue oxygen tensions. *Trans. Am. Soc. Artif. Organs* 2:41–48, 1956.
2. Harris, T.R., Nugent, M. Continuous arterial oxygen tension monitoring in the newborn infant. *J. Pediatr.* 82:929–939, 1973.
3. Clifton, J.S., Parker, D., Tseung, A.C.C. Galvanic cell transducers for the in-vivo measurement of oxygen tension. In Laughlin, J.S. (ed.), *Advances in Medical Physics, Second International Conference on Medical Physics,* Boston, Mass., 1971.
4. Parker, D., Key, A., Davies, R., et al. A disposable catheter-tip transducer for continuous measurement of blood oxygen tension in-vivo. *Biomed. Eng.* 6:313–317, 1971.
5. Parker, D., Soutter, L.P. In-vivo monitoring of blood PO_2 in newborn infants. In Payne, J.P. (ed.), *Current Status of Oxygen Measurements in Biology and Medicine.* London: Butterworth, 1975, pp. 269–283.
6. Soutter, L.P., Conway, M.J., Parker, D. A system for monitoring oxygen tension in sick newborn babies. *Biomed. Eng.* 10:257–260, 1975.
7. Reigel, K.P., Versmold, H.T. Intra-arterial vs. transcutaneous PO_2 monitoring in newborn infants—indications and limitations. *Biotelem. Patient Monit.* 6:32–43, 1979.
8. Wilkinson, A.R., Phibbs, R.H., Gregory, G.A. Improved accuracy of continuous measurement of arterial oxygen tension in sick newborn infants. *Arch. Dis. Child.* 54:307–310, 1979.
9. Finer, N.N., Stewart, A.R. Continuous transcutaneous oxygen monitoring in the critically ill neonate. *Crit. Care Med.* 8:319–323, 1980.
10. Potter, R.G. The multiple decrement life table as an approach to the measurement of use-effectiveness and demographic effectiveness of contraception. In: *Handbook for Service Statistics in Family Planning Programs,* 2nd edn. New York: Population Council, 1968, pp. 124–138.
11. Hahn, C.E.W., Brooks, W.N., Albery, W.J., Rolfe, P. O_2 and N_2O analysis with a single intravascular catheter electrode. *Anaesthesia* 34:263–266, 1979.

12. Severinghaus, J.W., Weiskopf, R.B., Nishimura, N., Bradley, A.F. O₂ electrode errors due to polarographic reduction of halothane. *J. Appl. Physiol.* 31:640–642, 1971.

13. Bates, M.L., Feingold, A., Dold, M.I. The effects of anesthetics on an in-vivo O₂ electrode. *Am. J. Clin. Pathol.* 64:448–451, 1975.

14. Brooks, W.N., Hahn, C.E.W., Foex, P., et al. On-line PO_2 and PN_2O analysis with an in-vivo catheter electrode. *Br. J. Anaesth.* 52:715–721, 1980.

15. Mokrohisky, S.T., Levine, R.L., Blumhagen, J.D., et al. Low positioning of umbilical artery catheters increases associated complications in newborn infants. *N. Engl. J. Med.* 299:561–564, 1978.

16. Wesstrom, G., Finnstrom, O., Stenport, G. Umbilical artery catheterization in newborns. I. Thrombosis in relation to catheter type and position. *Acta Paediatr. Scand.* 68:575–581, 1979.

17. Pollitzer, M.J., Soutter, L.P., Reynolds, E.O.R. Continuous monitoring of arterial oxygen tension in infants: four years of experience with an intravascular oxygen electorde. *Pediatrics* 66:31–36, 1980.

18. Rajani, K., Goetzman, B.W., Wennberg, R.P., et al. Effect of heparinization of fluids infused through an umbilical artery catheter on patency and frequency of complications. *Pediatrics* 63:552–556, 1979.

19. Conway, M., Durbin, G.M., Ingram, D., et al. Continuous monitoring of arterial oxygen tension using a catheter tip polarographic electrode in infants. *Pediatrics* 57:244–250, 1976.

20. Godfrey, S., Costeloe, K. Clinical use of an indwelling umbilical-artery electrode. *Lancet* 1:311–312, 1976.

21. Goetzman, B.W., Stadalnik, R.C., Bogren, H.G., et al. Thrombotic complications of umbilical artery catheters: a clinical and radiographic study. *Pediatrics* 56:374–379, 1975.

22. Miller, C., Clyman, R.I., Roth, R.S., et al. Control of oxygenation during the transport of sick neonates. *Pediatrics* 66:117–119, 1980.

23. Clarke, T.A., Zmora, E., Chen, J.H., et al. Transcutaneous oxygen monitoring during neonatal transport. *Pediatrics* 65:884–886, 1980.

24. Pollitzer, M.J., Whitehead, M.D., Reynolds, E.O.R., Delpy, D. Effect of electrode temperature and in-vivo calibration on accuracy of transcutaneous estimation of arterial oxygen tension in infants. *Pediatrics* 65:515–522, 1980.

16

New Concepts in the Treatment of Acute Respiratory Failure

Carl E. Hunt, M.D.*

Acute respiratory failure requiring ventilatory support is a major cause of morbidity and mortality in neonates with pulmonary dysfunction. The purpose of this Chapter is to summarize the current clinical status of two experimental modalities that may improve outcome: extracorporeal membrane oxygenation and postnatal surfactant replacement therapy. High-frequency ventilation, another experimental modality that may be beneficial in selected patient groups, is discussed in Chapter 18.

Extracorporeal Membrane Oxygenation

The use of extracorporeal membrane oxygenation (ECMO) is not a new treatment for severe respiratory failure. Based on the clinical experience obtained with intraoperative cardiopulmonary bypass, prolonged ECMO became feasible with the development of membranes and nonocclusive roller pumps that were significantly less traumatic to the cellular constituents of whole blood. The availability of a suitable technology led to the

*The author wishes to acknowledge Susan Seidler for her assistance in preparation of this manuscript.

formulation of the following questions 1) Will the use of ECMO reduce pulmonary oxygen toxicity in patients with severe respiratory failure? 2) Will ECMO reduce the effects of barotrauma in patients with severe respiratory failure? 3) In patients with severe respiratory failure, will ECMO improve survival? 4) In patients who might have been able to survive with only conventional ventilatory treatment, will ECMO reduce the associated morbidity?

After some initial promising results in individual patients and in uncontrolled clinical studies, a National Institutes of Health-supported collaborative, prospective control study was conducted in adults and older children (>12 years) with adult respiratory distress syndrome (RDS) [1]. The results of this study were discouraging because only 10 percent of the ECMO group survived, which was identical to the 10 percent survival rate in the control group. Although this was a well-designed study, the criteria for inclusion may have been too stringent to permit a fair assessment of the potential benefits of ECMO. That is, since most of the nonsurvivors in both groups already had pulmonary fibrosis before randomization, one can speculate that the outcome would have been significantly improved if ECMO had been initiated earlier in the clinical course.

More recent studies have suggested that ECMO can indeed improve outcome in adult RDS if applied early in the clinical course [2]. In addition, recent studies have also suggested a role for ECMO in improving outcome in severe neonatal respiratory failure due to RDS, meconium aspiration syndrome (MAS), diaphragmatic hernia, or persistent fetal circulation (PFC).

Bartlett et al. [3] recently reported their experience with ECMO in 45 moribund neonates: 14 with RDS, 22 with MAS, 5 with PFC including diaphragmatic hernia, and 4 with sepsis. Before beginning ECMO, all were receiving 100 percent O_2 and high-pressure ventilator assistance, most had one or more chest tubes, and all were considered to have a low potential for survival. The age at the onset of ECMO ranged from 10 hours to seven days (average, 41 hours). Venoarterial bypass was utilized, with cannulation of the right atrium via the jugular vein and of the aorta via the carotid artery. Heparin was infused continuously to maintain the activated clotting time at 200 to 300 seconds. ECMO flow rates of 100 to 120 ml/kg per minute (80 percent of cardiac output) permitted the lungs to then be placed at rest ($FI0_2$, 0.3; airway pressure, 16/3 cmH_2O; frequency, 10; I:E ratio, 1:1). ECMO was discontinued when lung function recovered or if irreversible organ failure supervened. Overall, 25 patients (55 percent) survived; among the clinical groups, survival was 43 percent with RDS, 68 percent with MAS, 60 percent with PFC, and 25 percent with sepsis. The average ECMO duration in the surviviors was 90 hours. The major complication, and the most common cause of death, was intracranial hemorrhage; 16 neonates (35 percent) had intracranial hemorrhage, and all but one died. The relationship between intracranial hemorrhage and ECMO is unknown, however, since this study was not controlled and the presence of intracranial hemorrhage was not ascertained before beginning ECMO. Of the 25 survivors, 20 (80 percent) were reported to be normal, healthy children with normal growth and development.

Hardesty et al. [4] also utilized ECMO in neonates with severe respiratory failure. After a successful outcome in two of three full-term infants with diaphragmatic hernia, they also successfully treated one preterm infant with severe RDS. As evidence of the efficacy and safety of ECMO, the RDS infant required ECMO for nine days, and treatment resulted in a successful outcome.

. The recent ECMO successes in neonates, albeit anecdotal and uncontrolled, provide a justification for prospective, control studies. Although an ECMO-related increase in survival rate is obviously desirable, the major potential benefit of ECMO may rather be a reduction in morbidity. Indeed, the low incidence of bronchopulmonary dysplasia among the 25 survivors in the series of Bartlett et al. (4 percent) suggests that the lung rest possible with ECMO may significantly lessen the associated lung injury caused by barotrauma or oxygen toxicity. Only a randomized study, however, will determine whether early initiation of ECMO and subsequent lung rest will significantly reduce the frequency and severity of bronchopulmonary dysplasia. Since the resources required for ECMO are considerable, the prospective studies will need to demonstrate a clear superiority for ECMO to justify such a commitment.

Postnatal Surfactant Replacement Therapy

ECMO can only be used as a treatment for fully established respiratory failure. Postnatal surfactant replacement therapy, however, may be of considerably greater clinical importance since, if the therapy is efficacious, severe respiratory failure will not develop. The following paragraphs will review the current status of postnatal surfactant replacement. Although most of the treatment studies have been short-term animal studies, a few preliminary clinical trials have now been completed.

Robertson [5] studied the response to tracheal instillation of natural surfactant in preterm rabbits. After treatment, each animal was ventilated for 10 minutes before sacrifice. Whereas control animals demonstrated bronchiolar necrosis and poor aeration of the terminal air spaces, in the treated animals the terminal air spaces were well expanded and the bronchiolar epithelium was intact. Adams et al. [6] administered natural surfactant by tracheal instillation to preterm lambs and then maintained them with assisted ventilation for two hours. Compared with twin controls, animals with the tracheal instillation of natural surfactant had 100% survival

211

for this two-hour study associated with stable blood gases on room air, compliant lungs with good pressure-volume relationships, well-aerated lungs at autopsy, and histologic evidence of good alveolar expansion with large amounts of free intraluminal phospholipid, normal lung surface tension measurements, no epithelial damage, and no hyaline membranes. In this short-term study, therefore, natural surfactant did protect the lungs from developing many features characteristic of RDS.

Jobe et al. [7] treated preterm lambs with natural surfactant by tracheal instillation, either before the first breath or after the development of significant respiratory failure. In the animals treated at birth, initial ventilation was dramatically improved compared with twin controls, but then progressively deteriorated; by eight hours these lambs were in severe respiratory failure. In the lambs treated after developing respiratory failure, ventilation improved significantly; this improvement, however, only lasted about three hours, and a second treatment was less effective. As summarized in a separate study in 120-day preterm lambs [8], the transient nature of the response to surfactant replacement in RDS may be caused by inhibitors of surfactant function that enter the airways and by immaturity of supporting lung structures.

Only a few clinical trials have been reported. Using an artificial surfactant developed in their own laboratory, Fugiwara et al. [9] treated 10 preterm infants with severe RDS by tracheal instillation. Although there was no control group, the improved ventilation, decrease in radiologic abnormalities, and 80 percent survival rate all suggested that tracheal instillation of this artificial surfactant might prove to be a useful treatment for severe RDS. Morley et al. [10] prepared an artificial surfactant as a dry powder, which was then blown down the endotracheal tube of preterm infants who required delivery room resuscitation and who were therefore at increased risk for severe RDS. The comparison group included comparable preterm infants born when one of the authors was not in the delivery room to administer the surfactant. The treated infants developed less severe RDS and all survived, whereas only 75 percent of the control group survived. Thus far, however, no prospective control study has confirmed the clinical efficacy of any artificial surfactant preparation in significantly improving morbidity and mortality from severe RDS.

The potential efficacy of postnatal surfactant replacement therapy for RDS is thus the subject of active experimental and clinical research. Many problems need to be resolved, however, before postnatal prevention of severe RDS can become a reality [11]. A fundamental problem with any type of exogenous replacement is that there is uncertainty about the physiologically essential components of surfactant in vivo. Although ongoing research efforts may eventually result in an artificial surfactant having the same primary surface properties as the complex natural surfactant, no such artificial mixture has yet been demonstrated in animal studies to be as efficacious as a natural surfactant mixture.

A second fundamental problem relates to whether protein is an essential component of any efficacious surfactant mixture. As the functional importance of protein to the surface tension-lowering properties of surfactant is still uncertain, and because of the potential antigenic risk of the protein component, surfactant preparations should preferably be protein free. Another potential problem with any natural surfactant complex will be to ensure sterility, including the absence of viruses as well as bacteria. This may be difficult to accomplish since heating might cause chemical hydrolysis as well as physical state changes in the lipids. Other important concerns include the following: the potential effect of exogenous surfactant on endogenous surfactant structure, synthesis, and secretion; the optimal delivery route, i.e., tracheal instillation, aerosolization, or a combination; the time course of therapy, i.e., single or multiple doses; and the optimal method for surfactant mixture preparation, i.e., sonication or vortexing.

In summary, the development of the optimal surfactant preparation for successful postnatal administration will require substantive new information regarding the biophysics and biochemistry of pulmonary surfactant. In the meantime, there is a population of infants with severe RDS whose morbidity and mortality risk from RDS is such that prospective well-controlled clinical trials are now justified. Pending further basic in vitro and experimental in vivo studies, it is not known whether an artificial or a natural extracted mixed lipid complex will be preferable, whether multiple doses will produce a more sustained result, and, finally, whether postnatal surfactant treatment will also be efficacious in acquired surfactant deficiency states. Additional clinical studies will thus need to be conducted to determine the potential role of surfactant replacement therapy in preventing or reversing respiratory failure in such diverse conditions as adult RDS, meconium aspiration, and diaphragmatic hernia.

References

1. National Heart Lung and Blood Institute and National Institutes of Health. *Extracorporeal Support for Respiratory Insufficiency.* Washington, D.C.: Department of Health, Education, and Welfare, 1980.
2. Gattinoni, L., Pesenti, A., Rossi, G.P., et al. Treatment of acute respiratory failure with low-frequency positive-pressure ventilation and extracorporeal removal of CO_2. *Lancet* 9:292–294, 1980.
3. Bartlett, R.N., Andrews, A.F., Toomasian, J.M., et al. Extracorporeal membrane oxygenation for newborn respiratory failure: forty-five cases. *Surgery* 92:425–433, 1982.
4. Hardesty, R.L., Griffith, B.R., Debski, R.F., et al. Extracorporeal membrane oxygenation: successful treatment of persistent fetal circulation following repair of congenital diaphragmatic hernia. 81:556–563, 1981.
5. Robertson, B. Treatment of the premature rabbit neonate with supplementary surfactant. *Prog. Respir. Res.* 15:269–278, 1981.

6. Adams, F.H., Towers, B., Osher, A.B., et al. Effects of tracheal instillation of natural surfactant in premature lambs. I. Clinical and autopsy findings. *Pediatr. Res.* 12:841–848, 1978.

7. Jobe, A., Ikegami, M., Glatz, T., et al. Duration and characteristic of treatment of premature lambs with natural surfactant. *J. Clin. Invest.* 67:370–375, 1981.

8. Jacobs, H., Jobe, A., Ikegami, M., et al. Premature lambs rescued from respiratory failure with natural surfactant: clinical and biophysical correlates. *Pediatr. Res.* 16:424–429, 1982.

9. Fugiwara, T., Chida, S., Watabe, Y., et al. Artificial surfactant therapy in hyaline-membrane disease. *Lancet* 55–59, 1980.

10. Morley, C.J., Miller, M., Bangham, A.D., Davis, J.A. Dry artificial lung surfactant and its effect on very premature babies. *Lancet* 64–68, 1981.

11. Notter, R.H., Shapiro, D.L. Lung surfactant in an era of replacement therapy. *Pediatrics* 68:781–789, 1981.

17

Respiratory Distress in the Infant of the Diabetic Mother

Philip G. Rhodes, M.D., and Daksha M. Patel, M.D.

It is now well appreciated that the infant of the diabetic mother (IDM) comes from a very abnormal intrauterine environment. Very early in gestation, congenital anomalies are commonly produced due to incompletely known factors [1,2]. The developing fetus is in an environment of high glucose and responds with high insulin production by the pancreatic beta cells [3]. Lipid metabolism is affected in a number of ways [4]. Liver functioning appears to be affected, and hemostasis is abnormal, with increased clotting ability most likely due to altered platelet function [5,6]. A distinct cardiac hypertrophy develops, resulting in cardiac failure that with time can resolve [7,8].

Once delivery has occurred the most usual life-threatening condition encountered by the IDM is that of respiratory distress related to pulmonary immaturity. The often-quoted article by Robert et al. examined retrospectively the incidence of hyaline membrane disease in IDMs compared with infants of other pregnancies [9]. It seems fairly well established that there is a marked increase in hyaline membrane disease in the IDM for any given gestational age. This is true even after controlling for the method of delivery and other variables that could influence the incidence of this disease. Considerable work has been done to establish the reason(s) for this increased incidence of respiratory disease. Much conflicting data has

215

been accumulated in various animal models with in vivo and in vitro studies. An attempt will be made in this discussion to present a reasonable summary of these data as well as our own work in this area in research for the cause of the increased pulmonary immaturity in the IDM. A complete review is not appropriate for this Chapter, and the reader is referred to other sources for more information [10,11].

Many different preparations of various animal models have been used for experimental studies of the IDM, including the rat, rabbit, and monkey. Because of the complexity of the in utero environment, there is a need for the many studies to determine the role of the various in utero abnormalities. One method of study has been to make the maternal animal model diabetic either before or during pregnancy through chemical destruction of the maternal beta cells. The results in rats have been somewhat confusing, with some fetal rats showing beta cell hypertrophy and others actually showing a decrease in beta cell number [12,13]. One explanation offered for the latter finding is that of insufficient time for beta cell hypertrophy [14]. There is also the same confusion regarding the rabbit model, and because of these differences it can be difficult to establish the final results of infant lung development in this model. There are, however, studies of hyperglycemia and enzyme activity and their effects on the development of the lung. In one rat model study the high-glucose milieu of the fetus seemed to prevent glycogen breakdown and the possible utilization of glucose for appropriate phosphatidyl choline production [15]. Therefore, hyperglycemia per se may play a role in decreased lung maturity in the IDM.

Much of the experimental data has been accumulated by looking at the effects of insulin or at least the effects of a high-insulin environment on pulmonary biochemical maturity. Again, the results are somewhat confusing, but certainly fascinating, at this point in time. The rabbit model has been used to determine some of the findings. We have used the rabbit model to determine the effects of insulin per se on pulmonary biochemical maturity [16]. Insulin was injected into fetal rabbits just before the time of lung biochemical maturity, with saline injected fetuses serving as controls. Figure 17–1 illustrates the results. Disaturated phosphatidyl choline was significantly increased in the lungs of insulin-injected fetal rabbits. This in vivo study supports the results of others showing that insulin itself seems to be a positive hormonal factor in pulmonary biochemical development [17]. There have been conflicting results when lung slices were used in vitro. Others have reported a decreased lecithin production in the presence of insulin [18]. Our data further show (Figure 17–2) that cortisol appears to have an additive effect with insulin in helping pulmonary biochemical maturation. However, actual lung function was not determined. In some interesting experiments on monkeys by Epstein et al., the fetuses

Figure 17–1

Effects of fetal insulin injection on lung surfactant. *(Data from Patel, D.M., Rhodes, P.G. Effects of insulin and hydrocortisone on lung tissue phosphatidyl choline in fetal rabbits in vivo. Diabetologia, 27:478–481, 1984.)*

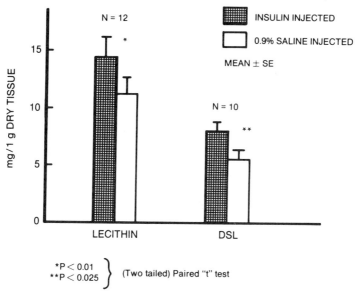

of streptozotocin-treated mothers appeared to have an increase in choline incorporation into lecithin in lung slices [17]. However, the fetal lung lecithin concentration was no different from that of controls. The investigators felt that this difference was most likely due to polyhydramnios with increased pulmonary lung fluid turnover and the inability to keep lecithin concentrations normal in spite of an increased production.

It is apparent then that, depending on experimental conditions, insulin may either induce lecithin production or inhibit it. The use of lung tissue from different animals has led to the same type of results. There is some information that insulin may inhibit enzymes in lecithin production or reduce the availability of glucose as a substitute for lecithin production. However, other studies show just the opposite results with insulin injections in vivo or with choline incorporation methodology in lung slices of monkeys.

In spite of all this varied information, it is important for the clinician to understand that strict control of the maternal diabetic state results in good outcome for the fetus and the newborn [19]. Good control before pregnancy may be important in decreasing the incidence of congenital malformations. Good control just after the onset of pregnancy will result in normal-sized infants with fewer metabolic disturbances. An increased

Figure 17–2

Combined effects of insulin and hydrocortisone on lung surfactant compared with insulin alone. *(Data from Patel, D.M., Rhodes, P.G. Effects of insulin and hydrocortisone on lung tissue phosphatidyl choline in fetal rabbits in vivo.* Diabetologia, 27:478–481, 1984.)

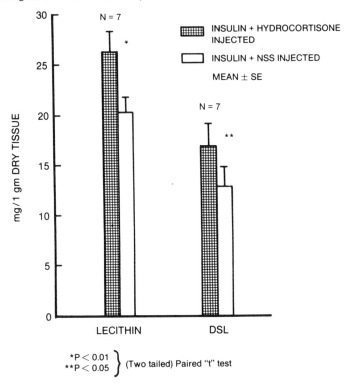

insulin production as a result of hyperglycemia from the mother could even result in hypoxia in utero [20].

If good control has not been achieved during pregnancy, then careful monitoring before and during labor is essential to decrease the incidence of asphyxia and to ensure the best possible start. Skilled resuscitation should be available upon delivery, and careful monitoring of metabolic functions should be started soon after birth. These infants often will have the combination of right-to-left shunting with an enlarged heart as a result of a myocardiopathy and then have hypocalcemia [21], hypoglycemia, and hyaline membrane disease combined. They may have renal vein thromboses and congenital anomalies that further complicate the management. Every effort should be made to ensure management at a tertiary care facility for these infants with complex problems.

References

1. Eriksson, U., Dahlstrom, E., Larsson, K.S., Hellerstrom, C. Increased incidence of congenital malformations in the offspring of diabetic rats and their prevention by maternal insulin therapy. *Diabetes* 30:1–6, 1982.
2. Mills, J.L. Malformations in infants of diabetic mothers. *Teratology* 25:385–394, 1982.
3. Persson, B., Heding, L.G., Lunell, N.O., et al. Fluid beta cell function in diabetic pregnancy. *Am. J. Obstet. Gynecol.* 144:455–459, 1982.
4. Andersen, G.E., Hertel, J., Kuhl, C., Molsted-Pedersen, L. Metabolic events in infants of diabetic mothers during first 24 hours after birth. *Acta Paediatr. Scand.* 71:27–32, 1982.
5. Ida, T., Sato, M., Yamaoka, Y., et al. Effect of insulin on mitochondrial oxidative phosphorylation and energy charge of the perfused guinea pig liver. *J. Lab. Clin. Med.* 87:925–933, 1976.
6. Stuart, M.J., Elrad, H., Graeber, J.E., et al. Increased synthesis of prostaglandin endoperoxides and platelet hyperfunction in infants of mothers with diabetes mellitus. *J. Lab. Clin. Med.* 94:12–17, 1979.
7. Gutgesell, H.P., Speer, M.E., Rosenberg, H.S. Characterization of the cardiomyopathy in infants of diabetic mothers. *Circulation* 61:441–450, 1980.
8. Wolfe, R.R., Way, G.L. Cardiomyopathies in infants of diabetic mothers. *Johns Hopkins Med. J.* 140:177–180, 1977.
9. Robert, M.F., Neff, R.K., Hubbell, J.P., et al. Association between maternal diabetes and the respiratory-distress syndrome in the newborn. *N. Engl. J. Med.* 294:357–360, 1976.
10. Frantz, I.D., Epstein, M.F. Fetal lung development in pregnancies complicated by diabetes. *Semin. Perinatol.* 2:347–352, 1978.
11. Pedersen, J. *The Pregnant Diabetic and Her Newborn,* 2nd ed. Baltimore, Md.: The Williams & Wilkins Co., 1977.
12. Cuezva, J.M., Burkett, E.S., Kerr, D.S., et al. The newborn of diabetic rat. I. Hormonal and metabolic changes in the postnatal period. *Pediatr. Res.* 16:632–637, 1982.
13. Swenne, I., Eriksson, U. Diabetes in pregnancy: islet cell proliferation in the fetal rat pancreas. *Diabetologia* 23:525–528, 1982.
14. Eriksson, U., Swenne, I. Diabetes in pregnancy: growth of the fetal pancreatic B cells in the rat. *Biol. Neonate* 42:239–248, 1982.
15. Gewolb, I.H. Barrett C., Wilson, C.M., Warshaw, J.B. Delay in pulmonary glycogen degradation in fetuses of streptozotocin diabetic rats. *Pediatr. Res.* 16:869–873, 1982.
16. Patel, D.M., Rhodes, P.G. Effect of insulin on pulmonary lecithin (L) and disaturated lecithin (DSL) in fetal rabbits (abstract). *Pediatr. Res.* 17:140A, 1983.
17. Epstein, M.F., Farrell, P.M., Chez, R.A. Fetal lung lecithin metabolism in the glucose intolerant rhesus monkey pregnancy. *Pediatrics* 57:722–728, 1976.
18. Neufeld, N.D., Sevanian, A., Barrett, C.T., Kaplan, S.A. Inhibition of surfactant production by insulin in fetal rabbit lung slices. *Pediatr. Res.* 13:752–754, 1979.

19. Miller, E., Hare, J.W., Cloherty, J.P., et al. Elevated maternal hemoglobin A_{1c} in early pregnancy and major congenital anomalies in infants of diabetic mothers. *N. Engl. J. Med.* 304:1331–1334, 1981.

20. Carson, B.S., Philipps, A.F., Simmons, M.A., et al. Effects of a sustained insulin infusion upon glucose uptake and oxygenation of the ovine fetus. *Pediatr. Res.* 14:147–152, 1980.

21. Cruikshank, D.P., Pitkin, R.M., Varner, M.W., et al. Calcium metabolism in diabetic mother, fetus, and newborn infant. *Am. J. Obstet. Gynecol.* 145:1010–1016, 1983.

18

Neonatal High-Frequency Ventilation: A Review

Stephen J. Boros, M.D.

High-frequency ventilation (HFV) is a relatively new method of mechanical ventilation that uses small tidal volumes, often less than the anatomical dead space, and extremely rapid rates (60 to 2400 breaths per minute [bpm]). This form of ventilation violates traditional concepts of how and why mechanical ventilators work. Tidal volumes less than the anatomical dead space, regardless of how fast they are delivered, should produce no alveolar ventilation and, hence, no gas exchange. The fact that gas exchange does indeed occur has captivated the present generation of pulmonary researchers.

The mechanisms by which high-frequency ventilators produce gas exchange are not clear. Some ventilators, because of their minimal compressible volumes, high flow rates, and direct deliveries may simply be more efficient systems for the rapid bulk delivery of small tidal volumes. By creating turbulence throughout the airways, HFV may enhance gas mixing and, hence, the distribution and diffusion of respiratory gases. Gas mixing, at any flow rate, is always greater during turbulent flow than during laminar flow. Rossing et al suggest that during HFV, gas mixing occurs through the entire tracheobronchial tree, creating a continuous CO_2 gradient from alveolus to atomosphere [1]. With this concept, there is no "dead space." Whatever the exact gas transport and exchange mechanisms, traditional theories no longer seem to apply.

There are several different methods of delivering HFV. At present, the nomenclature describing these techniques is inconsistent and, at times, confusing. The following is an attempt to define and simplify terms.

HFV: Delivery Methods

High-Frequency Positive-Pressure Ventilation (HFPPV) is HFV produced by a conventional ventilator. Contemporary infant ventilators can now cycle at rates up to 150 bpm. Most, however, operate effectively only up to rates of about 90 bpm. At rates above 90 bpm, relatively large compressible volumes and restricted flow rates severely limit the tidal volumes that these machines deliver. We recently tested five contemporary infant ventilators. All, save one, were capable of cycling at rates up to 150 bpm. Tidal volume and minute volume were measured as the rates were increased. In all, there was a maximum rate beyond which ventilator performance deteriorated and minute volume decreased. The maximum effective rates for the ventilators studied ranged from 75 to 100 bpm (Figure 18–1) [2]. A related clinical study by Brady et al compared the efficacy of various ventilator rates in infants with respiratory distress syndrome. At the more rapid rates, arterial oxygen tension, venous admixture, and the physiological dead space to tidal volume ratio worsened [3]. The optimum range of HFPPV appears to be 60 to 90 bpm.

High-Frequency Jet Ventilation (HFJV) delivers gas directly into the airways in short, high-flow, high-pressure bursts through a cannula or jet injector positioned within the airway. Jet ventilators have negligible compressible volumes and operate effectively at rates up to 400 bpm [4]. Tidal volumes are difficult to measure, but are assumed to be equal to or slightly greater than anatomical dead space. In addition to the tidal volumes delivered through the injector, gases from the surrounding atmosphere are entrained into the airway with each jet burst. The accelerated flow through the jet injector produces an area of negative pressure adjacent to the injector, entraining ambient gases and enhancing tidal volume. Jet ventilators do not have exhalation valves. Exhalation is always passive. Smith and others ventilated animals with HFJV at frequencies up to 600 bpm. At rates above 400 bpm, gas exchange was adequate; however, systemic vascular resistances increased, and heart rates and cardiac outputs decreased [5]. The optimum frequency range for HFJV appears to be 150 to 250 bpm.

Present HFJV injector, humidity, and airway pressure monitoring systems are crude. A recently developed triple-lumen endotracheal tube

Figure 18–1

Babybird I (BB 1), Babybird II (BB 2), Bourns BP200 (BP), Sechrist (SC), and Healthdyne (HD), were all maintained at constant peak inspiratory pressures of 25 cm H_2O, I:E ratios of 1:2, PEEP of 5 cm H_2O, and inspiratory flow rates of 10 liters per minute. Ventilatory rates were progressively increased from 25 to 150 bpm while minute volumes were measured. This figure graphs the minute volume each ventilator delivered at each given rate. (BB 1 could not maintain constant peak inspiratory pressures above 75 bpm at a flow rate of 10 liters per minute. Here, inspiratory flow was increased to 20 liters per minute.) *(From Boros, S.J., Bing, D.R., Mammel, M.C., et al. Using conventional infant ventilators at unconventional rates. Pediatrics 74:4, 487–494, 1984. Copyright American Academy of Pediatrics 1984.)*

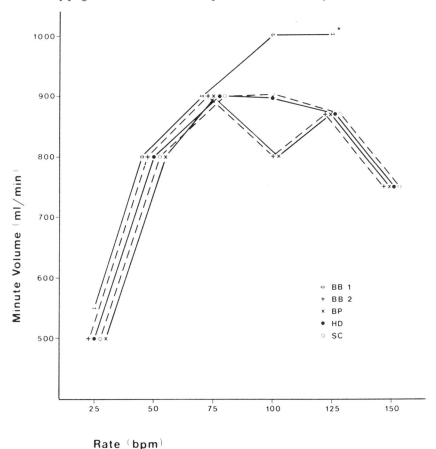

incorporates all these functions into one tube [6]. At present, clinical evaluations of this device are incomplete.

High-Frequency Oscillatory Ventilation (HFOV) is accomplished by using ventilators that are essentially airway vibrators. These devices vibrate a column of gas by moving a constant volume into and out of the airway. There is no bulk gas delivery [7]. Oscillations can be produced by electric piston pumps, rotating ball valves, or vibrating loudspeakers. Oxygen and humidity usually enter the system via a small tube attached at right angles to the delivery circuit. The tubing down stream from the patient is designed to have a greater impedance than the patient's airway, so oscillations are directed toward the patient. Frequency, amplitude of oscillations, distending pressure, and impedance of the down stream circuit can all be varied. HFOV appears to function best at rates greater than 900 bpm [4,7].

High-frequency ventilators, regardless of their design, have been shown to produce adequate gas exchange in a variety of species, including humans. Whether there is any advantage to this unorthodox form of mechanical ventilation remains to be seen.

HFV: Uses in Pathologic Conditions

HYALINE MEMBRANE DISEASE

Several studies of surfactant-deficient animals and a few recent clinical studies of surfactant-deficient neonates suggest that HFV may have a future in the treatment of hyaline membrane disease. Truog et al. compared HFOV and conventional mechanical ventilation in surfactant-deficient monkeys. Although there was little difference in oxygenation, both proximal airway pressures and arterial carbon dioxide tensions decreased significantly during HFOV [8].

Kolton et al. compared HFOV and conventional mechanical ventilation in surfactant-deficient rabbits [9]. At mean airway pressures greater than critical opening pressures, HFOV produced larger lung volumes and better oxygenation. These authors argue that the advantage of HFV lies in the dynamics of expiration. During HFOV, there are smaller proximal airway pressure swings and, hence, a more constant distending pressure. This constancy of pressure maintains larger lung volumes during expiration in a manner similar to positive end expiratory pressure. Because of the larger pressure swings during conventional mechanical ventilation, lung volumes recruited during inspiration cannot be maintained during expiration. Larger end tidal volumes may well account for the observed superiority of HFOV.

Kuehl et al. ventilated surfactant-deficient baboons with both conventional mechanical ventilation and HFOV. During HFOV, oxygenation improved, whereas arterial carbon dioxide tensions and mean airway pressures decreased. Despite the initial succes, all attempts at prolonged HFOV failed. All animals receiving HFOV for more than 4 to 6 hours developed diffuse atelectasis and eventually died [10]. A second experiment added a sigh to counteract atelectasis. Although the sighed animals were more stable, all developed significant pulmonary air leaks. No such air leaks occurred in a control group ventilated with conventional mechanical ventilation [11].

Marchak et al. were the first to successfully use HFOV in surfactant-deficient neonates. Eight infants with hyaline membrane disease were ventilated for periods ranging from 1 to 4 hours. In all, oxygenation was maintained, and arterial carbon dioxide tension decreased. There were no ill effects [12].

Frantz and co-workers compared HFOV and conventional mechanical ventilation in 10 infants with hyaline membrane disease. Each received HFOV at mean airway pressures comparable to CMV for approximately one hour. Gas exchange was adequate and, even though mean airway pressures were equivalent, there were smaller proximal airway pressure swings with HFOV [13, 14]. Again, there were no ill effects. To date, there have been no studies of prolonged HFV in neonates with hyaline membrane disease. Clearly, more clinical information is needed before this technique can be recommended as a reasonable alternative to CMV.

MECONIUM ASPIRATION SYNDROME

Mammel and co-workers alternated conventional mechanical ventilation and HFJV in a group of cats after each had aspirated 2 ml of human meconium per kg. At equivalent mean airway pressures, arterial oxygen tensions, alveolar-arterial oxygen differences, pulmonary artery pressures, and pulmonary vascular resistances all worsened during HFJV (Figure 18–2) [15]. A similar study by Karlson and DuRant comparing conventional mechanical ventilation and HFPPV had similar findings [16]. As of this writing, there appears to be no advantage to, or indication for, HFV in meconium aspiration syndrome.

DIFFUSE LUNG DISEASE–PULMONARY EDEMA

Intravenous oleic acid produces pulmonary capillary leaks and a progressive hemorrhagic pulmonary edema. It is often used to produce diffuse pneumonitis, pulmonary edema, or both, in laboratory animals. HFJV and HFOV have both been tested in this lung model.

225

Figure 18–2

Ten cats each aspirated 2 ml of 25 percent human meconium in saline per kg. Each cat was alternately ventilated with conventional mechanical ventilation and HFJV at equivalent mean airway pressures. This figure outlines the mean values for all animals ±1 standard error of the mean before and 15 minutes after each ventilator change. *(Modified from Mammel, M.C., Gordon, M.J., Connett, J.E., Boros, S.J. Comparison of high-frequency jet ventilation and conventional mechanical ventilation in a meconium aspiration model. J. Pediatr. 103:630–634, 1983.)*

EFFECT OF VENTILATOR CHANGE

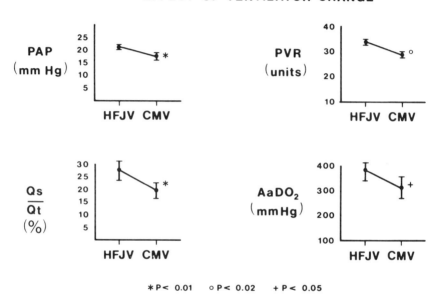

*P< 0.01   oP< 0.02   +P< 0.05

Stoddard et al. studied HFOV and conventional mechanical ventilation in dogs with oleic acid lung injuries. Although gas exchange was similar, higher mean airway pressures were required with HFOV. During HFOV, cardiac outputs were lower, whereas pulmonary artery pressures and pulmonary vascular resistances were significantly higher [17]. The exact opposite was observed by Carlon et al. during a similar HFJV study. Again, both ventilators produced adequate gas exchange. In this study, higher airway pressures were seen with conventional mechanical ventilation. Under these conditions, conventional mechanical ventilation produced significantly more hemodynamic impairment [18].

Kolton and co-workers compared HFOV and conventional mechanical ventilation in rabbits with oleic acid lung disease [9]. Oxygenation was better during HFOV, but only if it was preceded by a sustained lung inflation. During HFOV, sustained inflations produced immediate increases in arterial oxygen tensions and mean lung volumes. This did not occur during conventional mechanical ventilation. Kolton et al. believe these intermittent lung inflations better exploit the pressure-volume hysteresis of unstable lung units, resulting in larger mean lung volumes and better oxygenation. Again, the advantage of HFOV appears to lie in expiration. With conventional mechanical ventilation during much of the respiratory cycle the lung operates at volumes less than ideal for gas exchange. With HFOV, a more constant pressure distends the lung throughout the respiratory cycle, maintaining larger end tidal volumes.

The efficacy of HFOV and HFJV in diffuse lung disorders, such as pneumonia and pulmonary edema, is controversial. The results of recent studies are preliminary and, at times, contradictory. At present, the use of HFOV and HFJV in these conditions should be confined to laboratory animals or carefully controlled clinical studies.

PULMONARY AIR LEAKS

HFV has been uniquely successful in the treatment of experimental pulmonary air leaks in animals and seemingly intractable pulmonary air leaks in human patients.

Hoff et al. ventilated dogs with large bronchopleural fistulas with both HFOV and conventional mechanical ventilation. HFOV provided adequate gas exchange whereas conventional mechanical ventilation consistently resulted in life-threatening hypercarbia and acidosis [19]. Kuwik et al. also demonstrated that in large experimental bronchopleural fistulas, HFOV is an effective, indeed superior, form of mechanical ventilation [20].

Carlon at al. used HFJV in 16 adults with intractable pulmonary air leaks. Clinical and x-ray evidence of pulmonary air leaks improved in all, and eight patients ultimately survived. Three patients in this series developed unusual upper airway obstructions that were ultimately attributed to inadequate jet stream humidification [21].

Frantz and co-workers were the first to treat neonatal pulmonary air leaks with HFV. Five neonates with severe pulmonar interstitial emphysema were treated with HFOV. All promptly improved and, in all, pulmonary interstitial emphysema eventually resolved. Three patients ultimately survived [14].

Pokora et al. used HFJV in nine neonates with life-threatening bronchopleural fistulas or pulmonary interstitial emphysema. After HFJV, seven showed significant clinical and radiographic improvement (Figure 18–3). Five patients ultimately survived. Three infants in this series also developed bizarre tracheal obstructions [22]. These authors, like Carlon et al., attributed the airway obstructions to inadequate jet stream humidification [21,22].

Figure 18–3

Chest x-rays of a 1,300-g, 28-week infant before (A) and four hours after (B) HFJV. Pulmonary interstitial emphysema and gas trapped within the pulmonary ligament (arrow) decreased after HFJV. *(From Pokora, T., Bing, D., Mammel, M., Boros, S. Neonatal high-frequency jet ventilation.* Pediatrics *72:27–32, 1983. Copyright American Academy of Pediatrics 1983.)*

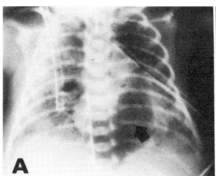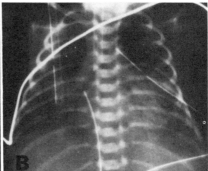

Why do pulmonary air leaks improve with HFV? In most situations, air leaks improve after HFV even though proximal airway pressures are little different than those delivered by conventional ventilators [22]. Some suggest, that during HFV, pressures rapidly equilibrate in the upper airway and deliver tidal volumes to the lower airways at a relatively constant distending pressure. This more constant pressure decreases the pressure differential between airway and intrapleural space and, in doing so, decreases the volume losses that commonly occur at peak inspiration during conventional mechanical ventilation [21]. A more constant distending pressure also eliminates the intermittent stretching of the lower airways, increasing the opportunity for self-repair. Whatever the exact mechanisms of action, HFV appears to be useful in the experimental and clinical treatment of major pulmonary air leaks. It was recently called the treatment of choice for major airway disruptions in adults [23].

HFV Complications

All treatments have risks as well as benefits. Any therapy said to be risk free has not been adequately studied. HFV is relatively new. In most situations, it was studied under very controlled circumstances and only for short periods of time. To date, there have been relatively few complications. However, preliminary HFV studies raised a number of clinically relevant questions that need answers.

Will HFV increase the risk of barotrauma? If HFV increases end tidal lung volumes at lower proximal airway pressures, it follows that it can also produce alveolar overdistention at lower proximal airway pressures. The maintenance of larger end tidal lung volumes requires higher alveolar pressures during expiration. Under such conditions, mean alveolar pressures will likely exceed mean proximal airway pressures [24]. Although such inadvertent or silent distending pressures are known to exist, there is presently no way to measure them directly. Until the question of whether inadvertent distending pressures develop during HFV is answered, patients receiving HFV probably should have their intrapleural or intraesophageal pressures continuously monitored.

Do high-frequency oscillations interfere with respiratory mucus production or mucociliary transport? In a recent study, Armengol et al. observed that the tracheal transport rates of radiolabeled particles were more retarded during HFOV than during conventional mechanical ventilation [25]. Nordin et al. noted that during HFJV tracheal transport rates were very different with different humidification systems. Unhumidified gases caused all mucociliary transport to cease within minutes. Excessive humidity also depressed mucolciliary transport and, over time, also caused it to cease [26]. HFV humidification is an important issue. It has not yet received the attention it deserves.

Several reports have linked tracheal injuries, tracheal obstructions, and necrotizing tracheitis to HFV. Carlon et al. and Pokora et al. both observed clinically significant tracheal obstructions and necrotizing tracheitis in patients treated with HFJV [21,22]. This damage was originally thought to be the result of inadequate humidification. Ophoven and co-workers tested this hypothesis in laboratory animals [27]. They compared the tracheobronchial histopathology seen following HFJV, using different humidity systems, to that seen following conventional mechanical ventilation. Humidity clearly influenced the pathology observed. However, regardless of the humidity system employed, HFJV always produced more tracheal damage. It appeared as though these tracheal injuries were iatrogenic complications unique to HFJV. Speculation was that these injuries were most likely the consequences of tissue trauma from the impact of high-speed, high-pressure jet streams. A series of recent clinical reports cast doubt on that assumption. These reports describe similar tracheal injuries in patients treated with HFPPV, HFOV, and rapid-rate manual ventilation [28,29]. Mammel et al. recently examined the tracheobronchial histopathology seen in animals following HFJV, HFPPV, and conventional mechanical ventilation [30]. In this study, both HFJV and HFPPV produced more tracheal damage than conventional mechanical ventilation. The histologic injuries produced by the two different forms of HFV were nearly identical.

HFV is an intriguing, potentially promising area of critical care medicine. Most investigations into this relatively new therapy are preliminary.

To date, most of these studies have posed interesting questions. They have yet to supply satisfying answers. Until the very basic issues of efficacy and safety are more clearly defined, this exciting form of experimental ventilatory therapy remains just that—an exciting new form of experimental therapy.

References

1. Rossing, T., Slutsky, A., Lehr, J., et al. Tidal volume and frequency dependence of carbon dioxide elimination by high frequency ventilation. *N. Engl. J. Med.* 23:1375–1378, 1981.

2. Boros, S.J., Bing, D.R., Mammel, M.C., et al. Using conventional infant ventilators at unconventional rates. *Pediatrics* 74:4, 487–492, 1984.

3. Brady, J., Deming, D., McCann, E. Is rapid ventilation better? (abstr.) *Clin. Res.* 31:133A, 1983.

4. Smith, R. Ventilation at high respiratory frequencies. *Anaesthesia* 37:1011–1018, 1982.

5. Smith, R., Klain, M., Babinski, M. Limits of high frequency percutaneous transtracheal jet ventilation using a fluid logic controlled ventilator. *Can. Anaesth. Soc. J.* 27:351–356, 1980.

6. Klain, M., Keszler, H., Kalla, R. New endotracheal tube for high frequency ventilation. (abstr.) *Crit. Care Med.* 9:191, 1981.

7. Gallagher, T., Klain, M., Carlon, G. Present status of high frequency ventilation. *Crit. Care Med.* 10:613–617, 1982.

8. Truog, W., Wright, K., Murphy, J., et al. Efficacy of high frequency oscillation in the treatment of experimental hyaline membane disease. (abstr.) *Am. Rev. Respir. Dis.* 125:195, 1982.

9. Kolton, M., Cattran, C., Kent, G., et al. Oxygenation during high frequency ventilation compared with conventional mechanical ventilation in two models of lung injury. *Anesth. Analg.* 61:323–332, 1982.

10. Kuehl, T., Meredith, K., Ackerman, N., et al. High vs. low frequency ventilation in the premature baboon with RDS. (abstr.) (Pediatr. Res. 16:295A, 1982.

11. Kuehl, T., Coalson, J., Ackerman, N., et al. Baroinjury associated with high frequency ventilation of baboon neonates with hyaline membrane disease. (abstr.) *Clin. Res.* 30:910A, 1982.

12. Marchak, B., Thompson, W., Duffy, P., et al. Treatment of RDS by high frequency oscillatory ventilation: a preliminary report. *J. Pediatr.* 99:287–292, 1981.

13. Frantz, I., Stark, A., Dorkin, H. Ventilation of infants at frequencies up to 1800 per minute. (abstr.) *Pediatr. Res.* 14:642, 1980.

14. Frantz, I., Stark, A., Werthammer, J. Improvement in pulmonary interstitial emphysema with high frequency ventilation. (abstr.) *Pediatr. Res.* 15;719, 1981.

15. Mammel, M.C., Gordon, M.J., Connett, J.E., Boros, S.J. Comparison of high frequency jet ventilation and conventional mechanical ventilation in a meconium aspiration model. *J. Pediatr.* 103:630–634, 1983.

16. Karlson, K.H., DuRant, R.H. A comparison of conventional ventilation and high-frequency positive pressure ventilation in experimental meconium aspiration syndrome. (abstr.) *Clin. Res.* 31:910A, 1983.
17. Stoddard, R., Minnick, L., Ackerman, N., et al. A comparison between high frequency and conventional mechanical ventilation in dogs with oleic acid lung injury. (abstr.) *Pediatr. Res.* 16:362A, 1982.
18. Carlon, G., Ray, C., Kvetan, V., Groeger, J. High frequency jet ventilation in oleic acid injured lungs. (abstr.) *Crit. Care Med.* 9:161, 1981.
19. Hoff, B., Smith, R., Wilson, E., et al. High frequency ventilation during bronchopleural fistula. (abstr.) *Anesthesiology* 55:A366, 1981.
20. Kuwik, R., Glass, D., Coombs, D. Evaluation of high frequency postive pressure ventilation for experimental bronchopleural fistula. (abstr.) *Crit. Care Med.* 9:164, 1981.
21. Carlon, G., Kahn, R., Howland, W., et al. Clinical experience with high frequency jet ventilation. *Crit. Care Med.* 9:1–6, 1981.
22. Pokora, T., Bing, D., Mammel, M., Boros, S. Neonatal high frequency jet ventilation. *Pediatrics* 72:27–32, 1983.
23. Carlon, G., Cole, R., Pierri, M., et al. High frequency jet ventilation: theoretical considerations and clinical observations. *Chest* 81:350–354, 1982.
24. Ackerman, N., Null, D., de Lemos, R. Airway pressures during high frequency ventilation. (abstr.) *Pediatr. Res.* 16:344A, 1982.
25. Armengol, J., Man, P., Logus, J., et al. Effects of high frequency oscillatory ventilation on canine tracheal mucous transport. (abstr.) *Crit. Care Med.* 9:192, 1981.
26. Nordin, U., Keszler, H., Klain, M. How does high frequency ventilation effect mucociliary transport? (abstr.) *Crit. Care Med.* 9:160, 1981.
27. Ophoven, J., Mammel, M., Gordon, M., Boros, S. Tracheobronchial histopathology associated with high-frequency jet ventilation. *Crit. Care Med.* 12:829–832, 1984.
28. Fox, W.w., Spitzer, A.R., Smith, V., et al. Tracheal secretion impaction during hyperventilation for persistent pulmonary hypertension of the neonate. (abstr.) *Pediatr. Res.* 18:323A, 1984.
29. Tolkin, J., Kirpalani, H., Fitzhardinge, P., et al. Necrotizing tracheobronchitis: a new complication of neonatal mechanical ventilation. (abstr.) *Pediatr. Res.* 18:391A, 1984.
30. Mammel, M.C., Ophoven, J.P., Gordon, M.J., et al. High-frequency ventilation produces inflammatory injuries in the proximal trachea. (abstr.) *Clin. Res.* 32:815A, 1984.

19

Extracorporeal Membrane Oxygenation for Newborn Respiratory Failure

Michael D. Klein, M.D., Alice French Andrews, M.D., and Robert H. Bartlett,*M.D.

Extracorporeal membrane oxygenation (ECMO) is cardiopulmonary bypass for prolonged periods of time in an intensive care unit setting. It is very much like using the heart-lung machine for open heart surgery in the operating room. The membrane in membrane oxygenation makes this possible since it is gentle enough on the blood to allow prolonged extracorporeal circulation (ECC). The standard oxygenator used in the operating room is a bubble oxygenator, which is quite efficient but is much harder on the blood. ECMO is a supportive and not a therapeutic measure; it implies a reversible underlying disease. ECMO can do two things: support the vital functions of children who will recover, and prevent further damage to the lung caused by high inspired oxygen concentrations and positive pressure ventilation.

*We acknowledge the many contributions, both direct and indirect, to this work of our collaborators in neonatology: Dietrich W. Roloff, M.D., Steve Donn, M.D., Roger Faix, M.D., and their fellows. We express our indebtedness to John M. Toomasian, C.C.P., and Cynthia A. Nixon, R.N., as well as the entire staff of ECMO technical specialists and nurses in the Holden neonatal intensive care unit at the University of Michigan Hospitals for their expert management of the patients in the University of Michigan series and their careful collection of the data on which much of this work is based. We also thank Michelle Hoffman for her careful preparation of the manuscript.

The Problem: Why Is ECMO Needed?

There were 434 admissions to the Holden Neonatal Intensive Care Unit at the University of Michigan Medical Center in Ann Arbor during 1982. Of these admissions, there were 66 deaths (14.5 percent); 250 (58 percent) of these children required mechanical ventilation for respiratory failure, and of these children there were 37 deaths (15 percent). Another 22 went on to develop bronchopulmonary dysplasia (BPD), and only six of these evenutally survived. Thus, in one year in one tertiary care center there were 37 children for whom mechanical ventilation was not adequate therapy for their respiratory failure. There were an additional 22 children who developed a complication of current treatment for respiratory failure. This is an indication for another approach to therapy.

History: The Development of ECMO

Many advances in basic science and applied technology have made ECMO possible. The first concerted attempts at ECC were the investigations of Alexis Carrel and the aviator, Charles Lindburgh [1]. Clinical ECC was begun by Gibbon [2] and opened the era of cardiac surgery. The use of an artificial pump and lung, however, was limited to one or two hours, not because of the pump, but because of the oxygenator, which severely alters blood cells and proteins [3,4]. Cardiac surgery progressed in the 1950s with the development of filming oxygenators [5,6] and later the bubble oxygenator [7]. The first membrane oxygenator built and used clinically was reported in 1956 by Clowes and his co-workers [8]. With the introduction of silicone rubber as a membrane for gas transfer [9], the membrane oxygenator became practical [10]. This oxygenator is gentle enough on the formed elements of the blood and its proteins to make long-term ECC practical.

The problems of coagulation and platelet loss, which occur during ECC, were carefully addressed beginning in 1967 with the studies of Ganz et al. [11,12]. Problems of blood surface interactions have formed an entire field of study [13,14]. The most important single advance in making ECC possible is probably the introduction of heparin, which was first clinically used as an anticoagulant in 1938 [15]. This keeps the blood in the device from clotting, but it also creates bleeding tendencies in the patient.

The first successful prolonged ECC for respiratory failure was reported in 1972 by Hill et al. [16]. Since that time several hundred patients have been treated with ECMO throughout the world. White et al. [17] treated three infants with neonatal respiratory failure with ECMO in 1970. Although there were no survivors, he was able to demonstrate satisfactory gas exchange. Our group has had the largest experience with neonatal

ECMO, first at Irvine, Calif., and now in Ann Arbor, Mich. In 1982 [18], we reported 45 neonates with respiratory failure treated with ECMO with 25 survivors. Also using ECMO for newborn respiratory failure are other groups in this country, including those at the University of Pittsburgh [19] and at the Medical College of Virginia [20]. The results have indicated that infants with a predicted mortality of 80 to 90 percent have a mortality of approximately 50 percent when treated with ECMO. The experience with adults has not been as good. In a nine-center prospective randomized study evaluating ECMO as therapy for acute respiratory failure in adults, the survival in patients receiving ECMO was 9.5 percent. The survival in the control group was 8.3 percent. Although respiratory gas exchange was well supported, long-term survival was not obtained [21]. This is probably due to the underlying natural history of the causes of respiratory failure in adults.

Indications For ECMO: Which Patients Can Be Successfully Treated?

In our combined Ann Arbor-Irvine experience, approximately 1,500 children with newborn respiratory failure required a ventilator and increased inspired oxygen concentrations, 150 were treated with maximal therapy: very high inspiratory pressure, inspired concentration of oxygen of 100 percent, vasodilator drugs such as tolazoline, reversed ratio of inspiratory time to expiratory time, and increased respiratory rate, in other words, whatever was considered, at the time, maximal ventilatory therapy. These are the children at risk for BPD. Among the 45 patients treated with ECMO, the underlying diseases were meconium aspiration syndrome in 22, infantile respiratory distress syndrome in 14, primary persistent fetal circulation in 5, and sepsis in 4.

The place where ECMO can be demonstrated to be of the most benefit is in those illnesses characterized by increased pulmonary artery hypertension. These children are usually otherwise healthy newborns over 2 kg. They include children with congenital diaphragmatic hernia and meconium aspiration syndrome as well as primary persistent fetal circulation. They do not have underlying parenchymal lung disease and often improve if acidosis and hypoxemia can be reversed.

Congenital diaphragmatic hernia is a particularly distressing disease for the pediatric surgeon since operation does correct the anatomic defect. In the first 24 to 48 hours after the operation, the children often look quite good. Many of them, however, become progressively hypoxemic and acidotic, with a mortality rate of 50 percent. The real problem appears to be pulmonary vasoconstriction with increased pulmonary artery pressure and a right-to-left shunt. Treatment with tolazoline to dilate the pulmonary artery has been attempted. Diaphragmatic hernia is the kind of problem that is amenable to ECMO therapy. The greatest experience with this disease has been at Pittsburgh. Weiner has presented data recently showing that ECMO can reverse this phenomenon [22].

Parenchymal lung diseases such as infantile respiratory distress syndrome (hyaline membrane disease) and streptococcal pneumonia do not respond as well to ECMO therapy, although there have been some successes. We ascribe this to the more variable natural history of these illnesses, which may not resolve in one to two weeks. Some children with parenchymal disease suffer barotrauma complications of ventilator therapy such as pneumothorax with persistent air leak. When these complications limit the ability of ventilator therapy to support them, ECMO is quite successful. Air leaks seal when the high inspiratory pressure, positive end expiratory pressure, and respiratory rate can be reduced. Children with parenchymal lung disease often weigh less than 2 kg, and this accounts for the diminished success in smaller babies.

Specific indications for a patient to receive ECMO are being developed from the accumulating experience. Our current practice is to select patients who in our experience in our nursery have a predicted 80 percent mortality risk with conventional management. They should be seven days of age or less, have no intraventricular hemorrhage, and have a "quality life potential." We have not considered children weighing less than 1 kg as candidates for ECMO since their underlying illnesses have not appeared amenable to this kind of treatment. The five criteria adopted for our current prospective controlled study illustrate which babies we would currently treat among those over 2 kg.

The first criterion is acute deterioration. This consists of an arterial oxygen tension (PaO_2) of less than 40 mmHg or a pH of less than 7.15 for greater than 2 hours.

The second criterion is a neonatal pulmonary insufficiency index that places the child in a risk category of 80 percent or greater predicted mortality. The index is calculated by using the inspired oxygen concentration and the arterial pH plotted against time [23,24]. This index has proved to be a valuable indicator of predicted mortality, although the specific numbers vary from institution to institution. Each nursery develops its own statistics by analyzing their experience.

The third indication is barotrauma. In this category children must meet four of seven criteria: pulmonary interstitial emphysema or pseudocyst formation, pneumothorax or pneuomediastinum, pneumoperitoneum, pneumopericardium, subcutaneous emphysema, and more than five chest tubes placed for air leak . The seventh is a mean airway pressure greater than 15 cm H_2O.

The fourth criterion includes children who have unresponsive pulmonary artery hypertension and two of the following three parameters for more than 3 hours: pH less than 7.40, hypotension, and PaO_2 of less than 55 mmHg.

The fifth indication is a child with a congenital diaphragmatic hernia who also has unresponsive pulmonary artery hypertension postoperatively as noted in the fourth criterion. In addition, if the inspired oxygen concentration (FiO_2) required to keep the preductal PaO_2 >80 mmHg is higher than 0.8, ECMO is indicated. Preoperatively ECMO may be valuable in patients with a diaphragmatic hernia if the pH is <7.2 or the PaO_2 is <50 mmHg.

Management of The Patient on ECMO

The standard venoarterial ECMO circuit is shown in Figure 19–1. Blood is drained from a catheter placed in the right atrium via the internal jugular vein. This blood drains by gravity through a servoregulating bladder to a pump. The bladder turns off the pump if the blood flow decreases so that

Figure 19–1
Circuit diagram for venoarterial ECMO.

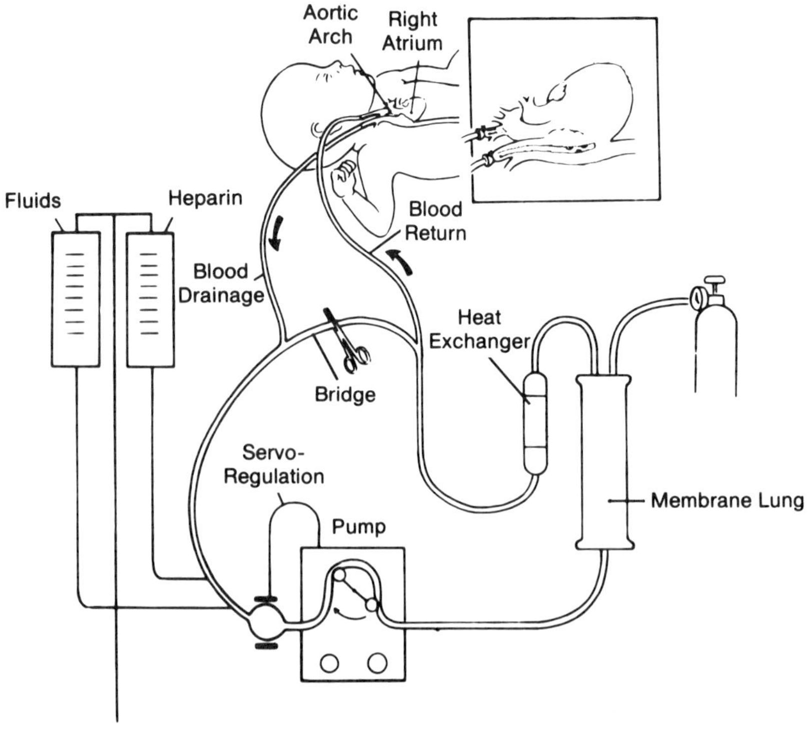

236

Figure 19–2

AP chest roentgenogram of a patient after cannulation for venoarterial ECMO. Umbilical vein and artery catheters come up from below. The venous drainage cannula reaches nearly to the diagram. The perfusion cannula ends at the entrance of the carotid artery into the aortic arch. A patent ductus arteriosus has been clipped.

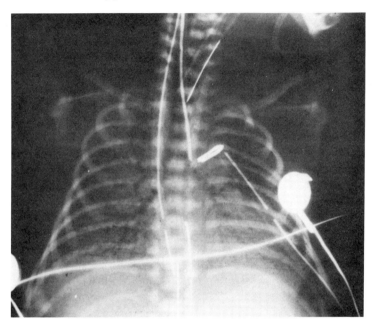

it does not suck air. The pump then propels the blood through the membrane lung and a heat exchanger and then to a cannula in the carotid artery placed at the level of the aortic arch. Heparin is continuously administered through a stopcock in the circuit, as are all fluids, parenteral nutrition, and medications.

The cannulation is done with local anesthesia in the neonatal intensive care unit with support from operating room personnel. These children are usually paralyzed and can be easily positioned with the neck extended and the head turned to the left. We make an incision along the border of the right sternocleidomastoid muscle and expose the carotid artery and internal jugular vein. Chest tubes are used as cannulas, and infants over 2 kg will accept a 14 or 16 venous cannula, which is positioned in the right atrium. Most patients will take an 8 or 10 cannula in the carotid artery, which we try to position at the level of its entrance into the aorta (Figure 19–2).

Once a child is on ECMO, an inspired oxygen concentration of 30 percent is usually sufficient. The pressures and rate can also be lowered.

Figure 19–3

AP chest films before (right) and after (left) venovenous ECMO. The venous drainage cannula extends to the diaphragm from the right internal jugular vein in the film on the right. The pulmonary artery monitoring catheter comes up from the groin. The perfusion cannula is in the distal iliac vein and is not visible in this roentgenogram. The increased lung density in this film is related to the decreased inspiratory pressures employed while the patient is on ECMO.

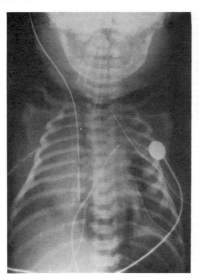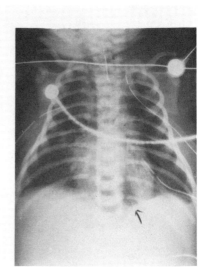

Once a child is on ECMO, the chest x ray usually appears worse since much less pressure is used to venitlate the baby, and there is much less aeration (Figure 19–3). The child no longer needs to be paralyzed and can breathe spontaneously and move. All patients are on antibiotics, and many continue on phenobarbital to control seizures. Monitoring includes arterial pressure through an umbilical artery line. Pulmonary artery pressure is often measured with a Swann-Ganz catheter, which is placed via a femoral vein by the cardiologist in the cardiac catheterization laboratory. Once a day there is a reference period when the child is taken off ECMO, and the ventilator settings are increased. Nutrition is maintained by using full parenteral nutrition administered via the ECMO circuit.

A child on ECMO uses two bed spaces in the neonatal intensive care unit. The nurse is a one-to-one intensive care nurse who manages the patient's usual needs. This includes dressings, vital signs, chest tubes, endotracheal tube, and suctioning. The nurse draws up and prepares all medications and fluids that are administered by the ECMO technical specialist (ECMO tech), who is at the bedside at all times while the patient is on ECMO. This person is responsible for measuring whole blood activated clotting time and controlling the infusion of heparin as well as controlling the flow and volume of the ECMO circuit. ECMO techs are nurses, respiratory therapists, or perfusionists who have a special interest in this technique. They are trained in both the classroom and the laboratory.

Blood flow through the device regulates the arterial oxygen tension. Usually children require 100 to 200 ml of blood flow per kg per minute to replace the function of their heart and lungs. The flow of gas (usually 100 percent oxygen) through the gas phase of the membrane lung regulates the $PaCO_2$ and by turning up the gas flow we can decrease the arterial saturation of carbon dioxide. Occasionally this is so low that the child does not breathe spontaneously, and we use carbogen (a mixture of 95 percent oxygen and 5 percent carbon dioxide). The blood volume is the best way to regulate the perfusion, and conversely the perfusion indicates when the blood volume is low. If we cannot maintain high enough blood flows through the device to oxygenate the patient, it is usually because the patient's blood volume is too low. Clinically what happens is that the servoregulator bladder begins to set off the alarm and turn off the pump. The ECMO tech then administers whole blood or plasma depending on the hematocrit. The flow can usually then be increased sufficiently for oxygenation.

Anticoagulation is maintained by titrating the patient with a constant infusion of heparin to an ACT of about 250 seconds (normal is about 100 seconds). We try to maintain the platelet count above 50,000 by using platelet transfusions. ECC of any kind removes platelets from the circulation by activating them and causing small platelet thrombi, which then break off of the membrane and are trapped in the body [25].

Figure 19–4 is a graphic presentation of an ECMO survivor who is a newborn with respiratory distress syndrome. At birth the alveolar-arterial oxygen difference (A-aDO_2 gradient) was over 400 mmHg, and it quickly rose to 600 mm Hg. Multiple chest tubes were required. Very high peak inspiratory pressures were required. The inspired oxygen concentration (FIO_2) was rapidly at 100 percent. ECMO was instituted late on the second day of life. The A-aDO_2 gradient dropped quickly, nearly to normal. The peak inspiratory pressures were decreased, and the FIO_2 could be decreased. The ECMO flow rates were between 100 and 150 ml/kg per minute early on and then decreased as the child was weaned. When ECMO was discontinued, the A-aDO_2 gradient increased for a brief time, but basically the peak inspiratory pressures did not have to be increased, nor did the FIO_2s, and the child was extubated and survived.

Some of the coagulation problems which occur can be demonstrated in this patient course shown in Figure 19–5. The platelet count began relatively low and was maintained with platelet transfusions. After ECMO the platelets recovered without further intervention. The fibrin degradation

Figure 19–4

Course of a child with respiratory distress syndrome who survived following treatment with venoarterial ECMO. *(From Bartlett, R.H., Gazzaniga, A.B. Fong, S.W., et al.: Extracorporeal membrane oxygenator (ECMO) support for cardiopulmonary failure: Experience in twenty-eight cases.* J. Thorac. Cardiovasc. Surg., 73(3):375, 1977. 1978.)

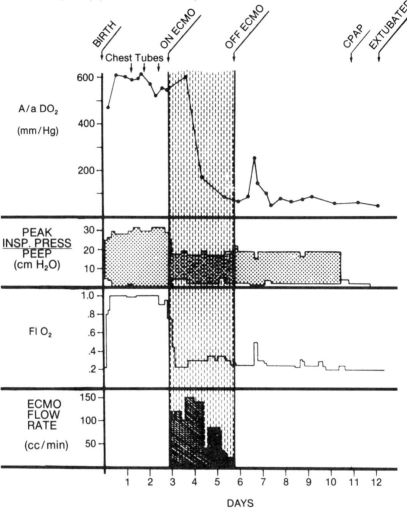

products were high before ECMO and dropped slowly during treatment with ECMO into the normal range. They did not rebound when ECMO was discontinued, so it was not the membrane lung that was removing the fibrin degradation products.

One of the problems often expressed concerning ECMO is that the right carotid artery is sacrificed. There have been no reported compli-

Figure 19–5

Platelet count and fibrin degradation products (f.d.p.) during course of patient treated with venoarterial ECMO.

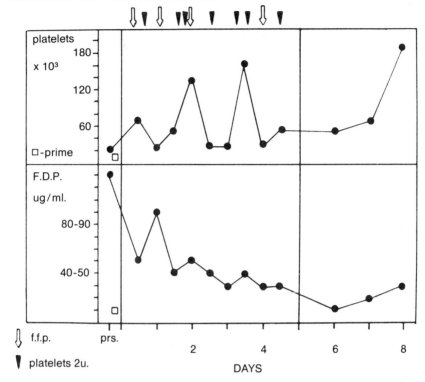

cations of carotid artery ligation. This is, however, still theoretically a problem. We have investigated the use of venovenous bypass, in which blood is drained from the right atrium but returned to a systemic vein [26,27]. This has the disadvantage of not supporting cardiac function, but it does have the theoretical advantage of returning oxygenated blood directly to the stream of blood going to the pulmonary artery and may help relieve the spasm in this vessel. The venovenous circuit in Figure 19–6 does not differ significantly from the venoarterial circuit other than having the return cannula placed in the common femoral vein. The groin dissection adds an hour to the length of the operative procedure because a separate incision is required and the femoral vein has multiple tributaries. Healing is not as rapid or as sure in the groin as in the neck, and the leg remains swollen for some time after the cannula is removed. There is also a potential problem of chronic venous disease in the operated leg.

Another problem of venovenous perfusion is incomplete mixing or recirculation, which occurs because oxygenated blood enters the vena

241

Figure 19–6

Circuit diagram for venovenous ECMO. *(From Bartlett, R.H., Andrews, A.F., Toomasian, J.M., Haiduc, N.J., Gazzaniga, A.B. Extracorporeal membrane oxygenation for newborn respiratory failure: forty-five cases. Surgery, 92(2):425, 1982.)*

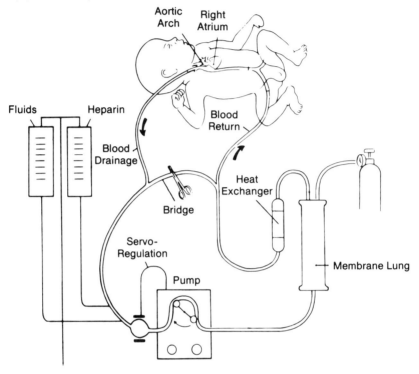

cava where it can be quickly drained by the cannula before circulating through the body. Fortunately, in both laboratory and clinical experience this has not been a major problem.

Figure 19–7 shows pressure changes that occur in the systemic and pulmonary circulations on venovenous ECMO. Before ECMO the pulmonary artery pressure was higher than systemic pressure. On ECMO this was reversed, and even after ECMO the pulmonary artery pressure continued to fall as the systemic pressure rose. Oxygen delivery on venovenous ECMO is presented in Table 19–1. The systemic arterial PO_2 remains high and the mixed venous PO_2 is stable or decreased while the patient is being supported on ECMO. In venovenous ECMO, however, the mixed venous PO_2 is very close to the systemic arterial PO_2 in contrast to venoarterial ECMO, where the mixed venous PO_2 is quite low. This results in a very small oxygen gradient across the membrane lung in venovenous ECMO, requiring higher blood flows through the circuit.

Figure 19–7
Systemic and pulmonary arterial pressure changes in a patient treated with venovenous ECMO.

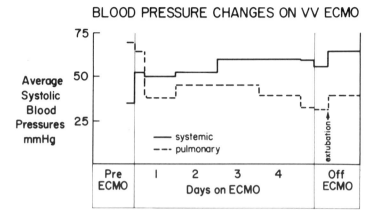

BLOOD PRESSURE CHANGES ON VV ECMO

Results of ECMO for Respiratory Failure in the Newborn

During two years at the University of Michigan we treated 21 patients, with 10 survivors; 17 of the patients were neonates and all 10 survivors were in this group. The average gestational age of the survivors was 39 weeks, and their birth weights ranged from 2,590 to 4,920 g. The mean age at which ECMO was begun was 77 hours. The average time on ECMO was 79 hours. The patients' diagnoses are displayed in Table 19–2 and include respiratory distress syndrome, meconium aspiration syndrome, primary persistent fetal circulation, hydrops fetalis, and polycythemia. Nine of these patients had persistent fetal circulation, either primary or secondary, and 12 patients had some form of barotrauma.

In addition to newborns with respiratory failure, we treated three patients immediately after repair of congenital heart disease and one older

Table 19–1
Comparison of Oxygenation
Parameters During Venoarterial (VA)
and Venovenous (VV) ECMO

Parameter	VA	VV
Pump flow (cc/kg/min)	90	131
O_2 delivery (cc/kg/min)	2.4	3.8
Arterial PO_2 (torr)	76	60
Mixed venous PO_2 (torr)	45	53

Table 19-2

Diagnoses in 21 Patients Treated with ECMO

Diagnosis	Patients	Survivors
Respiratory distress syndrome	7	2
Meconium aspiration syndrome	5	5
Persistent fetal circulation	2	2
Hydrops fetalis	2	0
Polycythemia	1	1
Secondary persistent fetal circulation	9	7
Barotrauma	12	6
Immediately post-repair congenital heart disease	3	0
Malignant histiocytosis	1	0

patient who had diffuse lung disease unresponsive to maximum ventilator management. None of our four nonnewborns survived. Those patients whose diseases were characterized by increased pulmonary artery pressures had the best survival.

Survival in patients undergoing venoarterial bypass was not as great as in those undergoing venovenous ECMO alone (Table 19-2). However, only the largest candidates were selected for venovenous bypass because the size of the femoral vein limits the size of the return cannula. Three patients were converted from venovenous to venoarterial bypass because we could not adequately oxygenate them, and two of these three survived.

We have performed three operations on patients while they were being supported with ECMO: two thoracotomies to control bleeding in one patient and ligation of a patent ductus arteriosus in another. One of these patients survived, and all three procedures went well in the neonatal intensive care unit with no complications related to the operation.

Of 21 patients, the total survivors are 10 (48 percent). If we limit this to the newborns only, the survival is 59 percent. If we limit the series to newborns without other fatal problems of which we were not aware at the time, the survival climbs to 71 percent. This omits one patient with uncorrectable congenital heart disease, one patient with no renal tissue, and one patient who had a cardiac arrest and died while being cannulated for ECMO. These survivals should be compared with the predicted survival of 20 percent based on data from the same nursery.

There are complications of ECMO (Table 19-3). Intracranial hemorrhage occurred in five patients, only one of whom survived. Intracranial hemorrhage on ECMO is often severe because of the heparinization. The incidence of intracranial hemorrhage on ECMO is similar to that in the same patients not treated with ECMO [18,28]. Only four patients had no complications. Four patients had seizure activity, and four had oliguria or anuria. Three oxygenator failures occurred, and only one of these pa-

Table 19–3

Survival in Venoarterial (VA)
and Venovenous (VV) ECMO

ECMO	Patients	Survivors
VA alone	8	3
VV alone	6	5
VV to VA	3	2

tients survived. There was one heat exchanger failure, one tubing rupture, one large retroperitoneal hematoma, one gastrointestinal hemorrhage, one cephalhematoma, and one hemothorax. Also occurring were hypercalcemia, hyperbilirubinemia, a torn fomoral vein during cannulation for venovenous ECMO, deafness, and significant maternal depression requiring psychiatric hospitalization.

The longest followup at the time of this survey was 2.5 years, and that child is entirely normal. Two of the 10 survivors have disinct problems. One has microcephaly and cerebral palsy, and one required rehospitalization three times for BPD.

New Horizons and Other Applications

There are other areas where ECMO may prove applicable. Older children with acute myocarditis occasionally die in heart failure before recovering.

Table 19–4

Complications Related to ECMO

Complication	Patients	Survivors
Intracranial hemorrhage	5	1
None	4	3
Seizures	4	3
Oliguria or anuria	4	2
Oxygenator failure	3	1
Heat exchanger failure	1	0
Tubing rupture	1	0
Retroperitoneal hematoma	1	0
Gastrointestinal bleed	1	1
Cephalahematoma	1	1
Hemothorax	1	1
Hypercalcemia	1	1
Hyperbilirubinemia	1	1
Torn femoral vein	1	0
Deafness	1	1
Maternal depression	1	1

Supporting their cardiac function may allow time for the disease to resolve. Some children with congenital heart disease are currently taken to the operating room while quite ill, hypoxic, and acidotic. Perhaps they could be placed on ECMO in the intensive care unit for 24 hours and then go to the operating room in better condition and not require additional cannulation for cardiopulmonary bypass. Small children with tracheobronchial anomalies, and injuries are currently a very difficult reconstructive problem. ECMO may enable an unhurried operation and recovery period without placing tubes or stents across a delicate anastomosis.

The future of ECMO may lie in the treatment of even smaller infants. We have not applied ECMO to the treatment of neonates weighing less than 1 kg but we are currently providing ECMO for infants between 1 and 2 kg. There is less success in this weight group because the underlying diseases of these children are more resistant to therapy and intracranial bleeding is more frequent and more severe. Perhaps, however, if ECMO were instituted earlier, better results could be obtained and BPD could be prevented by not using high inspired oxygen concentrations and high ventilator pressures. The solutions to the problems of treating smaller infants and those with parenchymal disease appear to lie in the areas of preventing hemorrhage by eliminating heparinization and encouraging earlier application of ECMO to prevent the development of complications of current ventilatory therapy. We are progressing toward the development of heparinless bypass by the use of wall-bonded heparin, which is showing great promise in the laboratory. We are also developing a techinque for single-vessel (the internal jugular vein) cannulation with a double-lumen catheter to avoid the morbidity that may be associated with cannulation of the femoral vein or carotid artery. In the future we may be able to treat respiratory failure intravenously the way we now treat nutritional failure.

References

1. Edwards, W.S., Edwards, P.D. *Alexis Carrel Visionary Surgeon*. Springfield, Ill.: Charles C. Thomas Co., 1974.
2. Gibbon, J.H., Jr. Artificial maintenance of circulation during experimental occlusion of pulmonary artery. *Arch. Surg.* 34:1105–1131, 1937.
3. Lee, W.H., Jr., Krumhaar, D., Fonkalsrud, E.W., et al. Denaturation of plasma proteins as a cause of morbidity and death after intracardiac operations. *Surgery* 50:29–39, 1961.
4. Dobell, A.R., Mitri, M., Galva, R., et al. Biologic evaluation of blood after prolonged recirculation through film and membrane oxygenators. *Ann. Surg.* 161:617–622, 1965.
5. Crafoord, C., Norberg, B., Senning, A. Clinical studies in extracorporeal circulation with a heart-lung machine. *Acta Chir. Scand.* 112:220–245, 1957.

6. Cross, F.S., Kay E.B. Direct vision repair of intracardiac defects utilizing a rotating disc reservoir oxygenator. *Surg. Gynecol.* Obstet. 104:711–716, 1957.

7. DeWall, R., Bentley, D.J., Hirose, M., et al. A temperature controlling (omnithermic) disposable bubble oxygenator for total body perfusion. *Dis. Chest* 49:207–211, 1966.

8. Clowes, G.H.A., Jr., Hopkins, A.L., Neville, W.E. An artificial lung dependent upon diffusion of oxygen and carbon dioxide through plastic membranes. *J. Thorac. Surg.* 32:630–637, 1956.

9. Kammermeyer, K. Silicone rubber as a selective barrier. *Ind. Eng. Chem.* 49:1685, 1957.

10. Kolobow, T., Bowman, R.L. Construction and evaluation of an alveolar membrane artificial heart lung. *Trans. Am. Soc. Artif. Intern. Organs* 9:238–243, 1963.

11. Ganz, H., Subramanian, V., Lillehei, C.W., Castaneda A.R. Problems in hemostasis during open heart surgery. VIII. On the in vivo turnover rate of plasminogen activator after cardiopulmonary bypass. *Surgery* 62:292–295, 1967.

12. Ganz, H., Castaneda, A.R., Subramanian, V.A., et al. Problems in hemostasis during open heart surgery. IX. Changes observed in the plasminogenplasma system and their significance for therapy. *Ann. Surg.* 166:980–986, 1967.

13. Varco, R.L. (conference chairman). Conference on Mechanical Surface and Gas Layer Effects on Moving Blood (San Diego, California, Jan. 1971). *Fed. Proc.* 30:1485–1488, 1971.

14. Bartlett, R.H., Andersen J.C. Blood-Surface interactions: An overview. In Stanley, J.C. (ed.), *Biologic and Synthetic Vascular Prostheses*. New York: Grune & Stratton, 1982.

15. Murray, G. *Surgery in the Making*. London: Johnson Publishers, Ltd., 1964.

16. Hill, J.D., O'Brien, T.G., Murray, J.J., et al. Prolonged extracorporeal oxygenation for acute post-traumatic respiratory failure (shock lung syndrome). *N. Engl. J. Med.* 286:629–634, 1972.

17. White, J.J., Andrews, H.G., Risemberg, H., et al. Prolonged respiratory support in newborn infants with a membrane oxygenator. *Surgery* 70:288–296, 1971.

18. Bartlett, R.H., Andrews, A.F., Toomasian, J.M., et al. Extracorporeal membrane oxygenation for newborn respiratory failure: forty-five cases. *Surgery* 92:425–433, 1982.

19. Hardesty, R.L., Griffith, B.P., Debski, R.J., et al. Extracorporeal membrane oxygenation. Successful treatment of persistent fetal circulation following repair of congenital diaphragmatic hernia. *J. Thorac. Cardiovasc. Surg.* 81:556–563, 1981.

20. Krummel, T.M., Greenfield, L.J., Kirkpatrick, B.V., et al. Clinical use of an extracorporeal membrane oxygenator in neonatal pulmonary failure. *J. Pediatr. Surg.* 17:525–531, 1982.

21. Zapol, W.M., Snider, M.T., Hill, D.J., et al. Extracorporeal membrane oxygenation in severe acute respiratory failure. *J. Am. Med. Assoc.* 242:2193–2196, 1979.

22. Wiener, E.S. Congenital posterolateral diaphragmatic hernia: new dimensions in management. *Surgery* 92:670–681, 1982.

23. Wetmore, N., McEwen, D., O'Conner, M., Bartlett, R.H. Defining indications for artificial organ support in respiratory failure. *Trans. Am. Soc. Artif. Intern. Organs* 25:459–461, 1979.
24. Cimma, R., Risemberg, H., White, J.J. A simple objective system for early recognition of overhelming neonatal respiratory distress. *J. Pediatr. Surg.* 15:581–585, 1980.
25. Andrews, A.F., Klein, M.D., Toomasian, J.M., et al. Venovenous extracorporeal membrane oxygenation in neonates with respiratory failure. *J. Pediatr. Surg.* 18:339–346, 1983.
26. Andrews, A.F., Toomasian, J., Oram, A., Bartlett, R.H. Total respiratory support with venovenous (VV) ECMO. *Trans. Am. Soc. Artif. Intern. Organs* 28:350–353, 1982.
27. Andrews, A.F., Bowerman, R.A., Toomasian, J.M., et al. Intracranial hemorrhage (IHC) in neonates on extracorporeal membrane oxygenation (ECMO). In: Ross Perinatal Intracranial Hemorrhage Conference. Columbus, Ohio: Ross Laboratories, 1982.
28. German, J.C., Worcester, C., Gassaniga, A.B., et al. Technical aspects in the management of the meconium aspiration syndrome with extracorporeal circulation. *J. Pediatr. Surg.* 15:378–383, 1980.

20

Perinatal Aspiration Syndromes

James H. Jose, M.D., and Richard L. Schreiner, M.D.

Meconium Aspiration

Appropriate obstetric and pediatric management of the high-risk mother and infant has led to a significant reduction in the incidence of meconium aspiration. An understanding of the etiology of this disease will help clinicians achieve the highest goal of health care: prevention.

ETIOLOGY

In utero passage of meconium occurs in 8 to 21 percent of live births [1–3]. Passage of meconium is most common in the term and postterm fetus, but has been reported in infants of less than 29 weeks of gestation [3]. The incidence is increased by factors that stress the uteroplacental capacity to nourish and oxygenate the fetus: toxemia, hypertension, maternal cardiovascular and respiratory disease, intrauterine growth retardation, and postterm gestation. The predisposition to acute or chronic asphyxia not only stimulates passage of meconium, but also induces gasping by the fetus. Asphyxia sufficiently severe to cause intrauterine gasping may account for the most severe instances of meconium aspiration syndrome (MAS) [4,5]. Gregory et al. did not find a significant correlation between the thickness of the meconium and the incidence of MAS [2]. Meis et al. found an increased incidence of MAS when there was heavy staining of the amniotic fluid noted before the active phase of labor and when any amount of meconium was first passed during active labor. Light meconium staining noted before active labor was rarely (0.6 percent) associated with MAS [3].

PATHOPHYSIOLOGY

Aspiration of meconium produces mechanical obstruction of the airways and chemical inflammation. Ball valve obstruction of the airways may cause air trapping, resulting in CO_2 retention, pneumothorax, pneumo-mediastinum, or pneumopericardium. Complete mechanical obstruction causes atelectasis with associated ventilation-perfusion mismatch (intra-pulmonary shunting). Chemical inflammation is not as abrupt in onset as is mechanical obstruction and probably develops over a 48-hour period [6]. This may then result in atelectasis with subsequent ventilation perfusion inequality.

The asphyxia that accompanies meconium aspiration may produce problems that increase the severity of parenchymal lung disease. Hypoxia and acidosis increase pulmonary vascular resistance and result in right-to-left shunts through the foramen ovale and ductus arteriosus (persistent fetal circulation). Asphyxial damage to the myocardium may result in systemic hypotension. The diminished cardiac contractility may make it even more difficult for the heart to compensate for the increased pulmonary vascular resistance.

PREVENTION OF PASSAGE OF MECONIUM

The prevention of fetal stress and asphyxia will decrease the likelihood that meconium will be passed or, once passed, that intrauterine aspiration will occur. Women who are at risk for uteroplacental insufficiency should be carefully monitored during pregnancy and should have fetal heart rate monitoring during labor. Fetal scalp blood samples for pH may be obtained when the fetal heart rate pattern is abnormal. Monitoring of the at risk and postdate pregnancy with biophysical profiles obtained by fetal ultrasound shows promise in the prevention of fetal asphyxia and consequent passage of meconium [7,8].

PREVENTION OF MECONIUM ASPIRATION

Perinatal suctioning of meconium-stained infants has been shown to greatly decrease the incidence of mechonium aspiration [1,2]. This practice is effective because before birth the fetus does not usually make sufficient respiratory efforts to move meconium into the small airways. Intrauterine meconium aspiration may occur, but is thought to occur only with very prolonged fetal asphyxia [4,5]. There is evidence that the mouth, pharynx, and trachea may contain a significant and even fatal dose of meconium; Gooding and associates found that 1.0 ml of a 50 percent meconium solution was uniformly fatal when instilled into the tracheas of newborn puppies [9]. We have found the dose-response curve in meconium aspiration to be very steep; newborn rabbits given 6 ml of a 10 percent meconium solution per kg will recover in less than 24 hours, whereas 8 ml/kg results in 100 percent mortality [10].

Figure 20–1
Immediately after delivery of the head, the oropharynx and nasopharynx are suctioned for meconium. *(From Schreiner, R.L., Kisling, J.A.,* Practical Neonatal Respiratory Care. *New York: Raven Press, 1982, p. 37.)*

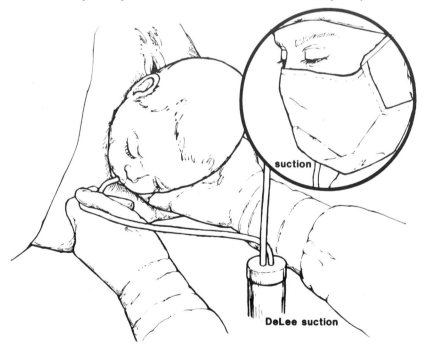

When meconium-stained amniotic fluid is detected, the obstetrician should be prepared to suction the mouth and nasopharynx before delivery of the chest. A bulb syringe is adequate for suctioning the mouth, whereas a DeLee suction catheter or a large (14-Fr) catheter connected to suction (40 to 80 cmH$_2$O) is preferred to clear the nose and oropharynx (Figure 20–1). The infant is then passed to another clinican who visualizes the vocal cords, ideally before respiratory efforts have been initiated. If meconium is seen at the cords, the trachea should be intubated and suction applied quickly (usually by mouth) while withdrawing the tube. The meconium is then blown out of the tube, and the process is repeated until the trachea is clear. An alternative method is to use a stiff 14-Fr catheter connected to wall suction (40 to 80 cmH$_2$O); the catheter is slowly withdrawn from the trachea while suction is applied. The infant's heart rate should be monitored during the procedure, and every effort should be made to clear the trachea before significant bradycardia occurs. One must balance the concerns of clearing the trachea with those of iatrogenic asphyxia. If there is no clinician with expertise in endotracheal intubation available, prolonged attempts at intubation with worsening asphyxia and bradycardia should be avoided; in this situation thorough suctioning of the oropharynx and nasopharynx should be completed, followed by bag and mask ventilation with 100 percent oxygen. Likewise, persistent efforts to clear the trachea in a vigorous, crying child who has already taken several breaths is unwise, as this may produce respiratory depression as well as trauma to the oropharyngeal area. In a depressed infant or an infant with respiratory distress, it may be worthwhile to suction the trachea even though the infant has already taken a number of breaths; indeed, in some infants fairly large amounts of meconium may be obtained from the trachea many minutes after delivery [11].

Some authorities advocate tracheal suctioning of all meconium-stained infants [2]. Gregory et al. found that 10 percent of their infants had tracheal meconium even though the pharynx was clear of meconium after suctioning by the obstetrician. Considering that one-third of their infants with tracheal meconium were sick even after tracheal suctioning, there would appear to be sufficient reason for intubating and suctioning the trachea of all meconium-stained infants. However, Carson and associates [1] performed tracheal suctioning only when pharyngeal meconium was present in 271 infants, and there were no cases of MAS when the pharynx was clear.

Tracheal suctioning should probably be performed under two conditions even when meconium is not seen in the pharynx: 1) when "pea soup" thick meconium is present; and 2) when the child is noted to have poor color, tone, and respiratory effort. In both cases there is a greater likelihood that a signficant dose of meconium is present in the trachea, and therefore direct visualization and suctioning of the trachea is indicated.

MANAGEMENT OF MECONIUM ASPIRATION

An infant who has low Apgar scores or respiratory distress in the delivery room should be admitted to the special care nursery. A chest x ray may help determine which infants require prolonged observation in that Gregory et al. found that two-thirds of their infants with abnormal chest radiographs had symptoms. Chest physiotherapy and suctioning of the oropharynx should be performed, but infants frequently need supplemental oxygen during this procedure to avoid hypoxia. Transcutaneous monitoring of the PO_2 will help prevent hypoxemia during physiotherapy as well as aid in further management of the infant's condition. Carson et al. performed tracheobronchial lavage on seven meconium-stained infants [1]. They found that iatrogenic wet lung disease occurred in five infants who had no meconium below the vocal cords. Burke-Strickland and Edwards used saline lavage and felt that it was beneficial, but did not have sufficient control subjects to confirm this impression [12,13]. The fact that meconium aspiration has been managed effectively without lavage has led most authors to conclude that lavage is not warranted in the management of meconium aspiration.

If hypoxemia cannot be managed by increasing the inspired oxygen, CPAP may be helpful; appropriate pressures to optimize oxygenation must be individually determined for each infant [14,15]. Positive end expiratory pressure and CPAP do not increase lung dead space (air trapping) early in the course of meconium aspiration in experimental animals [15], although this may not be the case as chemical pneumonitis becomes a factor several hours after aspiration [6]. Yeh et al. found that an increase in functional residual capacity occurred over the first three days of life in nonventilated infants with MAS [16]. This increased functional residual capacity was correlated with lower dynamic lung compliance, suggesting an overexpansion of the ventilated portions of the lung to the flattened portion of their pressure-volume curve. Positive end expiratory pressure may increase the functional residual capacity further, and Yeh et al. recommended that it be used with caution if hyperinflation is apparent clinically or radiographically. Due to decreased lung compliance, high inspiratory pressures are often necessary if mechanical ventilation is required [17]. Pneumothorax and pneumomediastinum occur in 10 to 20 percent of infants with meconium aspiration [2,18].

The infant with MAS requires attention to other organ systems in the newborn intensive care unit. Asphyxiated infants often experience hypotension, which may require treatment with infusion of saline or colloid and pressors. Fluids ultimately should probably be restricted as much as possible, however, to prevent cerebral and pulmonary edema, especially in the presence of acute renal failure. Severe metabolic acidosis may follow

253

asphyxia and should be treated with infusion of sodium bicarbonate. Blood glucose and calcium must be determined, and any abnormality must be corrected. Antibiotics are usually administered, since superimposed bacterial pneumonia is difficult to exclude. Steroids have often been used in the hope of ablating the chemical pneumonitis that occurs with meconium aspiration. Frantz et al. found that pneumonitis was decreased by steroids in neonatal rabbits who aspirated meconium, but there was an increased mortality among those animals receiving steroids [19]. A controlled trial of hydrocortisone in infants with MAS by Yeh et al. showed that an increased period of time was required in weaning from supplemental oxygen in treated infants [20]. They postulated that this was due to delayed clearance of meconium by macrophages after steroid treatment. Thus there is no evidence that steroids are beneficial in the treatment of MAS.

Pulmonary hypertention (persistent fetal circulation) frequently accompanies meconium aspiration, and it may be difficult to determine the extent to which it is responsible for the infant's respiratory distress. Evaluation of this factor may be aided by determining the degree of right-to-left shunt present. The shunt at the ductus arteriosus may be determined by comparison of the PO_2 of a blood sample from the right radial artery with one from an umbilical artery catheter. The shunt at the foramen ovale may be determined by echocardiography, using a peripheral injection of saline to trace the flow from the right to left atrium. It is helpful to determine as accurately as possible the relative significance of pulmonary hypertension as opposed to parenchymal lung disease if specific therapy for pulmonary hypertension is contemplated. The treatment of persistent fetal circulation may potentiate some of the complications of MAS; hyperventilation to lower the PCO_2 may aggravate air leaks, and pharmacologic treatment of pulmonary hypertension (e.g., tolazoline) may have adverse effects. Extracorporeal circulation with a membrane oxygenator is an experimental form of therapy that has been used with some success in infants with severe meconium aspiration [21].

Amniotic Fluid Aspiration

Schaffer and others [22–24] have described a syndrome in which respiratory distress in premature and term infants is presumably caused by aspiration of non-meconium-stained amniotic fluid, usually following an episode of fetal or neonatal asphyxia. The conclusion that the respiratory distress was secondary to amniotic fluid aspiration was supported by postmortem findings of squamous cells in the airways of infants dying of respiratory failure (Figure 20–2); however, squamous debris secondary to amniotic fluid aspiration has also been found in the lungs of infants dying of other causes [22]. Enthusiasm for this diagnosis appears to have waned

Figure 20–2

Alveoli (A) and bronchi and bronchioles (B) are filled with non-meconium-stained amniotic debris and squamae in an infant who died after severe asphyxia and respiratory distress complicated by bilateral pneumothoraces, pneumomediastinum, and subcutaneous emphysema. The amniotic fluid was not meconium stained. *(From Schreiner, R.L., Kisling, J. A., Practical Neonatal Respiratory Care. New York: Raven Press, 1982, p. 51.)*

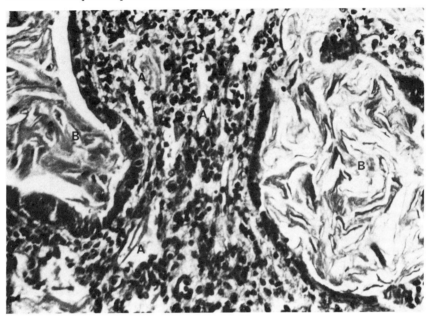

over the past several years, as an increased appreciation has developed for the role of asphyxia in producing surfactant deficiency, delayed clearance of lung water, and pulmonary hypertension (persistent fetal circulation). Further, there are no definite clinical or laboratory markers for the diagnosis of amniotic fluid aspiration. Many clinicians, however, continue to suspect that aspiration of noninfected, non-meconium-stained amniotic fluid is a significant cause of respiratory disease; thus, it is appropriate to consider the evidence pertinent to this.

The clinical picture of amniotic fluid aspiration usually involves a near-term or term infant with respiratory distress, possibly after an episode of in utero asphyxia. Some clinicians have noted a large amount of frothy fluid in the infant's mouth at delivery; some have claimed that this is amniotic fluid being aspirated by the infant [25], whereas others have suggested that this is fetal lung fluid being expelled by the infant. The chest x-ray may show increased perivascular markings, bilateral infiltrates, and hyperaeration as reflected by an increased anterior-posterior diameter,

Figure 20–3

Chest x ray of an infant with moderately severe respiratory distress. The amniotic fluid was not meconium stained; the white blood count and differential were normal; cultures of the infant were negative.

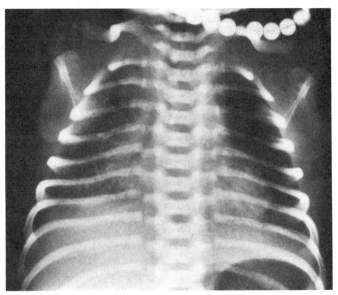

depressed diaphragm, and outward bulging of the pleura in the intercostal spaces (Figure 20–3). There appears to be a relatively high incidence of pneumomediastinum and pneumothorax.

Although the initial findings may be consistent with transient tachypnea of the newborn secondary to delayed resorption of fetal lung fluid, the moderate to severe nature of the respiratory distress and duration of symptoms for greater than 24 to 48 hours of life are not entirely compatible with this diagnosis. As amniotic fluid aspiration is to some degree a diagnosis of exclusion, most clinicians do not consider it unless other causes of neonatal respiratory distress are determined not to be present. Thus, if bacterial or viral infection, meconium aspiration, persistent fetal circulation, congenital heart disease, and polycythemia cannot explain respiratory distress in this clinical picture, some clinicians feel that the diagnosis of aspiration of non-meconium-stained, noninfected amniotic fluid should be considered.

The theory of perinatal aspiration of amniotic fluid supposes that aspiration occurs either in the intrauterine environment, possibly as a result of a series of intrauterine gasps, or during the process of delivery when the contents of the mouth and nasopharynx might be aspirated. Although the chemical composition of fetal lung fluid and amniotic fluid is similar in many respects, the two are not identical. Amniotic fluid has a higher pH, lower osmolality, higher protein concentration, and a relatively high concentration of cellular material that increases with advancing gestational age. The pathophysiologic mechanisms of injury might include airway obstruction by squamous cells, increased lung water, a washout of fetal pulmonary fluid with surfactant, or replacement of fetal lung fluid by a potentially noxious fluid with resultant chemical or mechanical damage.

Documentation of the existence of any aspiration syndrome requires proof that the substance aspirated is toxic and that the fetus or newborn can aspirate sufficient quantities to become ill. We investigated the toxicity of human amniotic fluid in the adult and newborn rabbit [10]. The newborn studies were performed on vaginally and cesarean delivered animals. Aspiration was induced by transtracheal puncture and, in the case of the cesarean delivered rabbits, this was accomplished before the first breath.

In the adult rabbits, arterial PO_2, PCO_2 and pH were determined over a 24-hour period, after which the lung weight and volume, a pressure-volume curve, and lung histology were obtained. Animals given 4 or 6 ml of human amniotic fluid or saline per kg showed a nearly identical response in all items of pulmonary function measured. A transient depression in oxygenation accompanied by mild atelectasis occurred in both the saline and amniotic fluid aspiration groups. Surprisingly, there was no correlation between the cellular content of the amniotic fluid aspirated and the post-aspiration PO_2 (Figure 20–4) or any other aspect of pulmonary function that was measured.

The newborn animals showed remarkably little respiratory compromise in response to aspiration of either saline or amniotic fluid. Vaginally delivered animals received a mean volume of 8 ml/kg, and cesarean delivered animals received a mean volume of 11 ml/kg. These amounts of fluid approach those shown to cause significant morbidity in laboratory studies of drowning in adult animals [26–28]. The newborn animals in our study showed no differences in respiratory rate, mortality, lung weight and volume, chest x-rays, and lung histology. The pressure-volume curves showed none of the expected air trappings that might occur if there were airway obstruction by squamous cells (Figure 20–5).

We concluded that human amniotic fluid was not a uniquely harmful substance. Similar amounts of 10 percent meconium solution given to newborn rabbits resulted in a 100 percent mortality. Although human amniotic fluid does not appear to add a toxic substance to the lung if aspirated, the question remains as to whether a series of fetal gasps might remove an essential substance such as surfactant. Sheldon et al. performed an extensive lung lavage of fetal sheep with their own amniotic fluid and did not find a decrease in surfactant content [29]. There was, however, a decrease in surfactant synthesis, which was interpreted as a toxic effect of the amniotic fluid of sheep. A significant washout of fetal lung liquid ap-

257

Figure 20–4

Lack of correlation between PO_2 and amniotic fluid epithelial cell count in newborn rabbits six hours after aspiration of amniotic fluid.

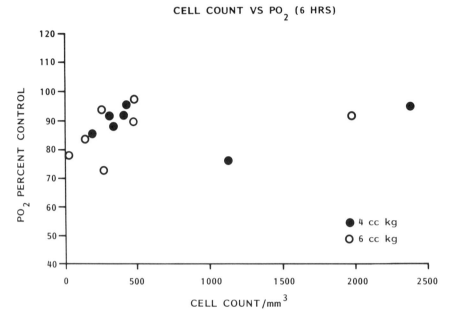

CELL COUNT VS PO_2 (6 HRS)

pears to be unlikely under normal conditions. Only during asphyxia is there sufficient gasping to exchange amniotic fluid with the 30 cc/kg of fetal pulmonary fluid normally present at birth. Judging from studies with fetal sheep, a minimum of nine minutes of asphyxia would be required to produce a 90 percent washout of the fetal pulmonary fluid [30]. Such a considerable degree of asphyxia would be expected to have profound effects on the fetus, and the effects of aspiration would probably be comparatively insignificant.

There may be aspects of fetal breathing yet to be elucidated that would allow the fetus to accumulate particulate matter from the amniotic fluid. Given the success of postnatal obstetric-pediatric suctioning of meconium in prevention of meconium aspiration, this seems unlikely. We thus surmise that the asphyxia that may accompany aspiration and consequent problems with clearance of fetal pulmonary fluid and surfactant production are more likely factors in neonatal respiratory disease attributed to the aspiration of amniotic fluid.

Neonatal Aspiration of the First Feeding

Although it has become common practice to feed the normal newborn infant within a few hours after birth, there continues to be controversy

Figure 20–5

Lung deflation curves *(percent total lung capacity (TLC) versus pressure)* in newborn rabbits after aspiration of saline or amniotic fluid in control animals.

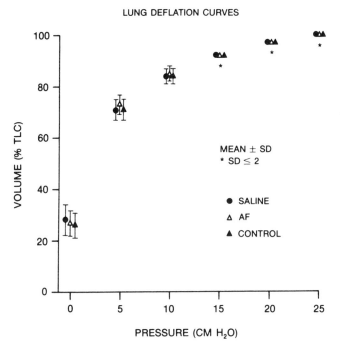

concerning the optimal composition of the first feeding. The goal of this early feeding is to provide nutrition early enough to prevent hypoglycemia while providing a substance that, if aspirated, would cause minimal pulmonary damage. Using rabbits as the experimental animal, Moran suggested that aspiration of a 12 to 50 percent glucose solution resulted in pulmonary edema; however, a 6 percent glucose solution did not cause significant pulmonary edema [31]. Thus, in the late 1950s a 5 percent glucose solution was recommended for the first feeding [32]. In 1970, Olson, using rabbits as the experimental animal, showed that aspiration of a 5 percent glucose solution or cow's milk formulas resulted in more profound clinical and pathologic changes than aspiration of sterile water; she recommended the use of sterile water as the first feed [33]. However, the effects of aspiration of water or glucose solutions mixed with gastric contents have not been investigated. We wondered whether aspiration of feedings of various composition but mixed with gastric juices, would have similar clinical and pathologic effects, and thus sterile water would probably offer no major advantages compared with 5 percent glucose solution (D_5W) as the first feeding [34].

Twenty New Zealand white rabbits were divided into five groups, four treatment groups and a control group. Treatment solutions consisted of sterile water, D_5W, gastric aspirates from an infant fed sterile water, and gastric aspirates from an infant fed D_5W. After aspiration of sterile water there was no significant fall in the PO_2. After aspiration of D_5W there was a marked decrease in the PO_2 with a slow return to control values by 24 hours. In the animals given either gastric aspirate-D_5W or gastric aspirate-sterile water, the PO_2 decreased and never returned to preaspiration levels during the study period. Postaspiration values of gastric aspirate-sterile water remained significantly ($P < 0.001$) below preaspiration at 24 hours. There was no significant postaspiration change in PCO_2 or pH in any of the treatment groups.

There was no pathologic effect of aspiration of sterile water or D_5W on histologic sections of lung tissue. In contrast, marked collapse and interstitial histiocytic response were seen after aspiration of gastric aspirate-sterile water or gastric aspirate-D_5W.

Mendelson stressed the importance of acidity in determining the extent of pulmonary injury when he showed that unneutralized liquid gastric contents caused an effect identical to 0.1 N HCl [35]. Subsequent investigators have confirmed Mendelson's findings and described a critical pH below which lung injury occurs [35–37]. This level seems to vary from species to species; for example, a pH of 1.7 has been suggested as critical for rats, and a pH of 2.1 to 2.4 has been suggested for rabbits [35], but Jones et al. have shown a mild but persistent and prolonged increase in capillary membrane permeability at pH 3 [37]. A critical pH of 2.5 has been suggested, but not proved, for humans [36,38].

The pHs of aspirated gastric fluids in our study were all between 2.5 and 3.2 (mean, 2.7), whereas the pHs of uncontaminated D_5W and sterile water were 4.5 and 5.0, respectively. The lower pH of the gastric aspirate may be responsible for the more prolonged decrease in the PO_2 values and the more marked pathologic changes. This may also explain the lack of clinical or pathologic differences between the two gastric aspirate groups. This finding is significant, since numerous investigators have found neonatal gastric pH values to be as low as 1.1 and commonly below 2.5 by six hours of age [39–41]. Our findings in animals who aspirated D_5W or sterile water are similar to those of Olson and others [33,35] which demonstrate that aspiration of liquids with a neutral pH cause transient clinical and mild pathologic changes.

DeCarlo et al. have reported that aspiration during the initial feedings may occur frequently in the newborn [42]. However, in our nursery clinical evidence of aspiration is relatively uncommon and appears to occur only after the initial feeding with regurgitation of gastric contents. This would eliminate any advantage of sterile water in comparison to D_5W. Sterile water rarely might be advantageous, for instance in infants with esophageal atresia where aspirates would not be contaminated with gastric contents.

However, hypoglycemia is a much more common occurrence in the normal newborn. Lubchenco and Bard found that 10 percent of normal full-term infants developed hypoglycemia (<30 mg/100 ml) by six hours of age. They also found that 18 percent of postterm infants and 25 percent of term infants who were small for gestational age developed hypoglycemia [43]. This transient hypoglycemia of the newborn might be averted by the administration of D_5W in an oral feeding.

We conclude that the advantages of sterile water for the initial feeding in normal infants seem to disappear if the aspirate contains gastric contents. Furthermore, the use of D_5W or formula as a first feeding may avert the much more common event of hypoglycemia.

References

1. Carson, B.S., Losey, R.W., Bowes, W.A., et al. Combined obstetric and pediatric approach to prevent meconium aspiration syndrome. *Am. J. Obstet. Gynecol.* 126:712–715, 1976.
2. Gregory, G.A., Gooding, C.A., Phibbs, H., Tooley, W.H. Meconium aspiration in infants: a prospective study. *J. Pediatr.* 85:848–852, 1974.
3. Meis, P., Hall, M., Marshall, J., Hobel, C. Meconium passage: a new classification for risk assessment during labor. *Am. J. Obstet. Gynecol.* 131:509–513, 1978.
4. Block, M., Kallenberger, D., Kern, J., Nepveu, D. In utero meconium aspiration by the baboon fetus. *Obstet. Gynecol.* 57:37–40, 1981.
5. Brown, B., Gleicher, N. Intrauterine meconium aspiration. *Obstet. Gynecol.* 57:26–29, 1981.
6. Tyler, D., Murphy, J., Cheney, F. Mechanical and chemical damage to lung tissue caused by meconium aspiration. *Pediatrics* 62:454–459, 1978.
7. Manning, F., Morrison, I., Lange, I., Harman, C. Antepartum determination of fetal health: composite biophysical profile scoring. *Clin. Perinatol.* 9:285–296, 1982.
8. Vintzileos, A.M., Campbell, W.A., Ingardia, C.J., Nochimson, D.J. The fetal biophysical profile and its predictive value. *Obstet. Gynecol.* 62:271, 1983.
9. Gooding, C.A., Gregory, G.A., Taber, P., Wright, R.R. An experimental model for the study of meconium aspiration of the newborn. *Radiology* 100:137–140, 1971.
10. Jose, J., Schreiner, R., Lemons, J., et al. The effect of human amniotic fluid aspiration on pulmonary function in the adult and newborn rabbit. *Pediatr. Res.* (In press.)
11. Gage, J., Taeusch, H., Treves, S., Caldicott, W. Suctioning of upper airway meconium in newborn infants. *J. Am. Med. Assoc.* 246:2590–2592, 1981.
12. Burke-Strickland, M., Edwards, N. Meconium aspiration in the newborn. *Minn. Med.* 56:1031–1035, 1973.
13. Burke-Strickland, M. Tracheobronchial lavage in small infants. *Minn. Med.* 56:287–289, 1973.

14. Fox, W., Berman, L.S., Downes, J.J., Peckham, G.J. The therapeutic application of end-expiratory pressure in the meconium aspiration syndrome. *Pediatrics* 56:214–217, 1975.
15. Truog, W.E., Lyrene, R.K., Standaert, T.A., et al. Effects of PEEP and tolazoline infusion on respiratory and inert gas exchange in experimental meconium aspiration. *J. Pediatr.* 100:284–290, 1982.
16. Yeh, T.F., Lilien, L.D., Barathi, A., Pildes, R.S. Lung volume, dynamic lung compliance, and blood gases during the first 3 days of postnatal life in infants with meconium aspiration syndrome. *Crit. Care Med.* 10:588–592, 1982.
17. Vidyasagar, D., Yeh, T.F., Harris, V., Pildes, R.S. Assisted ventilation in infants with meconium aspiration syndrome. *Pediatrics* 56:208–213, 1975.
18. Klaus, M. Cleansing the neonatal trachea. *J. Pediatr.* 85:853, 1974.
19. Frantz, I.D., Wang, N.S., Thach, B.T. Experimental meconium aspiration effects of glucocorticoid treatment. *J. Pediatr.* 86:438–441, 1975.
20. Yeh, T.F., Srinivasan, G., Harris, V., Pildes, R.S. Hydrocortisone therapy in meconium aspiration syndrome: a controlled study. *J. Pediatr.* 90:140–143, 1977.
21. German, J.C., Worcester, C., Gazzaniga, A.B., et al. Technical aspects in the management of the meconium aspiration syndrome with extracorporeal circulation. *J. Pediatr. Surg.* 15:378–383, 1980.
22. Avery, M.E., Fletcher, B.D., Williams, R.G. The lung and its disorders in the newborn infant. *Major Probl. Clin. Pediatr.* 1:275–283, 1981.
23. Leake, R.D., Gunther, R., Sunshine, P. Perinatal aspiration syndrome: its association with intrapartum events and anesthesia. *Am. J. Obstet. Gynecol.* 118:271–275, 1974.
24. Schaffer, A.J., Avery, M.E. *Diseases of the Newborn.* Philadelphia: The W.B. Saunders Co., 1977, pp. 116–122.
25. Pender, C.B. Respiratory distress in the newborn due to aspiration of amniotic fluid and its contents. *Resuscitation* 2:157–167, 1973.
26. Halmagyi, D.F.J. Lung changes and incidence of respiratory arrest in rats after aspiration of sea and fresh water. *J. Appl. Physiol.* 16:41–44, 1961.
27. Halmagyi, D.F.J., Colebatch, H.J.H. Ventilation and circulation after fluid aspiration. *J. Appl. Physiol.* 16:35–40, 1961.
28. Modell, J.H., Moya, F. Effects of volume of aspirated fluid during chlorinated fresh water drowning. *Anesthesiology* 27:662–672, 1966.
29. Sheldon, G., Brazy, J., Tuggle, B., et al. Fetal lamb lavage and its effect on lung phosphatidylcholine. *Pediatr. Res.* 13:599–602, 1979.
30. Howatt, W.F., Humphreys, P.W., Normand, I.C.S., Strang, L.B. Ventilation of liquid by the fetal lamb during asphyxia. *J. Appl. Physiol.* 20:496–502, 1965.
31. Moran, T.J. Pulmonary edema produced by intratracheal injection of milk, feeding mixtures and sugars. *Am. J. Dis. Child.* 86:45–50, 1953.
32. Nelson, W.E. *Textbook of Pediatrics,* 7th ed. Philadelphia: The W.B. Saunders Co., 1959, p. 304.
33. Olson, M. The benign effects on rabbits' lungs of the aspiration of water compared with 5% glucose or milk. *Pediatrics* 46:538–547, 1970.
34. Gresham, E.L., Kirby, W.C. Effects of neonatal gastric aspirates on the rabbit lung. *Pediatr. Res.* 10:461, 1976.

35. Wynne, J.W., Modell, J.H. Respiratory aspiration of stomach contents. *Ann. Intern. Med.* 87:466–474, 1977.
36. Teabeaut, J.R., II. Aspiration of gastric contents—an experimental study. *Am. J. Pathol.* 28:51–62, 1952.
37. Jones, J.G., Berry, M., Hulands, G.H., Crawley, J.C.W. The time course and degree of change in alveolar-capillary membrane permeability induced by aspiration of hydrochloric acid and hypotonic saline. *Am. Rev. Respir. Dis.* 118:1007–1013, 1978.
38. Vandam, L.D. Aspiration of gastric contents in the operative period. *N. Engl. J. Med.* 273:1206–1208, 1965.
39. Miclat, N.N., Hodgkinson, R., Marx, G.F. Neonatal gastric pH. *Anesth. Analg.* 57:98–101, 1978.
40. Ebers, D.W., Smith, D.I., Gibbs, G.E. Gastric acidity on the first day of life. *Pediatrics* 18:800–802, 1956.
41. Avery, G.B., Randolph, J.G., Weaver, T. Gastric acidity in the first day of life. *Pediatrics* 37:1005–1007, 1966.
42. DeCarlo, J., Jr., Tramer, A., Startzman, H.H., Jr. Iodized oil aspiration in the newborn. *Am. J. Dis. Child.* 84:442–445, 1952.
43. Lubchenco, L.O., Bard, H. Incidence of hypoglycemia in newborn infants classified by birth weight and gestational age. *Pediatrics* 47:831–838, 1971.

21

Bronchopulmonary Dysplasia

Philip, G. Rhodes, M.D., Glen R. Graves, M.D., and
Daksha M. Patel, M.D.

During the past 20 years much progress has been made in the care of infants with respiratory distress during the newborn period. In particular, improved care of newborns with hyaline membrane disease has resulted in lessened mortality in even more immature infants. In general, these results have occurred because of better respiratory support consequent to a better understanding of the disease process and its physiologic consequences. However, even with decreasing mortality there is a disturbing incidence of long-term complications of respiratory care. Chronic lung disease has occurred in a large number of infants as a consequence of respiratory care. Bronchopulmonary dysplasia is the particular term that has been used most in describing these infants with chronic lung disease [1]. In most cases these are infants who have had hyaline membrane disease, but in some cases this same chronic process has occurred in infants with meconium aspiration [2]. Table 21-1 gives a general description of the four stages of this disease process as described by Northway et al. [1]. In general, we and others have used stages three and four to describe the chronic process, whereas stages one and two are probably used to simply describe acute lung disease of great severity [3].

Northway and others have stressed high oxygen concentration and its toxicity in the causation of this chronic disease process [1,4]. However,

Table 21-1
Bronchopulmonary Dysplasia

Stage	Time (days)	Description
I	2–3	Hyaline membrane disease
II	4–10	Opacification
III	10–12	Blebs, pneumonia
IV	>15	Large blebs, scars

there has been much disagreement regarding this. Many feel that the process is the result of the combined effects of trauma related to pressure and delivery of oxygen at varying concentrations and not simply that of oxygen alone [5]. Direct airway trauma, primarily that of suctioning, may also play a part in this disease process. Changes in pulmonary interstitium resulting from a patent ductus arteriosus could also be important in contributing to chronic lung disease. A study by Moylan and Shannon indicates a prominent role of the effects of respiratory care and the endotracheal tube on the chronic disease process [6]. Thirty of 99 infants ventilated for hyaline membrane disease developed bronchopulmonary dysplasia, and of those 30 patients 12 had lower lobe (usually right) hyperinflation accompanied by upper lobe atelectasis. There is little question that the endotracheal tube itself contributes to airway pathology [7,8]. Similar lesions were reported by Miller et al., with autopsy results showing localized lesions in the right bronchi of obstructing granulation tissue [9]. Miller et al. ascribed these lesions to repeated trauma from routine suctioning.

That high environmental oxygen and the initial disease process play some role in the development of chronic lung disease is apparent from the studies by deLemos when he and coauthors ventilated lambs with room air and did not find chronic lung changes resulting from this [10]. The fact that the methodology of respiratory support plays a part in damaging lungs seems evident from reports of decreased chronic lung changes by ourselves and others using various ventilator care methods that decrease the amount of barotrauma delivered to infants with respiratory distress [2,11–13].

Because it was apparent that extremely few infants developed bronchopulmonary dysplasia findings in the absence of intubation and respirator care, various techniques of respirator management have been developed. Reynolds, et al. have introduced several modifications of respirator care, primarily decreasing peak pressures while lengthening the inspiratory time to achieve oxygenation with minimal change in CO_2 retention [14]. These investigators report a decrease in chronic lung changes with this methodology. We have reported a decreased incidence of chronic lung changes with the use of a mask in place of an endotracheal tube for the majority of infants requiring respirator support [2]. This, however, is a very difficult way of managing infants on the ventilator as it requires much nursing experience and skill. Subsequently, we have developed a protocol of care for infants with hyaline membrane disease who require the respirator [12]. The protocol emphasizes decreased overall pressures with minimal support. Intermittent mandatory ventilation is used on these infants at low rates. The indications for respirator care are apnea, oxygen needs of 100 percent, or an arterial pH below 7.20 associated with an elevated $PaCO_2$. The respirator rate is set at 20 to 28 per minute with an inspiratory time of 0.75 seconds and a peak inspiratory pressure of 18 cmH_2O. The positive end expiratory pressure is set at 4 cmH_2O at a flow of 5 to 10 L/minute. The respirator is a constant flow device allowing an intermittent mandatory ventilation (IMV) mode of operation (Baby Bird Respirator I or II; Bird Corp., Plam Springs, Calif.). During the past six months, all settings (inspiratory time, positive end expiratory pressure, mean airway pressure, peak inspiratory pressure, and rate) have been monitored electronically (Bird Mean Airway Pressure Monitor). Before that, mean airway pressure was calculated, inspiratory time was measured by a stop watch, the rate was counted, and peak inspiratory pressure and positive end expiratory pressure were measured by a manometer. Infants are cared for in the prone position, disturbed minimally (vital signs are taken from monitors), and not suctioned routinely. Suctioning is only performed when there is definite evidence of increased secretions. The hematocrit is kept at greater than 40 percent through packed red blood cell transfusion. The ductus arteriosus is ligated either medically or surgically by at least one week of age if its presence is demonstrated by contrast echo or by exam (murmur, increased pulse pressure, and enlarged heart). If the PaO_2 drops below 35 mmHg, the $PaCO_2$ is elevated, and there is a radiographic appearance of hyaline membrane disease, then peak pressure is raised 2 cmH_2O until the PaO_2 is again greater than 35 mmHg. The same procedure is followed if the pH drops below 7.20 and is associated with high oxygen needs or elevated $PaCO_2$ or both. Approximately 10 to 15 percent of the infants will become apneic or develop gasping respirations and are then placed on a respirator rate of 60 or more. Most of these infants are those less than 1,500 g who seem to have little respiratory reserve. Pressures are weaned back by 2 cmH_2O decrements as soon as the pH reaches 7.25 and the PaO_2 is greater than 60 mmHg. It is our belief that there is no way possible to achieve "normal blood gases" with severely diseased lungs without the dangers of overinflation, lung rupture, and barotrauma to those lung units that are at least partially functioning during this period of time. Because hyaline membrane disease is self-limited as long as no damage occurs, we feel that it is best to avoid the dangers of barotrauma and overinflation during the acute disease process. The survival rate of infants so cared for (respirator) is 79 percent overall, with a low incidence of bronchopulmonary dysplasia and pneumothorax (Table 21–2). The incidence of intraventicular hemorrhage is approximately 35 percent in infants

Table 21–2
Bronchopulmonary Dysplasia
(BFD) in Infants on Respirator for
Hyaline Membrane Disease

Number	BPD	Survival
168	6 (4%)	79%

less than 1,500 g among this population. This incidence no greater than that currently being reported [15,16]. Developmental problems are no different than those currently being reported in the very-low-birth-weight population. These results indicate that infants with hyaline membrane disease can survive the acute disease process with a minimum of chronic lung disease.

There is still much to be learned concerning appropriate care of newborns with hyaline membrane disease. Much more work is still needed in order to evaluate the most appropriate respirator care for these infants and the exact reasons for the lower incidence of bronchopulmonary dysplasma in those cared for with the described protocol. However, we believe that chronic lung changes and the acute trauma of pneumothoraces can be lessened when barotrauma is carefully limited.

The long-term follow-up of infants with bronchopulmonary dysplasia is an extremely difficult and expensive process. Careful monitoring of cardiac status through echocardiography can help determine oxygen needs [17,18]. Transcutaneous oxygen monitors can help in determining oxygenation status in the hospital and at home [19].

Innovative programs are needed and are being evaluted on different methods of long-term care that would decrease expense and family disruption. These infants are commonly in the hospital for six months to two years with their long-term oxygen needs and intermittent admissions for respiratory insufficiency [20]. Lung mechanisms do improve with age if these infants can be maintained [21]. Some are now being cared for in the home with a strong supportive program. The best answer to this problem is, of course, prevention of the disease process. More innovative ideas and research are needed for the long-term care of these difficult-to-treat infants.

References

1. Northway, W.H., Jr., Rosan, R.C., Porter, D.Y. Pulmonary disease following respirator therapy of hyaline-membrane disease. *N. Engl. J. Med.* 276:357–368, 1967.
2. Rhodes, P.G., Hall, R.T., Leonidas, J.C. Chronic pulmonary disease in neonates with assisted ventilation. *Pediatrics* 55:788–796, 1975.

3. Bancalari, E., Abdenour, G.E., Feller, R., Gannon, J. Bronchopulmonary dysplasia: clinical presentation. *J. Pediatr.* 85:819–823, 1979.

4. Boat, T.F. Studies of oxygen toxicity in cultured human neonatal respiratory epithelium. *J. Pediatr.* 85:916–919, 1979.

5. Philip, A.G.S. Oxygen plus pressure plus time: the etiology of bronchopulmonary dysplasia. *Pediatrics* 55:44–50, 1975.

6. Moylan, F.M.B., Shannon, D.C. Preferential distribution of lobar emphysema and atelectasis in brochopulmonary dysplasia. *Pediatrics* 63:130–134, 1979.

7. Blanc, V.F., Tremblay, N.A.G. The complications of tracheal intubation: a new classification with a review of the literature. *Anesth. Analg.* 53:202–213, 1974.

8. Joshi, V.V., Mandavia, S.G., Stern, L., Wiglesworth, F.W. Acute lesions induced by endotracheal intubation. *Am. J. Dis. Child.* 124:646–649, 1972.

9. Miller, K.E., Edwards, D.K., Hilton, S.. Acquired lobar emphysema in premature infants with brochopulmonary dysplasia: an iatrogenic disease? *Radiology* 138:589–592, 1981.

10. de Lemos, R., Wolfsdorf, J., Nachman, R., et al. Lung injury from oxygen in lambs: the role of artificial ventilation. *Anesthesiology* 30:609–618, 1969.

11. Taghizadeh, A., Reynolds, E.O.R. Pathogenesis of bronchopulmonary dysplasia following hyaline membrane disease. *Am. J. Pathol.* 82:241–258, 1976.

12. Rhodes, P.G., Graves, G.R., Patel, D.M., et al. Minimizing pneumothorax and bronchopulmonary dyslasia in ventilated infants with hyaline membrane disease. *J. Pediatr.* 103:634–637, 1983.

13. Stern, L., Ramos, A.D., Outerbridge, E.W., Beaudry, P.H. Negative pressure artificial respiration: use in treatment of respiratory failure of the newborn. *Can. Med. Assoc. J.* 102:595–601, 1970.

14. Reynolds, E.O.R. Effect of alterations in mechanical ventilator settings on pulmonary gas exchange in hyaline membrane disease. *Arch. Dis. Child.* 46:152–159, 1971.

15. Papile, L.-A., Burstein, J., Burstein, R., Koffler, H. Incidence and evolution of subependymal and intraventricular hemorrhage: a study of infants with birth weights less than 1,500 gm. *J. Pediatr.* 92:529–534, 1978.

16. Partridge, J.C., Babcock, D.S., Steichen, J.J., Han, B.K. Optimal timing for diagnostic cranial ultrasound in low-birth-weight infants: detection of intracranial hemorrhage and ventricular dilation. *J. Pediatr.* 102:281–287, 1983.

17. Halliday, H.L., Dumpit, F.M., Brady, J.P. Effects of inspired oxygen on echocardiographic assessment of pulmonary vascular resistance and myocardial contractility in bronchopulmonary dysplasia. *Pediatrics* 65:536–540, 1980.

18. Fouron, J.-C., Le Guennec, J.-C, Villemant, D., et al. Value of echocardiography in assessing the outcome of bronchopulmonary dysplasia of the newborn. *Pediatrics* 65:529–535, 1980.

19. Philip, A.G.S., Peabody, J.L., Lucey, J.F. Transcutaneous PO_2 monitoring in the home management of brochopulmonary dysplasia. *Pediatrics* 61:655–657, 1978.

20. Vohr, B.R., Bell, E.F., Oh, W. Infants with bronchopulmonary dysplasia. *Am. J. Dis. Child.* 136:443–447, 1982.

21. Morray, J.P., Fox, W.W., Kettrick, R.G., Downes, J.J. Improvement in lung mechanics as a function of age in the infant with severe bronchopulmonary dysplasia. *Pediatr. Res.* 16:290–294, 1982.

22

Congenital Abdominal Wall Defects

Michael D. Klein, M.D.*

Definition

Congenital abdominal wall defects are characterized by intraabdominal contents being present at birth outside the abdominal cavity and uncovered by normal skin. Omphalocele is the classic anomaly in this category. It consists of a large defect, centered at the umbilicus and covered with a translucent membrane. The contents of the hernia sac may include stomach, intestine, liver, and occasionally other abdominal organs (Figure 22–1). Another congenital abdominal wall defect is umbilical cord hernia. This is a small defect, centered at the umbilicus and also covered with a translucent membrane. In this case the sac contains only the midgut (Figure 22–2). The third anomaly in this group is gastroschisis (called ruptured cord hernia by some). This is also a small defect, but it is just to the right of the umbilical cord. There is no sac covering the herniated midgut, which

*I express my indebtedness to Jack H. Hertzler, M.D., who shared his large experience in treating children with congenital abdominal wall defects with me. It is out of our many conversations that my interest in, and many of my concepts of congenital abdominal wall defects developed. I also express graditude to Olive Grimm and Larry Stein, who collected and collated the data from the Children's Hospital of Michigan that form the factual basis for these concepts and to Michelle Hoffman for her careful preparation of the manuscript.

Figure 22–1

Omphalocele, lateral fold defect. The eviscerated abdominal contents are contained within a sac continuous with the umbilical cord. Both liver and intestine are present. The defect is large, and the rectus muscles insert broadly on the costal margin, leaving a depression just below the xyphoid.

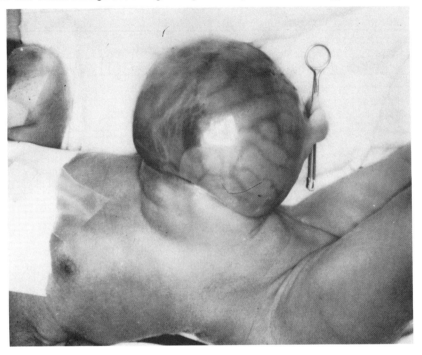

is usually edematous, matted, and firm. A portion of stomach or a gonad may also be herniated, but not the liver or other organs (Figure 22–3).

Not included in this group of anomalies is umbilical hernia, which is covered with normal skin and frequently closes spontaneously during infancy or early childhood.

The prune belly syndrome (also called congenital abdominal wall muscular deficiency syndrome) is not included with congenital abdominal wall defects. In this disorder the muscles are present, but there is a deficiency in the number of muscle cells and there is very little muscle tone. The same muscular deficiency is often present in other abdominal structures such as the ureters and bladder, leading to clinically significant problems.

Incidence

Congenital abdominal defects occur aproximately once in every 2,500 live births [1]. They are the most frequent congenital anomaly requiring op-

Figure 22-2

Umbilical cord hernia. The eviscerated abdominal contents are only midgut. They are covered by a translucent sac continuous with the umbilical cord. The defect is small, and the upper abdominal wall is normal, with the rectus muscles inserting near the midline at the xyphoid.

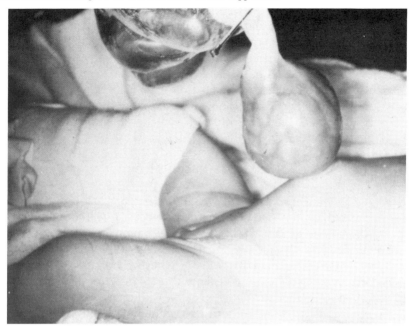

Figure 22-3

Gastroschisis or ruptured cord hernia. Midgut is eviscerated to the right of a normal umbilical cord. Most of the abdominal wall is normal. The intestine appears shortened, edematous, and matted together.

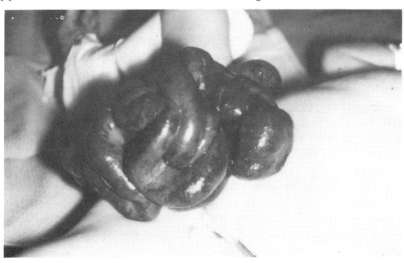

eration by a pediatric surgeon in the newborn period [2]. A change in the incidence of the several types of congenital abdominal wall defects is occurring [3,4], with gastroschisis becoming more frequent. Gastroschisis was formerly thought to be a rare anomaly [5,6]. Hagemeyer [7] reviewed the world literature in 1955 and found 10 cases with 4 survivors. Examining reports from the world literature after 1960, there are 786 cases of congenital abdominal wall defects, of which 38 percent are gastroschisis. In the series from the Children's Hospital of Michigan from 1958 to 1963, 22 percent were gastroschisis, whereas from 1964 to 1979, 45 percent were gastroschisis [8]. Other reports show an even more dramatic shift away from omphalocele and umbilical cord hernia and toward gastroschisis [3,9].

Historical Perspective

Congenital abdominal wall defects were first described in the 16th century [10]. In the 19th century the first treatment successes were reported [11–13]. By the middle of this century reports of multiple successful repairs were published [14–17]. Initially, the mortality of such defects treated surgically was 40 to 50 percent [18]. In 1967, Schuster [19] reported a method of obtaining early fascial closure of these defects using prosthetic material. This addition to therapeutic choices, along with improved neonatal care for the control of temperature, artificial ventilation, and total parenteral nutrition, has resulted in improved survival rates of 60 to 90 percent [4,8,20–23]

Embryology and Clinical Correlation

Many theories of embryogenesis of congential abdominal wall defects have been proposed. All are based on an understanding of normal human anatomy and embryology and speculate on what developmental aberration might have occurred. Most clinicians now agree with Duhamel's [24] interpretation of abdominal wall formation, which is a result of the German embryologic research of the 1920s and 1930s [25–27]. Duhamel postulated that the underlying cause of omphalocele was the failure of the migration of the primary body folds, which occurs when the flat disc embryo forms an enclosed body cavity (Figure 22-4). This results in an actual lack of abdominal wall and a large (greater than 4 cm) defect. The eviscerated abdominal contents are contained in a sac of amnion and chorion extending from the gaping body wall to the umbilical cord. The rectus muscle insertions are widely separated on the costal margins and not in the midline. The sac contents include liver, small bowel, and colon as well as other abdominal organs on occasion. The folding of the embryonic disc to en-

272

Figure 22–4

Abdominal wall folding, three to four weeks gestation. A) The flat disc embryo with the heart in front of the head and the bladder behind the sacrum. B) Folding occurs both laterally and at the caudal and cephalic ends. The yolk sac is continuous with the primitive gut. C) Pleuroperitoneal canals have formed and then been divided by the septum transversum or diaphragm which comes with the cephalic fold. The yolk sac will be resorbed, and the gut will have a primitive attachment to this through the vitelline duct.

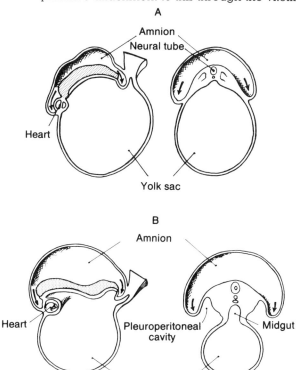

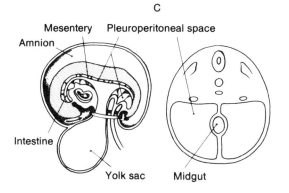

Figure 22–5

Omphalocele, caudal fold defect. There is an infraumbilical omphalocele and an imperforate anus. The intussuscepted ileum appears in the midline, and a portion of exstrophied bladder is on either side of the intussuscepted ileum. *(From Klein, M.D., Koloske, A.M., Hertzler, J.H. Congenital defects of the abdominal wall. J. Am. Med. Assoc. 245:1643–1646, 1981.)*

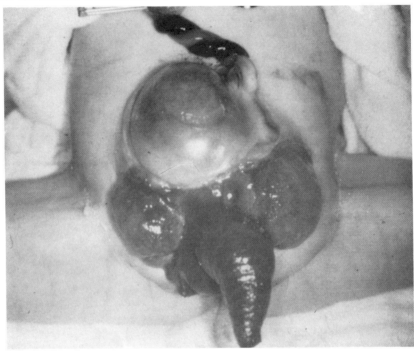

close the body cavity occurs between three and four weeks after fertilization, when organogenesis is most active [28,29]. This, any insult affecting these folds could be expected to result in anomalies of other organ systems. Children with omphaloceles do actually have an increased incidence of other anomalies, as high as 70 percent in some series [8].

Whereas the classic omphalocele is a failure of the lateral embryonic folds to enclose the pleuroperitoneal canals, there are also caudal and cephalic somatic folds. In the disc embryo, the heart is in front of the brain, and the bladder is behind the sacrum. As these folds occur the bladder is carried forward with the anterior abdominal wall, and the heart and diaphragm are similarly brought around. Failure of caudal fold migration results in a vesicointestinal fissure or cloacal exstrophy. This anomaly includes an infraumbilical omphalocele, exstrophy of the bladder, and imperforate anus (Figure 22–5). Failure of cephalic fold migration results in a syndrome described by Cantrell et al. [30] including a supraum-

Figure 22–6

Omphalocele, cephalic fold defect. There is a supraumbilical omphalocele. A sternal cleft and pericardial and diaphragmatic defects allow the heart to be outside the body wall. *(From Klein, M.D., Koloske, A.M., Hertzler, J.H., Congenital defects of the abdominal wall. J. Am. Med. Assoc. 245:1643–1646, 1981.)*

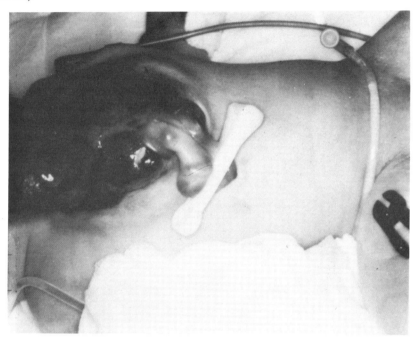

bilical omphalocele, a sternal cleft, an intracardiac anomaly, and pericardial and diaphragmatic defects (Figure 22–6). Successful reconstruction of caudal fold defects is possible by a series of operative procedures. However, there have been very few reported survivors with cephalic fold defects, primarily due to obstruction to the great vessels from attempts to reposition the heart within the thorax and the associated intracardiac anomalies.

Children with an umbilical cord hernia have an apparently normal abdominal wall with a slightly enlarged umbilical ring. Small bowel alone is present in a translucent hernia sac at the base of the cord. Benson et al. [17] separated this from other congenital abdominal wall defects. They postulated that this anomaly represents a failure of the normally herniated, elongating midgut to return to the abdominal cavity from the umbilical celom (Figure 22–7). This event normally occurs at about 10 to 12 weeks after fertilization, when organogenesis is nearly complete.

Figure 22–7

Midgut herniation, 6 through 12 weeks of gestation. A) The umbilical ring and body wall has been formed. The midgut is a straight tube connected to the yolk sac by the vitelinne or omphalomesenteric duct. B) Elongation of the midgut occurs resulting in herniation into the umbilical celom. C) The yolk sac involutes, and the midgut begins to return to the abdominal cavity, where it will rotate and fix to the posterior abdominal wall. D) The midgut has returned to the abdominal cavity, and the umbilical celom is obliterated.

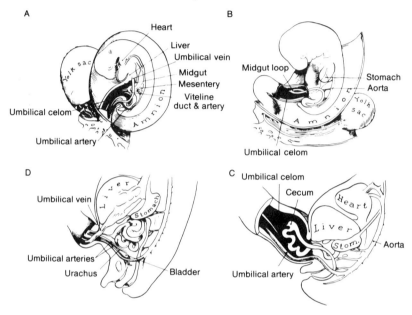

These children may be expected to have relatively few associated congenital anomalies.

There are many theories advanced to explain the embryogenesis of gastroschisis. I find most satisfying the proposal that the primary problem is agenesis of the umbilical celom, which normally forms in the connecting stalk (umbilical cord) during the sixth week after fertilization to allow for the herniation of the elongating midgut. When there is no cavity for the midgut, it ruptures out through the base of the cord. This occurs preferentially to the right through the defect remaining where the right umbilical vein resorbs before herniation occurs and just after the primary folds are completed. The resorbtion of this vein leaves some weakness in that portion of the umbilicus (Figure 22–8). The child with gastroschisis has a nearly normal abdominal wall with the rectus muscles inserting normally at the xyphoid. Children with gastroschisis are often premature, perhaps because the presence of intestine in the amniotic fluid is a stimulus for the uterus to empty [31]. They have fewer associated anomalies than chil-

Figure 22–8

Development of gastroschisis or ruptured cord hernia. The umbilical celom has not formed. The elongating intestine ruptures out to the right of the umbilical cord through the fascial defect left by the resorbing right umbilical vein. The intestinal loops then lie free within the amniotic fluid.

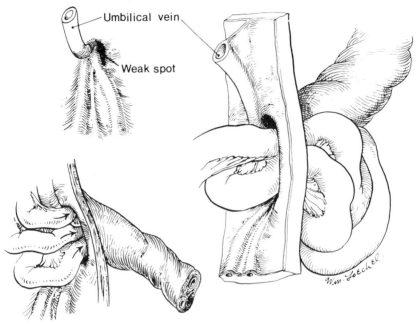

dren with omphalocele, probably because the insult occurs later in embryogenesis. The intestine is indurated and edematous from floating in amniotic fluid [32].

Many agents, including dexamethasone, have been demonstrated to create abdominal wall defects in the offspring of experimental animals [33–35)]. On examining the specimens most of these abdominal wall defects induced by teratogens appear to be gastroschisis.

All children with congenital abdominal wall defects must be considered to have a malrotation. The intestine has never returned to the abdominal cavity from the physiologic herniation into the umbilical celom, and therefore cannot have rotated and fixed to the posterior abdominal wall.

Antenatal diagnosis of congenital abdominal wall defects has become possible with ultrasound, although this cannot as yet distinguish between the varieties unless the liver is clearly visualized in the defect [36]. Congenital abdominal wall defects are associated with false-positive alpha-fetoprotein levels when this test is used for the antenatal diagnosis of myelodysplasia [37,38]. It has been unclear whether elevated alpha-fetoprotein in maternal serum and amniotic fluid detects all abdominal defects or only gastroschisis.

Evaluation and Treatment of Infants with Congenital Abdominal Wall Defects

The difficulty in treating babies with omphalocele is evidenced by the high mortality before current neonatal intensive care techniques. When the membrane is intact, there is no immediate danger. The mass gives the patient a larger surface area, and heat loss can be significant. Fluid tends to accumulate in the eviscerated bowel and liver, and the blood volume must be maintained with at least twice maintenance intravenous fluids [39]. An orogastric or nasogastric tube adequate for decompression (10-Fr sumped tube) should be placed immediately to suction to prevent distension of the bowel loops. A digital rectal examination is helpful in evacuating meconium from the distal bowel. Sepsis is a serious risk, and broad-spectrum intravenous antibiotics are required. As with all newborns it must be documented that 1 mg of vitamin K has been administered to prevent hemorrhagic disease of the newborn. The child should be assessed for other congenital anomalies, and management of these should be begun.

The baby can go to the operating room as soon as reasonably possible. There is no advantage in delaying the procedure, and any delay compounds the difficulties of maintaining temperature and blood volume as well as exposing the child to the risk of sac rupture or separation and ensuing sepsis. Attempts to treat patients with omphalocele by painting the sac with antiseptic solutions [40,41] have been employed when current prosthetic materials and artificial ventilation were not available. This method of treatment may still be required if an intracardiac defect demands repair before abdominal closure, but the complications of separation of the sac from the abdominal wall and sepsis are frequent, and the process of total coverage often takes months and not weeks.

The first operative procedure successful for large omphaloceles was a skin closure in which the sac is excised and flaps of skin are dissected up, often all the way around to the back, and used to cover the bowel [42]. A secondary procedure is then necessary to close the remaining hernia. This can be hazardous, with loops of bowel densely adherent to the skin. In addition it is often not successful, as the bowel continues to grow in the skin sac outside the abdominal cavity. The abdominal cavity does not enlarge enough to prevent replacement at the time of the secondary procedure. To overcome this, Schuster [19] developed the prosthetic closure. The material used for this closure has changed, but Schuster's principles are still maintained. The sac is excised, and the prosthesis (usually a Dacron mesh incorporated in a silicone rubber sheet) is sutured to the fascia and then to itself. The skin is not closed, and the child can return to the neonatal intensive care unit. The prosthesis is gradually tightened until the abdominal cavity enlarges. The child can then be returned to the operating room to have the prosthesis removed and a fascial closure performed. Wesley et al. [43] have devised an important addition to this technique. By monitoring the intragastric pressure with a water manometer through the nasogastric or gastrostomy tube, the prosthesis may be tightened more rapidly than was originally thought possible, often twice a day. This allows it to be removed in three to seven days and greatly reduces the chances for separation and sepsis. Additional intraoperative procedures such as appendectomy, gastrostomy, Meckel's diverticulectomy, and Ladd's procedure are not performed at the time of abdominal wall closure.

Skin flap closure can be successful if all of the intestine is replaced first and the liver is then reduced beneath the costal and rectus margins. Then postoperatively the patient can be fitted with an abdominal binder that serves to provide physiologic intraabdominal pressure as a stimulus for growth of the intraabdominal cavity in the same way that Schuster's prosthesis does. Usually, between six months and two years of age the child can return to have the residual ventral hernia repaired. The rectus muscles can never be totally apposed in the midline superiorly because of their lateral attachment on the costal margin. Fortunately, the liver closes this defect effectively.

Many omphaloceles can now be closed primarily employing a combination of operative techniques and postoperative care procedures. Muscle relaxants are employed during anesthesia, and the abdominal wall is manually and gently but forcefully stretched. A gastrostomy is not used, since this takes up almost one fourth of the abdominal cavity. In the postoperative period artificial ventilation is often required, and care must be taken to observe the patient for signs of vena caval or renal vein obstruction. If there is a saphenous intravenous line placed to gravity, it will often slow down and stop as the intraabdominal pressure becomes dangerously high. Sometimes replacement of the liver in the abdomen acutely angulates the hepatic veins at the vena cava with resulting hypotension and acidosis. Use of gradual reduction with a prosthesis is then definitely indicated. Usually the tightness and edema of the abdominal wall resolve over three to seven days.

Postoperative care requires careful attention to fluid status. These children often require large amounts of fluid in the first 24 to 48 hours postoperatively and then begin to diurese rapidly. Nasogastric suction and antibiotics are maintained, and the patient is weaned from the ventilator as rapidly as possible. The intestine in the omphalocele is usually quite normal, having been protected from the amniotic fluid by the sac, so that feeding can begin when signs of intestinal motility appear.

The management of gastroschisis follows closely the principles outlined for omphalocele, with some exceptions. It is more difficult to prevent heat loss in patients with gastroschisis, since the bowel loops are not covered by a sac. It is important not to use saline-soaked gauze alone to cover the intestine initially. The evaporative heat loss is greater than the heat provided during the short time the saline is warm. The gauze can be wrapped with plastic food wrap to reduce evaporation, or more simply, the child can be placed in a plastic bag such as a bowel bag up to the axillae. Gastroschisis can almost always be closed primarily without skin flaps or a prosthesis because abdominal wall formation is normal [44]. The bowel in gastroschisis is definitely abnormal due to the chemical peritonitis from prolonged exposure to the amniotic fluid. These patients will need intravenous nutrition for two weeks or more [45]. In gastroschisis, associated gastrointestinal anomalies such as atresias are not treated during the initial procedure because of the indurated and edematous nature of the bowel wall. If an atresia is noted at the time of gastroschisis repair (and often it cannot be seen as the loops are so matted together), the abdomen is closed, nasogastric suction is maintained, and hyperalimentation is instituted. Two to three weeks later, when the bowel is more normal in character and the abdominal wall and cavity have adapted, a second procedure can be carried out to deal with the atresia. Patients with gastroschisis do not have the incidence of associated anomalies that the patients with omphalocele do, but they are more often premature or small for gestational age with their own particular problems. Babies with an omphalocele that ruptures during delivery combine the problems of omphalocele with many of those of gastroschisis.

Umbilical cord hernias can be treated very much like simple umbilical hernias. The midgut returns nicely to the abdominal cavity, the sac is excised, and rectus edges are dissected out and closed. A cosmetically acceptable umbilicus can usually be created.

References

1. Lindham, S. Omphalocele and gastroschisis in Sweden 1965–1976. *Acta Paediatr. Scand.* 70:55–60, 1981.
2. Ravitch, M.M., Barton, B.A. The need for pediatric surgeons as determined by the volume of work and the mode of delivery of surgical care. *Surgery* 76:754–763, 1974.
3. Moore, T.C. Gastroschisis and omphalocele: clinical differences. *Surgery* 82:561–568, 1977.
4. Mayer, T., Black, R., Matlak, M.E., Johnson, D.G. Gastroschisis and omphalocele. *Ann. Surg.* 192:783–787, 1980.
5. Bernstein, P. Gastroschisis, a rare teratological condition in the newborn. *Arch. Pediatr.* 57:505–513, 1940.

6. Warkany, J. *Congenital Malformations: Notes and Comments.* Chicago, Year Book Medical Publishers, 1981, pp. 758–764.
7. Hagemeyer, W. Uber eine Gastroschisis. *Zentralbl. Chir.* 80:1987–1991, 1955.
8. Klein, M.D., Hertzler, J.H. Congenital defects of the abdominal wall. *Surg. Gynecol. Obstet.* 152:805–808, 1981.
9. Klein, M.D., Kosloske, A.M., Hertzler, J.H. Congenital defects of the abdominal wall. *J. Am. Med. Assoc.* 245:1643–1646, 1981.
10. Lycosthenes, W.C. *Prodigiorum ac Ostentorum Chronicon.* Basle: H Petri, 1557, p. 596.
11. Hey, W. *Practical Observations in Surgery.* London: Cadell & Davis, 1803.
12. Visick, A. An umbilical hernia in the newly born child. *Lancet* 1:829, 1873.
13. Olshausen, R. Zur Therapie der Nabelschnurhernien. *Arch. Gynak.* 29:443, 1887.
14. Herbert, A.F. Hernia funiculi umbilicalis, with report of three cases. *Am. J. Obstet. Gynecol.* 15:86–88, 1928.
15. Gross, R.E. Blodgett, J.B. Omphalocele (umbilical eventration) in the newly born. *Surg. Gynecol. Obstet.* 71:520–527, 1940.
16. O'Leary, C.M., Clymer, C.E. Umbilical hernia. *Am. J. Surg.* 52:38–43, 1941.
17. Benson, C.D., Penberthy, G.C., Hill, G.C. Hernia into the umbilical cord and omphalocele (amniocele) in the newborn. *Arch. Surg.* 58:833–847, 1949.
18. Hutchin, P. Somatic anomalies of the umbilicus and anterior abdominal wall. *Surg. Gynecol. Obstet.* 120:1075–1090, 1965.
19. Schuster, S. A new method for the staged repair of large omphaloceles. *Surg. Gynecol. Obstet.* 125:837–850, 1967.
20. Hasse, W., Maholo, P. Omphalocele and gastroschisis. *Prog. Pediatr. Surg.* 13:71–73, 1979.
21. Stringel, G., Filler, R.M. Prognostic factors in omphalocele and gastroschisis. *J. Pediatr. Surg.* 14:515–519, 1979.
22. Fonkalsrud, E.W. Selective repair of neonatal gastroschisis based on degree of visceroabdominal disporportion. *Ann. Surg.* 191:139–144, 1980.
23. Helardot, P., Foucard, C., Bienaymé, J. L'omphalocele: une malformation curable. *J. Gynecol. Obstet. Biol. Reprod. (Paris)* 9:267–272, 1980.
24. Duhamel, B. Embryology of exomphalos and allied malforamtions. *Arch. Dis. Child.* 38:142–147, 1963.
25. Pernkopf, E. Die Entwicklung der Form des Magendarm Kanales beim Menschen. II. Die weitene Ausbildung der form des Mitteldarmes und des Pankreas angefangen vom Zeitpunkt des Auftretens der ersten Dunn darmschlingen. *Z. Gesamte Anat.* 77:1–143, 1925.
26. Politzer, G., Sternberg, H. Über die Entwicklung der ventralen Körperwand und des Nabelstranges beim Menschen. *Z. Gesamte Anat.* 92:279–379, 1930.
27. Sternberg, H., Politzer, G. Über die formale Genese derFehlbildungen des Nabelstranges und der ventralen Körperwand, nebst Beschreibung eines ein-schlugigen Falles. *Beitr. Pathol. Anat.*, 88:150–192, 1931.
28. Witschi, E. Characterization of developmental stages: I. Man. In Altman, P. L., Dittmer, D.S. (eds.), *Biology Data Book,* 2nd edn. Bethesda, Md.: Federation of American Societies for Experimental Biology, 1972, pp. 176–178.
29. Moore, K.C. *The Developing Human,* 2nd ed. Philadephia, The W. B. Saunders Co., 1977.

30. Cantrell, J.R., Haller, J.A., Jr., Ravitch, M.M. A syndrome of congenital defects involving the abdominal wall, sternum, diaphragm, pericardium and heart. *Surg. Gynecol. Obstet.* 107:602–614, 1958.
31. Colombani, P.M., Cunningham, M.D. Perinatal aspects of omphalocele and gastroschisis. *Am. J. Dis. Child.* 131:1386–1388, 1977.
32. Sherman, N.J., Asch, M.J., Isaacs, H., Jr., Rosenkrantz, J.G. Experimental gastroschisis in the fetal rabbit. *J. Pediatr. Surg.* 8:165–169, 1973.
33. Vannier, B., Jequier, R., Jude, A. Sensibilitié du rat Wistar à láction teratogene de la dexaméthasone. *C. R. Soc. Biol. (Paris)* 163:1269–1272, 1969.
34. Lane, G.A., Nahrwold, M.L., Tait, A.R., et al. Anesthetics as teratogens: nitrous oxide is fetotoxic xenon is not. *Science* 210:899–901, 1980.
35. Thompson, D.J., Molello, J.A., Strebing, R.J., Dyke, I.L. Reproduction and teratological studies with 1-(2-chloroethyl)-3-cyclohexyl-1-nitrosourea (CCNU) in the rat and rabbit. *Toxicol. Appl. Pharmacol.* 34:456–466, 1975.
36. Canty, T.G., Leopold, G.R., Wolf, D.A. Maternal ultrasonography for the antenatal diagnosis of surgically significant neonatal anomalies. *Ann. Surg.* 194:353–365, 1981.
37. Young, J.L., Crawford, J.W. Omphalocele and raised alpha-fetoprotein in maternal serum. *Br. J. Obstet. Gynaecol.* 84:578–579, 1977.
38. Wald, N.J., Cuckle, H.S., Barlow, R.D., et al. Early antenatal diagnosis of exomphalos. *Lancet* 1:1368–1369, 1980.
39. Philippart, A.I., Canty, T.G., Filler, R.M. Acute fluid volume requirements in infants with anterior abdominal wall defects. *J. Pediatr. Surg.* 7:553–558, 1972.
40. Ahlfeld, F. Der Alkohol bei der Behandlung inoperabeler Bauch Bruche. *Monatsschr. Geburtsh. Gynaekol.* 10:124–125, 1889.
41. Grob, M. Conservative treatment of exomphalos. *Arch. Dis. Child.* 38:148–150, 1963.
42. Gross, R.E. A new method for surgical treatment of large omphaloceles. *Surgery* 24:277–292, 1948.
43. Wesley, J.R., Drongowski, R., Coran, A.G. Intragastric pressure measurement: a guide for reduction and closure of the silastic chimney in omphalocele and gastroschisis. *J. Pediatr. Surg.* 16:264–270, 1981.
44. Filston, H.C. Gastroschisis—primary fascial closure. *Ann. Surg.* 197:260–264, 1983.
45. Touloukian, R.J., Spackman, T.J. Gastrointestinal function and radiographic appearance following gastroschisis repair. *J. Pediatr. Surg.* 6:427–434, 1971.

23

Neonatal Polycythemia/ Hyperviscosity

Edward A. Liechty, M.D., and Richard L. Schreiner, M.D.

Neonatal polycythemia/hyperviscosity is relatively common in newborns, although until recently it had received little attention in the pediatric literature. Sequelae secondary to polycythemia/hyperviscosity may be severe, but most infants appear asymptomatic and have a normal outcome. The relationship between an elevated hematocrit (polycythemia) and elevated blood viscosity (hyperviscosity) is complex. Although a hematocrit is easily determined in any laboratory, the capability to determine blood viscosity is unavailable in most hospitals. The purpose of this chapter is to review the incidence, etiology, clinical presentation, and treatment of polycythemia as well as the relationship between polycythemia and hyperviscosity, the methods of measuring viscosity, and the results of the few long-term follow-up studies of infants with polycythemia/hyperviscosity.

Polycythemia

INCIDENCE

The incidence of polycythemia varies according to the definition accepted, site and time of blood sampling, and laboratory method for determination of the hematocrit. Cord blood hemoglobin concentration averages about

Figure 23-1

Changes in venous hematocrit and whole blood viscosity with increasing postnatal age. *(Modified from Shohat, M., Salomon, H., Reisner, M.B., et al. Neonatal Polycythemia: II. Definition related to time of sampling.* Pediatrics *73:11-13, 1984.)*

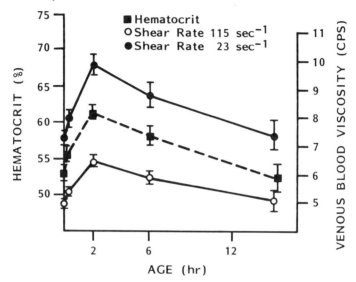

17 mg/dl; hemoglobin values from the umbilical artery are about 0.5 mg/dl higher. During the first two to four hours after birth a redistribution of plasma water occurs, which decreases total blood volume and plasma volume, whereas red cell volume remains stable (Figure 23-1). This results in an increase in the hemoglobin concentration and the hematocrit. This effect is most pronounced in infants who have received an excessive placental transfusion at birth.

There are also significant differences in hemoglobin concentration and hematocrit between simultaneously obtained venipuncture and capillary samples. The capillary values average 5 to 10 percent greater than the venipuncture samples, although there is no clinically useful relationship (Figure 23-2). The greatest discrepancies are in premature infants, especially those of less than 30 weeks gestation, infants with acidosis, and infants with poor vascular perfusion. Postnatally there is persistence of the capillary-venous hematocrit and hemoglobin difference for up to 10 weeks in premature infants and 4 to 6 weeks in full-term infants [1].

In addition to these physiologic variations in hematocrit and hemoglobin concentrations, there are also variations among different laboratory methods. The packed red cell volume determined by the microhematocrit method is slightly but consistently higher than the hematocrit determined

Figure 23–2

Scatter plot of simultaneously determined capillary and venipuncture hematocrit measurements. Note that while the capillary values are in general greater, the variability precludes clinical usefulness. *(Modified from Linderkamp, O., Klose, H. J., Betke, K., et al. Increased blood viscosity in patients with cyanotic congenital heart disease and iron deficiency.* J. Pediatr. *95:567–569, 1979.)*

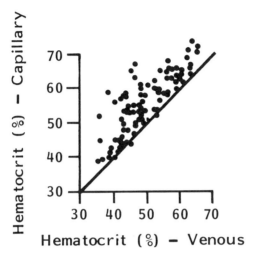

by an automated electronic particle counter. The slope of the correlation regression line is 10 percent greater than identity; thus, although the absolute differences between the two methods tend to be small, the greatest divergence is seen at higher hematocrit measurements. No such systematic differences are seen between hemoglobin concentrations determined by hemoglobinometers and electronic particle counters [2].

When polycythemia is defined as a hematocrit from a "central" (e.g., antecubital) vein greater than 65 percent, the incidence is approximately 1 to 4 percent of all live-born infants (Table 23–1). Although the majority of these infants are appropriately grown for gestational age, a dispropor-

Table 23–1
Incidence of Polycythemia[a]

Study	Reference	Incidence (%)
Rawlings	[4]	0.8
Wirth et al.	[3]	4
Stevens and Wirth	[5]	1.8
Ramamurthy	[6]	2.2

[a] Definition of polycythemia is a hematocrit ≥ 65 percent on peripheral venous blood.

tionate number have some abnormality of intrauterine growth. In studies conducted in Denver [3] and at sea level [4–6], approximately 20 percent of polycythemic infants have been small for gestational age, and an additional 20 percent have been large for gestational age, with 60 percent appropriately grown for gestational age.

ETIOLOGY

The etiology of polycythemia may be related to either increased fetal erythropoiesis or to passive transfusion of blood to the infant (Table 23–2). Maternal smoking may decrease uterine blood flow, thereby reducing tranplacental oxygen transfer [7], and may also result in elevated fetal carbon monoxide levels, reducing the oxygen-carrying capacity of fetal blood; both of these aberrations of fetal oxygenation may increase erythropoiesis.

The incidence of hyperviscosity is approximately 15 to 20 percent in the infant who is small for his gestational age [8]. Although the precise pathogenetic relationships responsible for this incidence are not clear, it seems reasonable to postulate suboptimal oxygen supply to the fetus as the primary factor. Placental oxygen transfer depends upon several factors, including relative uterine and umbilical blood flows, oxygen-carrying capacities, partial pressures of oxygen and carbon dioxide, and oxygen diffusability [9]. Maternal hypertensive vascular diseases may decrease uterine blood flow. Placental villitis may decrease oxygen diffusability.

Table 23–2
Etiology of Polycythemia

Increased erythropoiesis
    "Placental insufficiency"
    Maternal vascular disease
    Congenital infections
    Preeclampsia
Maternal smoking
Trisomies 13, 18, 21
Maternal hypoxemia (e.g., heart disease)
Congenital adrenal hyperplasia
Neonatal hyperthyroidism
Fetal hyperinsulinemia/hyperglycemia
    Maternal diabetes
    Beckwith's syndrome
Passive transfusion
    Delayed cord clamping
    Maternal-fetal transfusion
    Twin-twin transfusion

Placental infarctions, shunts, or abruptions decrease surface area available for oxygen diffusion. Any of these factors may act to decrease transplacental oxygen flux. The fetus attempts to compensate by increasing its hemoglobin concentration and oxygen-carrying capacity, which would tend to increase umbilical extraction of oxygen. This pathogenetic scheme remains speculative; however, erythropoietin release has been demonstrated in fetal lambs made acutely hypoxic, and elevated erythropoietin levels have been found in polycythemic intrauterine growth-retarded infants [10]. In addition, abnormalities of placental weight, surface area, and thickness of capillary basement membrane are often found in placentae of intrauterine growth-retarded infants.

Infants of diabetic mothers may have an increased incidence of polycythemia, which may, in part, be responsible for the increased incidence in infants of diabetic mothers of several complications, such as renal vein thrombosis, peripheral thrombosis [11], and excessive bilirubin production [12]. Elevated erythropoietin levels have been demonstrated in infants of

Table 23–3
Fetal Hypoxemia and Polycythemia

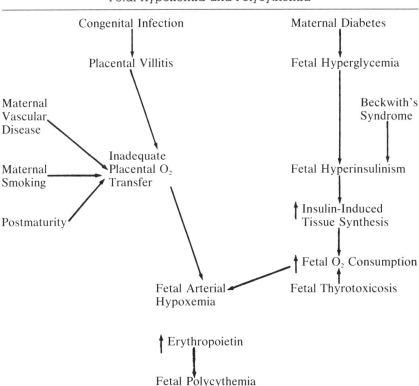

diabetic mothers, as well as in insulin-infused rhesus monkey fetuses [13]. The fetal monkeys also had greater extramedullary hematopoiesis compared with controls. Phillips et al. have also demonstrated arterial hypoxemia [14], elevated erythropoietin concentrations [15], and increased fetal oxygen consumption [16] in fetal lambs made hyperglycemic by glucose infusion. Thus it is speculated that in the diabetic pregnancy increased fetal oxygen consumption induced by fetal hyperglycemia or hyperinsulinemia or both may result in arterial hypoxemia, erythropoietin secretion, and polycythemia. Whether this pathogenetic sequence is operative in fetuses with hyperinsulinemic states from other causes, such as Beckwith's syndrome, is also speculative.

Table 23–3 outlines a speculative sequence by which several seemingly varied etiologic factors all may lead to the final common point of fetal hypoxemia with subsequent polycythemia.

The second general etiology of polycythemia includes transfusion of blood from the placenta (delayed cord clamping), mother (maternal-fetal transfusion), or a cofetus (twin-to-twin transfusion).

Blood Viscosity

Most clinical signs of polycythemia are thought to relate to the increase in the viscosity of the blood. Viscosity is defined as the resistance to flow generated when one "layer" of a fluid flows over another layer. This is often conceptualized as the "thickness" of the fluid. Newton described it as a lack of slipperiness between adjacent layers of fluid. The viscosity of a liquid is roughly analagous to the concept of friction between two solid surfaces.

It is the relationship of viscosity to blood flow that is of interest to physicians. The mathematical relationships were first defined by Poiseuille's law, which states that flow is directly proportional to the pressure drop across a given length of tubing, and inversely proportional to the viscosity of the fluid, as in equation 1 [17].

$$\text{Flow} = (P_1 - P_2)\, r^4/8\eta L \tag{1}$$

where $(P_1 - P_2)$ is the pressure gradient across the system, r is the tube (vessel) radius, L is the tube (vessel) length, and η is the viscosity of the liquid under study. This equation is analagous to the equation $y = ax + b$, which describes a straight line. If the pressure drop across the system and the tube radius and length remain constant, their product defines the slope of this line. Flow and viscosity are, therefore, reciprocally related in a linear fashion. Likewise, if viscosity is constant, the flow and the pressure change across the system are directly related to a linear fashion.

The viscosity of a liquid is quantitated by measurement of the forces

Figure 23–3

Simplified drawing of Wells-Brookfield viscometer. The fluid is placed in the cup; the revolutions per minute of the spindle (cone) determines the shear rate. The torque of the system is measured by the calibrated spring and related to shear stress. Viscosity is then determined as shear stress/shear rate.

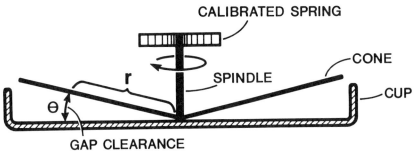

generated as flow increases. The movement of different layers of fluid relative to each other is called shearing, and the rate at which this is accomplished is called the shear rate. The resistive force opposing flow is called the shear stress. The ratio of these two parameters (shear stress and shear rate) is defined as viscosity.

The Wells-Brookfield viscometer is the most common instrument used for the measurement of shear stress, and thus viscosity (Figure 23–3) [18]. In brief, this instrument consists of a cone rotating within a small cup that holds the liquid being tested. The tip of the cone rests on a small jeweled point, which is taken to impart negligible resistance to rotation. Thus, any resistance to rotation of the cone is due to the resistive forces of the liquid. The shear rate in this system is defined as in equation 2 in Table 23–4 and can be varied by changes in the revolutions per minute (N in equation 2 in Table 23–4). This relationship simplifies to shear rate = 2.06 N/s. Thus, a shear rate of 11.5/s, the rate of shear thought to be operative in small venules and thus often used in clinical studies, is obtained by a cone speed of 5.6 revolutions per minute, whereas a shear rate of 230/s is obtained by a comparatively rapid 111 revolutions per minute.

The torque or angular momentum necessary to overcome the resistive forces of the liquid is measured by means of a calibrated spring mounted on the instrument drive shaft. This spring is connected to a long pointer that overrides a numbered dial rotating in phase with, but not connected to, the drive shaft. In the absence of a test sample that pointer remains at the zero point of the dial; when a sample is added to the cone, any deflection of the pointer is related to the torque applied to the cone to overcome the resistive forces of the test liquid. This torque determination is then mathematically related to the shear stress generated by the following equation.

Table 23–4

Definition of Shear Rate and Viscosity

Shear rate $= \dfrac{\text{peripheral velocity (cm/s)}}{\text{gap clearance (cm)}}$ Equation (2)

$= \dfrac{(2\pi r)(N/60) \text{ cm/s}}{r \text{ sine } \Theta \text{ cm}}$

$= 2.06 \text{ N/s}$

where N = cone speed in revolutions per minute

    r = radius from apex of cone to point on cone where peripheral velocity is determined

The viscosity is defined as:

$\dfrac{\text{shear stress}}{\text{shear rate}} = \dfrac{\text{dyne/cm}^2}{1/s} = \dfrac{\text{dyne s}}{\text{cm}^2} = \text{poise}$

The centipoise, the most commonly used unit, equals 100 poise.

For Newtonian fluids, viscosity is constant over the range of shear rates, implying that shear stress necessarily increases linearly as shear rate increases. Blood, however, has anomolous viscosity and flow properties and is known as a non-Newtonian fluid (as are most fluids with suspended particles) [17]. Although plasma viscosity is an important factor in whole blood viscosity, the suspended erythrocytes are quantitatively much more important. In addition, they impart the anomolous rheologic

Figure 23–4

Effect of shear rate on viscosity *in vitro* at a fixed hematocrit, demonstrating the dramatic increase in viscosity at lower rates of shear.

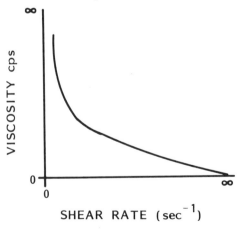

properties to the blood, primarily by their ability to deform and realign themselves as shear stress increases, as well as by the formation of multicell aggregates, the size of which depends on the shear rate.

Erythrocytes in whole blood at rest form large multicell aggregates that increase the fluid's resistance to flow. At low rates of shear, insufficient shear stress is generated to break up these aggregates; as shear rate and thus shear stress increase, these aggregates are broken into smaller and smaller particles that impart less resistance to flow. Therefore, measured whole blood viscosity is higher at low shear rates and decreases as shear rate is increased (Figure 23–4). This behavior of whole blood is markedly different from that of a Newtonian fluid, which demonstrates a constant measured viscosity over all shear rates.

Erythrocyte aggregation is enhanced at higher hematocrit values; thus at any given shear rate the viscosity will be higher with a higher hematocrit (Figure 23–5). The viscosity change is approximately linear until the hematocrit reaches 65 percent, at which point the viscosity increases in an exponential fashion. It is for this reason that a hematocrit of 65 percent or greater is generally considered to be synonymous with hyperviscosity.

The deformability of the erythrocyte also affects the measured viscosity because as flow velocity increases, the red cell membranes deforms and aligns its major axis with the flow, thus decreasing viscosity. Red cells rendered artificially nondeformable and resuspended in a nonaggregating medium do not demonstrate this decreased viscosity with higher

Figure 23–5

Effect of hematocrit on viscosity *in vitro,* showing the increased viscosity with increasing hematocrit, especially when the hematocrit is greater than 65 percent. In addition, the higher viscosity and the more pronounced effect of an increased hematocrit on viscosity are seen with low shear rates.

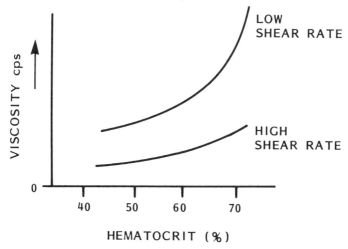

291

shear rates. The red cells of newborns are inherently less deformable than those of adults [19]. Thus, in spite of the neonate's lower plasma viscosity, the elevated hematocrit and rigid erythrocytes tend to increase the apparent whole blood viscosity [20–23].

There are several potentiators of this viscosity, which include low temperature, abnormalities of osmolality, abnormal erythrocyte membranes or hemoglobin, and acidosis [22], all of which appear to act by decreasing cell deformability. Hyperproteinemic states not only increase plasma viscosity, but also increase whole blood viscosity by potentiating red cell aggregation. This is especially true for hyperfibrinogenemia.

What happens in vivo is less predictable. Shear rates vary at the different components of the vascular system, being highest in the large vessels and lowest in the capillaries and small venules. Thus, one might expect the viscosity to increase in the small vessels. Fahraeus and Lindqvist first

Figure 23–6

Effect of decreasing tube diameter on apparent viscosity. Numbers 1, 2, and 3 represent physiologic samples of whole blood. Number 4 was centrifuged, and portion of plasma was removed to increase the hematocrit. *(Modified from Fahraeus, R., Lindqvist, T., The viscosity of the blood in narrow, capillary tubes.* Am. J. Physiol. *96:562–568, 1931.)*

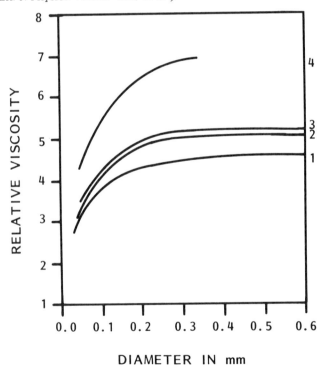

demonstrated in vitro that this is not true; as the diameter of the tube is decreased, the apparent viscosity also decreases to approach that of plasma in tubes less than 0.3 mm (Figure 23–6) [24]. This phenomenon is due to the decreased cell-to-cell interaction in the smaller tubes. Indeed, in the capillary bed, where the vessel diameter is less than the red cell diameter, blood flow is "single file," i.e., a bolus of plasma followed by a single, deformed erythrocyte, followed by a second bolus of plasma [25]. In these vessels there is virtually no cell-to-cell interaction, and flow may be unrelated to Poiseuille's determinants, but rather be dependent on factors that determine red cell deformability [26].

Most clinical studies of hyperviscosity syndromes report viscosity measurements at shear rates of $11.5-^1$, the rate throught to be operative in the venules [26] and where erythrocyte cell-to-cell interaction has large effect on measured viscosity. Whether this measurement reflects the in vivo situation is not clear. Experiments in a maximally vasodilated skeletal muscle bed of the dog [27] and in the cat mesenteric bed [28] have demonstrated the validity of the Fahraeus-Linqvist effect in vivo; this is apparently due to migration of the red blood cells to the fast axial stream and a decrease in the microvascular (small vessel) hematocrit relative to systemic (large vessel) hematocrit. These experiments would indicate that erythrocyte aggregates, and thus the hematocrit, are of minimal importance in determining microvascular blood flow. Rather, the ability of the cell to deform and pass through the small capillaries may be of greatest importance [22].

Other workers have demonstrated a decrease in cerebral blood flow velocity [29] and decreased urine output (presumably from lowered renal perfusion) [30] with polycythemia, both of which increase after isovolemic hemodilution. An increase in maximal blood flow to the lower extremity after isovolemic hemodilution has also been demonstrated in polycythemic infants, although no change was observed in resting blood flow [31]. Interpretation of these studies is difficult, as hemodilution will decrease the oxygen-carrying capacity of the blood in proportion to the decrease in hemoglobin concentration, and these organ systems autoregulate blood flow to maintain constant oxygen delivery.

Signs of Polycythemia/Hyperviscosity

The majority of clinical signs attributed to polycythemia are thought to relate to either poor organ perfusion or elevated red blood cell mass. The most common signs are listed in Table 23–5 [32]. In addition to these findings, there have also been case reports of peripheral infarction [33], testicular infarction [34], frank congestive heart failure, acute renal failure [35], necrotizing enterocolitis [36], and cerebral infarction [37]. Whether

Table 23–5
Clinical Signs Attributed to
Polycythemia/Hyperviscosity

Plethora/ruddiness
Jaundice
Peripheral cyanosis
Respiratory distress
Congestive heart failure
Poor feeding
Lethargy
Jitteriness, irritability
Seizures

these complications are due to polycythemia/hyperviscosity per se or to the underlying pathology that resulted in polycythemia is often difficult to determine.

Ramamurthy et al. investigated the relatively common clinical signs of polycythemia—lethargy, cyanosis, pallor, tachycardia, tremors, tachypnea, and jaundice—and their correlation to the measured viscosity. They found that there was no difference between hyperviscous and normoviscous polycythemic infants with a single symptom, nor was any one of the above symptoms predictive of hyperviscosity; an infant with two or more symptoms was likely to be hyperviscous [32]. However, 16 of the 54 infants had other clinical disorders that might also account for the observed symptoms.

Laboratory abnormalities may occur in polycythemic infants. Hypoglycemia is a frequent finding [38,39]; thus, a glucose concentration should be performed. If a whole blood glucose is obtained, it must be remembered that this value is less than the plasma glucose, and the difference between the whole blood and plasma glucose increases as the hematocrit increases. Various abnormalities of the coagulation system may also be seen in infants with polycythemia. These include thrombocytopenia, circulating fibrin monomer, and increased intravascular thromboplastin activity, which, in one study, resolved after isovolemic hemodilution [40]. Another study showed normal prothrombin time, activated partial thromboplastin time, fibrinogen, and plasminogen levels, but an increased incidence (20 percent) of thrombocytopenia in polycythemic infants with no effect of partial exchange transfusion on these laboratory findings [41].

Radiologic signs of pulmonary plethora and cardiomegaly have also been described [42,43] and have been reported to improve after therapy. One group noted these changes in premature infants who had received an excessive placental transfusion and were symptomatic at lower hematocrits than were comparable full-term infants. They suggested that the symptoms were due to hypervolemia rather than polycythemia.

Diagnosis and Treatment

Infants with abnormalities of intrauterine growth, infants from multiple births, infants of diabetic mothers, and infants with symptoms compatible with polycythemia should have a hematocrit performed. If the blood is obtained from a "capillary" source (heel, toe, finger) and the hematocrit is greater than 65 to 70 percent, a ventipuncture from a large-caliber vein such as an antecubital or scalp vein should be performed. A hematocrit of 65 percent or greater is a reasonable definition of polycythemia.

Whether to routinely screen asymptomatic infants with normal intrauterine growth is more problematic. In many nurseries a heel stick hematocrit is obtained at two or eight hours of age; if this hematocrit is above a predetermined level (65 to 70 percent), a peripheral venipuncture for a "central" hematocrit is performed. Although the heel stick hematocrit is nearly always higher than that obtained from a peripheral or central vein, the linear correlation is poor and not clinically useful [32]. However, routine venipuncture for all infants is not practical. Thus, the practitioner must decide how important it is to diagnose polycythemia in asymptomatic infants.

Although polycythemia is not synonymous with hyperviscosity, few hospitals have the equipment necessary for determination of viscosity; therefore a presumptive diagnosis of hyperviscosity must be based on the hematocrit. Ramamurthy et al. have demonstrated that an umbilical venous hematocrit of 63 percent or greater generally predicts hyperviscosity defined as an umbilical venous viscosity greater than 14.6 centipoise (cps) at a shear rate of 11.5/s (Figure 23–7) [32]. This represents a value greater than 3 standard deviations above the mean for cord blood determinations on normocythemic infants. Of the infants with an umbilical venous hematocrit less than 63 percent, only two exhibited viscosity measurements greater than 14.6 cps. However, the data of Ramamurthy et al. demonstrates that an antecubital hematocrit of 65 percent or greater is a poor predictor of hyperviscosity, since 33 of 55 (60 percent) infants with an antecubital hematocrit of 65 percent or greater had an umbilical vein viscosity measurement within the normal range; 16 of 55 (29 percent) were within 2 standard deviations of the normal mean. Thus, if hyperviscosity rather than polycythemia is the physiologic criterion upon which one desires to perform a partial exchange transfusion, a significant number of infants will be subjected to the procedure needlessly. Ramamurthy suggests that when an infant is suspected of polycythemia/hyperviscosity syndrome, either because of symptoms or results of a screening test, a scalp vein or antecubital venipuncture should be performed for determination of the hematocrit. If this is greater than 65 percent, an umbilical venous hematocrit should be obtained; if this is 63 percent or greater, the infant can be presumed to be hyperviscous.

Our clinical approach is slightly different, as we exclude the umbilical

Figure 23–7

Data of Ramamurthy et al. showing that an umbilical venous hematocrit of 63 percent or greater is predictive of hyperviscosity. The shadowed area represents normal range of viscosity. *(Modified from Ramamurthy, R.S., Brans, Y.W., Neonatal polycythemia. I. Criteria for diagnosis and treatment.* Pediatrics *68:168–174, 1981.)*

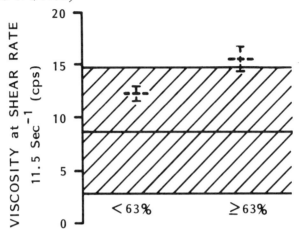

venous hematocrit. If the venous (scalp or antecubital vein) blood sample has a hematocrit greater than 65 percent, we make a presumptive diagnosis of polycythemia/hyperviscosity. We realize that his approach will erroneously label as hyperviscous those infants who have an elevated antecubital hematocrit, but an umbilical venous hematocrit and viscosity within the normal range. However, since we intervene only in infants who are symptomatic or have an antecubital hematocrit greater than 70 percent (Table 23–6), this seems to be a reasonable compromise compared with the actual measurement of viscosity or determination of the hematocrit from umbilical venous blood, which would require an invasive procedure.

The accepted therapy for the polycythemia/hyperviscosity syndrome is isovolemic hemodilution or partial exchange transfusion. During this procedure a volume of blood is removed in small aliquots and replaced volume for volume with a colloid or cyrstalloid solution. The amount to be exchanged is calculated to dilute the blood to a desired hematocrit, generally 50 to 55 percent (equation 4). An estimate of the volume for exchange to produce the desired hematocrit is given by the formula:

$$\text{Volume (ml) to be exchanged} = \text{BV} \times \frac{(\text{Hct}_{obs} - \text{Hct}_{des})}{\text{Hct}_{obs}} \quad (4)$$

where BV is the blood volume of infant (assume 100 ml/kg), Hct_{obs} is the hematocrit at beginning, and Hct_{des} is the desired hematocrit (generally

Table 23–6
Guidelines for Management of Polycythemic Infants

Antecubital Hematocrit (%)	Symptoms	Recommendation
< 65	Asymptomatic	Observe
	Symptomatic	Consider hyperfibrinogenemia, abnormal erthrocyte deformability, acidosis
65–70	Asymptomatic	Observe closely, follow glucose concentration, neurologic examination
	Symptomatic	Partial exchange transfusion
> 70		Partial exchange transfusion

50 to 55 percent). A blood volume of 100 ml/kg is a reasonable approximation, although the blood volume varies with birth weight and with red cell mass.

A sample calculation for a 3-kg infant with an initial hematocrit of 65 percent is:

$$\text{exchange volume} = 3 \text{ kg} \times 100 \text{ ml kg} \times \frac{(65\% - 55\%)}{(65\%)} = 46 \text{ ml}$$

This method of calculation assumes that the decrease in hematocrit is linear with each exchange cycle, which is not strictly true, but for practical purposes is acceptable. An alternative method for determining exchange volume is to utilize a nomogram devised by Berman et al. [44].

The exchange transfusion may be performed via the umbilical vein or the umbilical artery with in-out cycles of approximately 5 percent of total blood volume, each through the common catheter. Recent concern regarding possible mesenteric hemodynamic derangements during exchange transfusion that might predispose to ischemia and necrotizing enterocolitis has prompted some investigators to recommend the use of peripheral arteries and veins, generally with blood withdrawal through a radial artery and simultaneous colloid infusion through a medium caliber vein. At present, no evidence exists to determine which method is optimal.

Partial exchange transfusion will reliably lower the infant's hematocrit and nearly always lowers the in vitro viscosity [32]. In addition, partial exchange transfusion causes an apparent decrease in extracellular water and interstitial water while increasing intracellular water [45]. Thus the effects of partial exchange transfusion are not limited to lowering hematocrit and viscosity, but the procedure also affects body water distribution.

297

Outcome

When it is decided to perform an invasive procedure with a small but real risk, some beneficial effects to the patient should be expected. A partial exchange transfusion will improve some of the short-term symptoms, including a decrease in the abnormal rate of glucose utilization [46], an increase in renal glomerular filtration rate [30,47], an increase in cerebral blood flow velocity [29] (and possibly cerebral blood flow), and a diminution of the radiologic evidence for pulmonary congestion. Although the significance of these physiologic alterations for the asymptomatic infant is not known, there is little doubt that they benefit the symptomatic infant.

It is the asymptomatic infant who poses the greatest dilemma to the practitioner. One is presumably trying to prevent the complications, mostly neurologic that might, but also might not, occur if the infant is not treated. Some idea of the risks and benefits to the patient must be known before a decision can be reached.

The risks of a partial exchange transfusion are significant, although their rate of occurrence is low, especially if one maintains meticulous attention to careful technique. Primarily the complications are those that may occur with any instrumentation of a central vessel, including infection, thrombosis, and air embolism. Air embolism can lead to rapid death in the newborn infant; therefore, one must be careful that the umbilical vein is occluded by either catheter, umbilical tape, or a purse-string suture at all times. This is especially true during catheter withdrawal, which leaves a tract directly to the ductus venosus. Partial exchange transfusions may predispose to necrotizing enterocolitis.

Several, but not all [38,48], investigators have noted a higher incidence of long-term neurologic dysfunction in polycythemic/hyperviscous infants compared with control infants. These have included spastic diplegia, hemiparesis, athetosis, and seizure disorders. Black et al. also documented a higher incidence of neurologic complications when hypoglycemia was present in addition to polycythemia [49].

Several investigators have found improvement in subtle neurologic function after partial exchange transfusion compared with matched hyperviscous controls who were observed only. Goldberg, et al. noted a significantly higher percentage of abnormal results on the Brazelton examination at both 72 hours and at two weeks of age in the nonexchanged group, whereas the exchanged infants attained scores equal to nonhyperviscous infants by 72 hours. However, on the Prectl examination no difference could be detected between the exchanged and non-exchanged infants [50]. Black et al. found no differences in neurologic examinations at one year in exchanged infants compared with nonexchanged infants, but there was a higher incidence of abnormalities at two years in the nonexchanged group [49].

van der Elst et al. found no significant differences in the neurologic assessment and developmental scores attained at eight months in a comparison of hyperviscous infants randomly assigned to partial exchanged transfusion or observation, and all were said to have normal development for their age. The exchanged group did have more symptoms in the neonatal period, so it is not clear whether the groups were comparable [51].

Although it seems prudent to treat the infant with clinical signs or laboratory abnormalities of polycythemia, the proper therapy for the asymptomatic polycythemic infant is less clear, as the benefits of such prophylactic therapy are still speculative. Each physician must develop his or her own set of guidelines for the mangement of such infants. Our approach is outlined in Table 23–6. Asymptomatic infants demand close attention, especially in regard to glucose homeostasis, level of arousability and feeding patterns.

References

1. Rivera, L.M., Rudolph, N. Postnatal persistence of capillary-venous differences in hematocrit and hemoglobin values in low-birth-weight and term infants. *Pediatrics* 70:6, 1982.
2. Penn, D., Williams, P.R., Dutcher, T.F., Adair, R.M. Comparison of hematocrit determinations by microhematocrit and electronic particle counter. *Am. J. Clin. Pathol.* 72:71–74, 1979.
3. Wirth, F.H., Goldberg, K.E., Lubchenco, L.O. Neonatal hyperviscosity. I. Incidence. *Pediatrics* 63:833–836, 1979.
.4 Rawlings, J.S., Pettett, G., Wiswell, T.E., Clapper, J. Estimated blood volumes in polycythemic neonates as a function birth weight. *J. Pediatr.* 101:594–599, 1982.
5. Stevens, K., Wirth, F.H. Incidence of neonatal hyperviscosity at sea level. *J. Pediatr.* 97:118–119, 1980.
6. Ramamurthy, R.S. Neonatal polycythemia and hyperviscosity state of the art. *Perinatol./Neonatol.* 2:38–40, 1979.
7. Buchan, P. Cigarette smoking in pregnancy and fetal hyperviscosity. *Br. Med. J.* 286:1315, 1983.
8. Hakanson, D.O., Oh, W. Hyperviscosity in the small-for-gestational age infant. *Biol. Neonate* 37:109–112, 1980.
9. Longo, L.D., Hill, E.P., Power, G.G. Theoretical analysis of factors affecting placental O_2 transfer *Am. J. Physiol.* 222:730–739, 1972.
10. Widness, J.A., Garcia, J.A., Oh, W., Schwartz, R. Cord serum erythropoietin values and disappearance rates after birth in polycythemic newborns. *Pediatr. Res.* 16:218A, 1982.
11. Ward, T.F. Multiple thromboses in an infant of a diabetic mother. *J. Pediatr.* 90:982–984, 1977.
12. Stevenson, D.K., Bartoletti, A.L., Ostrander, C.R., Johnson, J.D. Pulmonary excretion of carbon monoxide in the human infant as an index of bilirubin production. II. Infants of diabetic mothers. *J. Pediatr.* 94:956–958, 1979.

13. Widness, J.A., Susa, J.B., Garcia, J.F., et al. Increaseed erythropoiesis and elevated erythropoietin in infants born to diabetic mothers and in hyperinsulinemic rhesus fetuses. *J. Clin. Invest.* 67:637–642, 1981.

14. Philipps, A.F., Dubin, J.W., Matty, P.J., Raye, J.R. Arterial hypoxemia and hyperinsulinemia in the chronically hyperglycemic fetal lamb. *Pediatr. Res.* 16:653–658, 1982.

15. Philipps, A.F., Widness, J.A., Garcia, J.F., et al. Erythropoietin elevation in the chronically hyperglycemic fetal lamb. *Proc. Soc. Exp. Biol. Med.* 170:42–47, 1982.

16. Philipps, A.F., Porte, P., Sabinsky, S., Raye, J.R. Effects of chronic fetal hyperglycemia upon oxygen consumption in the ovine uterus and conceptus (abstr.) *Pediatr. Res.* 17:294A, 1983.

17. Roos, A. Poiseuille's Law and its limitations in vascular systems. *Med. Thorac.* 19:224–238, 1962.

18. Wells, R.E., Denton, R., Merrill, E.W. Measurement of viscosity of biologic fluids by cone plate visicometer. *J. Lab. Clin. Med.* 57:646–656, 1961.

19. Gross, G.P., Hathaway, W.E. Fetal erythrocyte deformability. *Pediatr. Res.* 6:593–599, 1972.

20. Foley, M.E., Isherwood, D.M., McNicol, G.P. Viscosity, haematocrit, fibrinogen, and plasma proteins in maternal and cord blood. *Br. J. Obstet. Gynaecol.* 85:500–504, 1978.

21. Chien, S. Determinants of blood viscosity and red cell deformability. *Scand. J. Clin. Lab. Invest.* 41(Suppl. 156):7–12, 1981.

22. LaCelle, P.L., Week, R.I. Contribution of normal and pathologic erythrocytes to blood rheology. *Prog. Hematol.* 7:1–31, 1971.

23. Riopel, L., Fouron, J.C., Bard, H. Blood viscosity during the neonatal period—role of plasma and red blood cell type. *J. Pediatr.* 100:449–453, 1982.

24. Fahraeus, R., Lindqvist, T. The viscosity of the blood in narrow capillary tubes. *Am. J. Physiol.* 96:562–568, 1931.

25. Prothero, J. Burton, A.C. The physics of blood flow in capillaries. I. The nature of the motion. *Biophys. J.* 1:566–579, 1961.

26. Wells, R., Schmid-Schobein, H., Bygdeman, S. Analysis of viscous deformation of the red cell and its effect upon microvascular flow. 5th European Conference Microcirculation, Gothenburg, 1968, Karger, 1969. *Bibl. Anat.* 10:92–98, 1969.

27. Gustafsson, L., Appelgren, L., Myrvold, H.E. The effect of polycythemia on blood flow in working and non-working skeletal muscle. *Acta Physiol. Scand.* 109:143–148, 1980.

28. Lipowsky, H.H., Kovalcheck, S., Zweifach, B.W. The distribution of blood rheological parameters in the microvasculature of cat mesentery. *Circ. Res.* 43:738–749, 1978.

29. Rosenkrantz, T.S., Oh, W. Cerebral blood flow velocity in infants with polycythemia and hyperviscosity: effects of partial exchange transfusion with plasmanate. *J. Pediatr.* 101:94–98, 1982.

30. Aperia, A., Bergqvist, G., Broberger, O., et al. Renal function in newborn infants with high hematocrit values before and after exchange transfusion. *Acta. Pediatr. Scand.* 63:878–884, 1974.

31. Bergqvist, G., Zetterstrom, R. Submaximal blood flow and blood viscosity in newborn infants. *Acts. Pediatr. Scand.* 64:253–256, 1975.
32. Ramamurthy, R.S., Brans, Y.W. Neonatal polycythemia. I. Criteria for diagnosis and treatment. *Pediatrics* 68:168–174, 1981.
33. Papageorgiou, A., Stern, L. Polycythemia and gangrene of an extremity in a newborn infant. *J. Pediatr.* 81:985–987, 1970.
34. Jung, A., McGaughey, H.R., Matlack, M. Neonatal testicular infarction and polycythemia. *J. Urol.* 123:781–782, 1980.
35. Herson, V., Raye, J.R., Rowe, J., Philipps, A. F. Acute renal failure associated with polycythemia in a neonate. *J. Pediatr.* 100:137–139, 1982.
36. Leake, R.D., Thanopoulos, B., Nieberg, R. Hyperviscosity syndrome associated with necrotizing enterocolitis. *Am. J. Dis. Child.* 129:1192, 1975.
37. Amit, M., Camfield, P.R. Neonatal polychythemia causing multiple cerebral infarcts. *Arch. Neurol.* 57:109–100, 1980.
38. Black, V.D., Lubchenco, L.O., Luckey, D.W., et al. Developmental and neurologic sequelae of neonatal hyperviscosity syndrome. *Pediatrics* 69:426–431, 1982.
39. Creswell, J.S., Warburton, D., Susa, J.B., et al. Hyperviscosity in the new born lamb produces perturbation in glucose homeostasis. *Pediatr. Res.* 15:1348–1350, 1981.
40. Rivers, R.P.A. Coagulation changes associated with a high hematocrit in the newborn. *Acta Pediatr. Scand.* 64:449–456, 1975.
41. Katz, J., Rodriguez, E., Mandani, G., Branson, H. Normal coagulation findings, thrombocytopenia, and peripheral hemoconcentration in neonatal polycythemia. *J. Pediatr.* 101:99–102, 1982.
42. Saigel, S., Wilson, R., Usher, R. Radiologic findings in symptomatic neonatal plethora resulting from placental transfusion. *Radiology* 125:185–188, 1977.
43. Wesenberg, R.L., Rumack, C.M., Lubchenco, L.O., et al. Thick blood syndrome. *Radiology* 125:181–183, 1977.
44. Berman, B., Krieger, A., Naiman, J. A new method for calculating volumes of blood required for partial exchange transfusion. *J. Pediatr.* 94:86–89, 1979.
45. Thornton, C., Shannon, D., Hunter M., et al. Body water estimates in neonatal polycythemia. *J. Pediatr.* 102:113–117, 1983.
46. Leake, R.D., Chan, G., Zakaudden, S. Glucose utilization in hyperviscosity. *Pediatr. Res.* 10:412, 1976.
47. Kotagal, U., Kleinman, L. Effect of acute polycythemia on newborn renal hemodynamics and funtion. *Pediatr. Res.* 16:148–151, 1982.
48. Gross, G., Hathaway, W., McGuaghey, H. Hyperviscosity in the neonate. *J. Pediatr.* 82:1004–1012, 1973.
49. Black, B., Lubchenco, L.O., Koops, B.L., Poland, R.L. Neonatal hyperviscosity: randomized study of partial plasma exchange in altering long term outcome. (abstr.) *Pediatr. Res.* 16:279A, 1982.
50. Goldberg, K., Wirth, F.H., Hathaway, W.E., et al. Neonatal hyperviscosity., II. Effects of partial plasma exchange. *Transfusion* 69:419–425, 1982.
51. van der Elst, C.W., Molteno, C.D., Malan, A.F., de V. Heese, H. Management of polycythemia in the newborn infant. *Early Hum. Dev.* 4:393–403, 1980.

24

Retinopathy of Prematurity

Graham E. Quinn, M.D.*

Retrolental fibroplasia (RLF), or as it is now more commonly called, retinopathy of prematurity (ROP), is still an area of active concern for neonatologists, ophthalmologists, and other physicians caring for premature infants. Since the first description by Terry [1], controversy concerning etiology, susceptibility, prognosis, and therapy has been wide ranging and intensive. In spite of continued efforts of the scientific and medical community to eradicate this disorder, Phelps [2] estimated that 546 infants in the United States were blinded from ROP in 1979. The public health consequences of these blind children are enormous, and it is incumbent on us to observe with care the incidence of the disorder in our nurseries and to undertake thoughtful, controlled investigation of medical or surgical management of those afflicted infants. It is the purpose of this chapter to describe my basic understanding (and ignorance) of the disease process, present the classification system that we use in our nurseries, and review current modes of therapy.

Historical Perspective

Severe cicatricial RLF was devastatingly frequent in the early 1950s, when oxygen was routinely given without monitoring to prematurely born infants. Campbell [3] published the first papers suggesting a causal relationship of high oxygen treatment and ROP [3], and such studies stimulated much fervent investigation. The first controlled clinical trial was undertaken in Washington, D.C., by Patz et al. [4], and this was followed by a multicentered study organized by Kinsey [5]. This group found, among other things, that the incidence of cicatricial ROP in the routine oxygen group was 3.5 times that of the oxygen-curtailed group. A severe curtailment of oxygen therapy ensued, and the incidence of ROP as seen by the direct ophthalmoscope dropped dramatically by the late 1950s.

However, a high price was paid for the "cure" of ROP. In 1960, Avery and Oppenheimer [6] documented an increased mortality from hyaline membrane disease during a period of oxygen curtailment (1954 through 1958) compared with uncurtailed oxygen use (1944 through 1948). Cross [7] also estimated that, for every case of blindness prevented in the United Kingdom, an excess of 16 deaths were seen from restricted oxygen use.

Now the neonatologists were faced with administering a level of oxygen that would maintain life and still not cause ROP. In the early 1970s, the technology for blood gas measurements rapidly improved, and this capability led to another collaborative study to consider what were "safe" levels of oxygen for the premature infant [8]. The study showed that birth weight, gestational age, and time in oxygen correlated well with the development of ROP, but that blood gases (including PaO_2) did not reliably correlate. It was speculated that continuous monitoring might be needed to answer this problem.

Other theories as to the cause of ROP have been discussed since the original description [1], and indeed it was not known until the careful observations of Owens and Owens [9] that eyes that later developed ROP were normal at birth. This ruled out ROP as a congenital anomaly. At about this time, also, Heath suggested that the term "retinopathy of prematurity" would most accurately describe the findings in these infants [10].

Considerable attention has been given lately to the possible effect of the naturally occurring antioxidant, vitamin E (alpha-tocopherol) in preventing blinding ROP. In the 1940s, Owens and Owens [11], pointing out that premature neonates have defective fat absorption, postulated that vitamin E deficiency could contribute to the development of ROP. In their initial study, alternate infants weighing 1,360 g or less were given supplemental vitamin E as soon as they began oral feeding. Owens and Owens reported that of 73 infants who received no vitamin E, 17 developed ROP, whereas only 1 of 23 vitamin E-treated babies developed the condition.

There followed a period where several centers tried to confirm these findings, but were unable to do so. It is of note here that during this time unmonitored oxygen therapy was becoming more widely available and, as oxygen therapy was implicated as "the cause" of ROP and its control the "cure," routine vitamin E therapy was gradually discontinued.

Other modes of therapy were tried in the early years. Reese et al. [12] suggested the efficacy of adrenocorticotropin and cortisone, but controlled trials concluded that their use was ineffectual.

Retinal Vascularization

Before four months of gestation, the retinal elements receive their blood supply by diffusion from the choroid, which has vessels of large caliber and rapid blood flow. At around four months, a mesenchymal ridge ("vanguard") appears near the disc and progresses to the ora serrate. Ashton [13] observed that this advancing edge trails behind it a primitive capillary network that gradually remodels into mature arteries and veins with an interposed capillary network. This primitive vascular network is the "rearguard." The orderly progression of vascular tissue to the ora serrata is largely completed by birth in humans. Toyofuku et al. [14] and Ashton [15] observed some variation of vascular completion between 38 and 44 weeks of gestation. It should be noted here that most of this vascular growth occurs at an intrauterine arterial pressure of oxygen of 20 to 25 mmHg [16].

Abnormal Retinal Vascularization

In sustained hyperoxic states (for the premature newborn, room air is a state of hyperoxia), the orderly sequence of vascular growth is disrupted, and eventually irreversible vessel closure results. This is the vasoobliterative phase [17]. Based on the fluorescein angiographic records of Flynn et al. [18], it appears that the obliterated vessels are the newly formed capillaries just posterior to the advancing ridge. Kretzer et al. [19] recently reported that the major insult is confined to the spindle cells under present conditions.

This sets the stage for clinically detectable ROP. Ashton [20] beautifully demonstrated that the location of the vasoproliferation is intimately tied to the area where the vasoobliteration occurs. for instance, if vascularization has proceeded to the far periphery when the vasoobliterating insult occurs, then the proliferative phase will occur in that region. He also showed in kittens that vasoproliferation would follow occlusion of capillaries by glass ballotini, [21], i.e., without exposure to oxygen. Similarly, vasoproliferation has occurred in anencephalus [22] and "congenital" retrolental fibroplasia [23]. Such studies and observations suggest that the proliferative phase of ROP is not oxygen dependent, but rather a response to anoxia resulting from disturbance of retinal blood flow.

In a scheme proposed by Flynn et al. [18], the obliteration of the

304

capillary meshwork leads to the union of the advancing mesenchyme and the remaining arteries and veins to form a demarcation line. The normal gradual blending of vascularized into avascular retina is no longer apparent, and there is now a clinically apparent abrupt termination of vascularized retina. This demarcation line is silver-white and, on fluorescein angiography, fills rapidly with dye and leaks profusely. The vessels leading to this structure are dilated and tortuous. This line, in progressive ROP, thickens and becomes elevated above the plane of the retina, and there is neovascularization along it up into the vitreous. These proliferative vessels set the stage for vitreoretinal traction and may be quite extensive.

Particular attention should be paid to the vessels of the posterior pole, if they appear normal in caliber and configuration, then the child probably has mild disease. If the vessels are modestly to markedly tortuous and dilated, we would classify the infant as having "plus" disease [24] to reflect our concern for this more active condition with greater potential for long-term damage. Also frequently seen in "plus" disease are iris vessel engorgement at the pupillary margin with resistance to dilation and increasing vitreous haze, probably reflecting leakage of serous material from the new vessel proliferation.

As the fibrovascular proliferation into the vitreous progresses, vitreous hemorrhage may occur from these fragile vessels, and the retina may be pulled from the retinal pigment epithelium by traction of the vitreous bands. This may ultimately lead to the complete detachment of the retina.

It is important that the clinician observing this disorder remain acutely aware that the individual infant may undergo regression at any point before retinal detachment. Regression means an end of the active vasoproliferation and gradual remodeling of the vascular architecture with vessels growing within the retinal plane toward the ora serrata. It is heralded by a change of color of the demarcation line or ridge from white to pink or red [18] and vascularized retina peripheral to the line itself. It need not occur in all areas at the same pace or time.

Regression may progress to either complete remodeling and clinical normality of the peripheral retina or to scar formation, setting up mechanisms for dragging of the retina as the scar contracts. If the retina is dragged directly temporal, then macular heterotropia will result. If more severe, a tenting up of the retina into a fold may occur. Most severe would be a retinal detachment, either partial or total, occurring during this cicatricial phase of the disease.

Classification—Active ROP

The clinical observation of ROP in the infant is not technically difficult and has been greatly enhanced by the use of the indirect ophthalmoscope since the 1960s. With current instrumentation, one is able to observe milder, more peripheral forms of the disease and document accurately the location and extent of involvement. What is lacking is a uniform classification system used by all observers so that communication among ophthalmologists can be facilitated. Several logical schemes have been proposed [25–30]; and there is currently an international group meeting to propose a new uniform classification. It is imperative that we use easily communicable grades to evaluate responses to therapy modes and evaluate regional differences among populations.

I would like to review briefly the active and cicatricial grading of ROP that we use at The University of Pennsylvania Neonatal Complex Nurseries [31].

Grade 1 ROP shows abnormal intraretinal vessels with arborization or tuftlike formations. The zone between vascularized and avascular retina is vague and indistinct. The vessel abnormalities may be quite subtle and are often difficult to see due to persistant vitreous haze.

Grade 2 ROP has the clear finding of the demarcation line of Flynn et al. [18], and the retinal vessels stop abruptly at this line. There is now a clear distinction between the pinkish vascular retina and the white glistening peripheral retina. The demarcation line is usually observed in the superotemporal region, but may be segmented or circumferential.

In Grade 3 ROP, the demarcation line thickens above the retinal plane, and true neovascularization into the vitreous space takes place. Once again, the involvement may be segmental, and extraretinal involvement maybe tiny budlike formations just posterior to the ridge which have little longterm consequence, or the involvement may be large formations resembling sausages along the ridge.

We use "plus" disease to suggest a more rapidly progressive, virulent, and ominous form of the disease, and we find this especially useful in early ROP. If there is moderate to marked posterior pole vascular dilation and tortuosity in association with the findings of grades 1, 2, or 3 ROP, then we are much more concerned about his child's ultimate visual prognosis. For example, a child with a demarcation, no extraretinal neovascularization, and posterior vascular tortuosity would have 2 + ROP. This is in close agreement with the Japanese classification, which defines a type I, II, and intermediate form of ROP [29].

Grade 4 ROP has as its hallmark a retinal detachment posterior to the demarcation line, and hemorrhage into vitreous is common at this point. Resolution from this point is quite unlikely; indeed we have not observed it. The detachment may be serous or tractional.

Grade 5 ROP is a total retinal detachment or fibrovascular overgrowth and probably should be blended into cicatricial disease, since scarring and vitreoretinal traction lead to it.

Approximately 80 percent of infants with grades 1 and 2 ROP will spontaneously regress [27]. Regression is also fairly frequent in grade 3 ROP, but distinctly uncommon in grade 3 + ROP.

Classification—Cicatricial Disease

Cicatricial disease is the unpredictable and variable outcome of the acute vasoproliferative process. We divide its findings into five categories of increasing severity. Unless there is a retinal fold, we defer cicatricial grading of the eye until one year from due date and view the eye with vascular remodeling as having transitional ROP.

Grade 1 cicatricial disease is a constellation of findings. The vision is usually correctable to 6/6, although myopia and anisometropia are common. The retinal findings are fine, cloudlike vitreoretinal membranes and irregular pigmentation of the retinal pigment epithelium along the previous demarcation line. Kushner [32] reported patients with similar findings.

Grade 1 + cicatricial disease has dense vitreoretinal fibrosis that may appear as an elevated white plaque. Vision is correctable 6/12 at least, but myopia is moderate to severe and anisometropia is more common.

Grade 2 cicatricial disease has a wide range of visual acuities from 6/12 to 6/30 with evere myopic correction. There is distortion of the posterior pole vessels, which tug toward a dense peripheral scar. Because this scar is almost always temporal, the tug results in displacement of the macula (macular heterotopia). The degree of visual compromise is generally related to the extent of macular drag.

In Grade 3 cicatricial disease, the vision is rarely better than perception of hand motion, since there is a retinal fold extending from the optic disc to the peripheral scar with marked dragging of retinal tissue.

Patients with Grade 4 or 5 cicatricial disease have light perception at best and show partial or total retrolental membranes, respectively.

Predicting Ocular Morbidity

We have found a quadrant summing system useful to describe the extent of active disease and to predict the likely ocular morbidity for an individual eye. The information is obtained from the retinal drawing sheet of the highest observed activity of ROP for an infant. The eye is graded as the highest observed acute ROP in any quadrant, and the number of quadrants involved with that grade or activity in any other quadrant is noted (Table 24–1). Posterior pole vascular dilatation and tortuosity ("plus" disease) adds one or two points depending on whether two or four quadrants are involved (generally all four quadrants are involved). Extraretinal neovascularization with posterior vascular tortuosity in a quadrant causes its

Table 24–1
Quadrant Summary Score

A. Add the grades for each quadrant highest acute stage ROP.
B. Add 0.5 for each quadrant with posterior pole vascular tortuosity.
C. Double the quadrant score when extraretinal neovascularization with posterior vascular tortuosity is present.
D. Triple the quadrant score when a retinal detachment is present in any quadrant.

score to be doubled, and any retinal detachment in a quadrant leads to tripling the score.

For example (Table 24–2), a child with grade 3 ROP in one quadrant, a demarcation line in the second, and fully vascularized retina in quadrants 3 and 4 (nasal quadrants) would have a score of 5, whereas a child with posterior dilation and tortuosity and the same retinal findings would score 10.5. This doubling of the score reflects adequately our increased clinical concern. In the few examples given, I have not tried to predict every possible combination, but just a few clinically likely schemes that might be observed in the nursery. Indeed, for most of these examples, there are corresponding patients from the files of my colleagues, D.B. Schaffer, M.D., and L.H. Johnson, M.D., and it does appear that the scores of the children correlate well with the ocular morbidity score at one year from due date (Schaffer, Quinn, and Johnson, unpublished data).

Such "computer-friendly" ways of grading clinical situations are essential in the evaluation of modes of prophylaxis or treatment of conditions that are rare and may indeed vary somewhat in incidence from one pop-

Table 24–2
Quadrant Grading of ROP

ROP highest grade	# Quadrants involved	Sample eye by quadrants				Sum score
		I	II	III	IV	
2	2	2	2	0	0	4
2	2	2	2	1	1	6
2 +	4	2.5	2.5	2.5	2.5	10
3	1	3	2	0	0	5
	1	3	3	2	2	10
3 +	1	3.5	2.5	0.5	0.5	10.5
	2	3.5	3.5	2.5	1.5	18
	4	3.5	3.5	3.5	3.5	28
4	1	4	3.5	3.5	3.5	33
	4	4	4	4	4	48

ulation to another. Controlled clinical trials from disparate institutions must be available to compare data easily and with confidence.

Vitamin E and ROP

The current controversy concerning vitamin E therapy for infants at risk for ROP reflects many of the current difficulties in communication in complex clinical situations. As mentioned above, vitamin E was initially thought to decrease the incidence of cicatricial disease when administered early to premature infants [9], and Johnson et al. [33] decided to reexamine this question in 1974. Using a derived mean severity score, they found significantly less severe disease and a lower incidence overall in the treated versus the control babies of less than 2000 g at birth. The disease was not eradicated, but its devastation was diminished by supplementing babies with vitamin E. At this time vitamin E relative to polyunsaturated fatty acids was low in nursery formulas.

Since those initial trials, the clinical E nutrition of the premature infants has markedly improved [34].

Additional support for using vitamin E came from the laboratory work of Phelps and Rosenbaum using kittens [35]. Kittens can be induced to have vasoproliferation with oxygen therapy, but they do not develop cicatricial disease. However, these investigators reported a significant decrease in retinal pathology in those animals treated with vitamin E during and after oxygen exposure. They found that neovascularization could be decreased when vitamin E was given after the oxygen insult.

These promising results led to widespread interest in vitamin E supplementation as a way of helping these unfortunate infants. Several double-blind, randomized control trials were undertaken [36–38], and some have been completed. Hittner et al. [39] reported that oral vitamin E given to infants greater than 1,500 g from birth resulted in a significant decrease in extraretinal neovascularization with posterior pole dilation and tortuosity. They derived these results from 50 vitamin E-treated babies (100 mg per day) and 51 controls (5 mg/kg per day) and eliminated from consideration all infants who died before four weeks of age. At birth the plasma vitamin E levels for both groups in this study were between 0.3 and 0.4 mg/100 ml, approximately one-half that reported by Johnson in premature infants born in 1978 [34]. Hittner et al. [39] also derived an RLF score based on such factors as gestational age, birth weight, level and duration of oxygen sepsis, and intraventricular hemorrhage. At three weeks of age, this score could be calculated, and Hittner et al. used it to predict the likelihood of developing severe ROP.

Admittedly, the number of infants in Hittner's study is small, and two larger clinical trials are underway. (One of these trials is underway at the nurseries of The University of Pennsylvania Neonatal Complex.) Before we make any movement toward prophylactic treatment of large numbers of infants with vitamin E, we must have more information concerning the risk/benefit ratio, and we await these larger studies with concern. Phelps [40] addressed this issue in detail recently and recommended waiting for the results of safety and side-effect evaluations.

Surgical Treatment of ROP

Some surgical treatments have been used in the vasoproliferative phases of acute ROP. Photocoagulation or cryotherapy of the proliferating vessels has been performed, but to date no prospective clinical trial has proven its value. Kingham [27] reported disappointing results from cryosurgery on 14 eyes of 12 infants. He urged caution in subjecting these tiny infants to a surgical procedure. Perhaps the largest series is reported by Nagata and Yamagishi [41], where zenon-arc photocoagulation was used at the point of severe progression of extraretinal new vessels (stage IIIb), and it was felt efficacious. Almost all infants received bilateral therapy. Sasaki et al. [42] also employed cryocautery and felt it useful.

McPherson [43] and Tasman [44] have pioneered the surgical management of tractional retinal detachment in the very young child with ROP. Vitrectomy has also been attempted, with disappointing results [45]. Certainly there is a place for these procedures in eyes that would be lost otherwise, but once again, by treating surgically before significant retinal detachment, we may be subjecting these high-risk infants to unnecessary surgery. Controlled, multicentered trials based on a uniform classification are essential to answer these efficacy and safety questions.

The Ophthalmologist in the Nursery

In 1974, the American Academy of Pediatrics recommended that "a person experienced in retrolental fibroplasia (ROP) should examine the eyes of all infants born at less than 36 weeks gestation, or weighing less than 2000 g, who have received oxygen therapy." They also felt that the examination need not take place until discharge from the nursery and at six months of age [46].

At our current state of knowledge, these guidelines would seem to subject large numbers of babies to unnecessary examinations, especially the premature child over 1,500 g who has a relatively uncomplicated course. Hittner et al. [39] and Palmer [47] demonstrated that ROP is most likely to be observed between 6 and 10 weeks of age and that, for screening purposes, two examinations during that period would yield most of the low-grade ROP and allow identification of those few infants at risk for severe disease. This seems a logical approach in the nursery for screening, but would be inadequate to evaluate treatment and to correlate visual outcome with active disease. For these purposes, weekly examinations would be the minimal gap necessary in my mind. This requires a much larger manpower commitment than is currently available in most intensive care nurseries.

The ophthalmologist has an obligation also to convey to the parents the status of the infant's eyes and the reason for observation. As he is seeing the child in consultation for a neonatologist, basic information concerning the reason for consultation should come from that source, with ophthalmologic input at the referring physician's request. When significant visual compromise is expected, the ophthalmologist must be involved in appropriate referral to agencies for the visually handicapped.

Conclusion

I have outlined for you my understanding of the disease processes in ROP, a system of classification that we use at Children's Hospital of Philadelphia, and current therapeutic considerations. The current controversy concerning vitamin E is not resolved in my mind, and therapy must be approached with circumspection. Further work is under way.

Acknowledgment

The author would like to thank his colleague, Lois Johnson, M.D., for reviewing this manuscript and making several suggestions.

References

1. Terry, T.L. Extreme prematurity and fibroplastic overgrowth of persistent vascular sheath behind each crystaline lens: a preliminary report. *Am. J. Ophthalmol.* 25:203–208, 1983.
2. Phelps, D.L. Retinopathy of prematurity: an estimate of vision loss in the United States—1979. *Pediatrics* 67:924–925, 1981.
3. Campbell, K. Intensive oxygen therapy as a possible cause of retrolental fibroplasia. A clinical approach. *Med. J. Aust.* 2:48–50, 1951.
4. Patz, A., Hoeck, L.E., de la Cruz, E. Studies on the effect of high oxygen administration in retrolental fibroplasia: nursery observation. *Am. J. Ophthalmol.* 35:1248–1253, 1952.
5. Kinsey, V.E. Retrolental fibroplasia. *Arch. Ophthalmol.* 56:481–543, 1956.
6. Avery, M.E., Oppenheimer, E.H. Recent increase in mortality from hyaline membrane disease. *J. pediatr.* 57:553–558, 1960.
7. Cross, K.W. Cost of preventing retrolental fibroplasia. *Lancet* 2:954–956, 1973.

8. Kinsey, V.E., Arnold, H.J., Kalina, R.E., et al. PaO$_2$ levels and retrolental fibroplasia: a report of the cooperative study. *Pediatrics* 60:665–668, 1977.

9. Owens, W.C., Owens, E.U. Retrolental fibroplasia in premature infants. *Am. J. Ophthalmol.* 32:1–4, 1949.

10. Heath, P. Pathology of the retinopathy of prematurity: retrolental fibroplasia. *Am. J. Ophthalmol.* 34:1249–1259, 1951.

11. Owens, W.C., Owens, E.U. Retrolental fibroplasia in premature infants. *Am. J. Ophthalmol.* 32:1631–1637, 1949.

12. Reese, A.B., Locke, J.C., Silverman, W.A., Day, R.L. Results of use of corticotropin (ACTH) in treatment of retrolental fibroplasia. *Arch. Ophthalmol.* 47:551–555, 1952.

13. Ashton,N. Oxygen and the growth and development of retinal vessels. In Kimura, S.J., Caygill, W.N. (eds.) *Vascular Complications of Diabetes Mellitus.* St. Louis: C.V. Mosby Co., 1967, pp. 3–32.

14. Toyofuku, H., Yoshizumi, M., Kairada, K., Tanouie, F. Peripheral retinal vessels in the normal newborn. *Acta Soc. Ophthalmol. Jpn.* 80:962–966, 1976.

15. Ashton, N. Retinal angiogenesis in the human embryo. *Br. Med. Bull.* 26:103–106, 1970.

16. Phelps, D.L., Rosenbaum, A.L. Observations of vitamin E in experimental oxygen-induced retinopathy. *Ophthalmology* 86:1741–1748, 1979.

17. Ashton, N., Ward, B., Serpell, G. Effect of oxygen on developing retinal vessels with particular reference to the problem of retrolental fibroplasia. *Br. J. Ophthalmol.* 38:397–432, 1954.

18. Flynn, J.T., Cassady, J., Essner, D., et al. Fluorescein angiography in retrolental fibroplasia: experience from 1969–1977. *Ophthalmology* 86:1700–1723, 1979.

19. Kretzer, F.L., Hittner, H.M., Johnson, A.T., et al. Vitamin E and retrolental fibroplasia: ultrastructural support of clinical efficacy. *Ann. N.Y. Acad. Sci.* 393:145–166, 1982.

20. Ashton, N. Retrolental fibroplasia. *Am. J. Ophthalmol.* 39:153–159, 1955

21. Ashton, N., Henkind, P. Experimental occlusion of retinal arterioles. *Br. J. Ophthalmol.* 49:225–234, 1965.

22. Cogan, D.G. Development and senescence of the human retinal vasculature. *Trans. Ophthalmol. Soc. U.K.* 83:465–489, 1963.

23. Karlsberg, R.C., Green, W.R., Patz, A. Congenital retrolental fibroplasia. *Arch. Ophthalmol.* 89:122–123, 1973.

24. Quinn, G.E., Schaffer, D.B., Johnson, L.H. Classification of retinopathy of prematurity as a predictive tool: a re-evaluation. In: Syllabus from Retinopathy of Prematurity Conference, Washington, D.C., Dec. 4–6, 1981, vol. 1, Columbus, Ohio: Ross Laboratories, 1981, pp. 303–317.

25. Payne, J.W., Patz, A. Current status of retrolental fibroplasia. *Am. Clin. Research.* 11:205–221, 1979.

26. McCormick, A.Q. Retinopathy of prematurity. *Curr. Probl. Pediatr.* 7:3–28, 1977.

27. Kingham, J.D. Acute retrolental fibroplasia. *Arch. Ophthalmol.* 95:39–47, 1973.

28. Reese, A.B., King, M., Owens, W.C. A classification of retrolental fibroplasia. *Am. J. Ophthalmol.* 36:1333–1335, 1953.

29. Uemura, Y. Current states of retrolental fibroplasia. *Jpn. J. Ophthalmol.* 21:366–378, 1977.

30. Schaffer, D.B., Johnson, L., Quinn, G.E., Goggs, T.R. A classification of retrolental fibroplasia to evaluate vitamin E therapy. *Opthalmology* 86:1749–1760, 1979.
31. Quinn, G.E., Schaffer, D.B., Johnson, L.H. Classification of retinopathy of prematurity. *Am. J. Ophthalol.* 94:744–749, 1982.
32. Kushner, B.J. Strabismus and amblyopia associated with regressed retinopathy of prematurity. *Arch. Ophthalmol.* 100:256–261, 1982.
33. Johnson, L., Schaffer, D., Boggs, T.R., Jr. The premature infant, vitamin E deficiency and retrolental fibroplasia. *Am. J. Clin. Nutr.* 27:1158–1173, 1974.
34. Johnson, L. Retrolental fibroplasia: a new look at an unresolved problem. *Hosp. Pract.* 16(1):109–121, 1981.
35. Phelps, D.L., Rosenbaum, A.L. Vitamin E in kitten oxygen induced retinopathy. II. Blockage of vitreal neovascularization. *Arch. Ophthalmol.* 97:1522–1526, 1979.
36. Puklin, J.E., Simon R.M., Ehrenkranz, R.A. Influence on retrolental fibroplasia of intramuscular vitamin E during respiratory distress syndrome. *Ophthalmology* 89:96–103, 1982.
37. Finer, N.N., Schindler, R.F., Grant, G. Effect of intramuscular vitamin E in the frequency and severity of retrolental fibroplasia: a controlled trial. *Lancet* 1:1087–1091, 1982.
38. Milner, R.A., Watts, J.L., Paes, B., Zipursky, A. RLF in 1500 gm. neonates: part of a randomized clinical trial of the effectiveness of vitamin E. Retinopathy of Prematurity conference syllabus, Washington, D.C., Dec. 4–6, 1981, vol. 2, pp. 703–716.
39. Hittner, H.M., Godio, L.B., Rudolph, A.J., Retrolental fibroplasia: efficacy of E in a double-blind clinical study of preterm infants. *N. Engl. J. Med.* 305:1365–1371, 1981.
40. Phelps, D.L. Vitamin E and retrolental fibroplasia in 1982. *Pediatrics* 70:420–425, 1982.
41. Nagata, M., Yamagishi, N. Treatment of acute proliferative. Retinopathy of Prematurity Conference Syllabus, Washington, D.C., Dec. 4–6, 1981, vol. 2, pp. 772–790.
42. Sasaki, K., Yamashita, Y., Maekawa, T., Adachi, T. Treatment of retinopathy of prematurity in active stage by cryocautery. *Jpn. J. Ophthalmol.* 20:384–395, 1976.
43. McPherson, A. Retinal detachment surgery in very young premature infants with acute retrolental fibroplasia: 25 new cases. Retinopathy of prematurity conference syllabus, Washington, D.C., Dec. 4–6, 1981, vol. 2, pp. 701–801.
44. Tasman, W. Retinal detachment in retrolental fibroplasia. *Albrecht von Grafes Arch. Klin. Ophthalmol.* 195:129–139, 1975.
45. Treister, G., Machemer, R. Results of vitrectomy for rare proliferative and hemorrhagic disease. *Am. J. Ophthalmol.* 84:394–412, 1977.
46. James, L.S., Lanman, J.T. (eds.), History of oxygen therapy and retrolental fibroplasia. Pediatrics 57 (Suppl. 4): 591–637, 1978.
47. Palmer, E.A. Optimal timing of examination for acute retrolental fibroplasia. In: Syllabus from Retinopathy of Prematurity Conference, Washington, D.C., Dec. 4–6, 1981, vol. 1, Columbus, Ohio: Ross Laboratories, 1981, pp. 282–302.

25

Congenital Eye Infections

Graham E. Quinn, M.D.

Congenital ocular infections present as a wide spectrum of ocular abnormalities in the newborn period. A majority of infections are acquired via transplacental transmission of the infective agent, but retrograde infection may occur in premature rupture of membranes, and infection may be transmitted during vaginal delivery

The extent and type of ocular abnormality is greatly influenced by the age of the fetus at infection. However, the virulence of the organism, its affinity for certain tissues, and the distribution of the agent within the human organism play a large part in the visual outcome for an individual eye. In general, the earlier the insult, the greater the malformation or disruption manifest in the eye. Infections acquired near or during birth tend to present as inflammatory processes.

The TORCH syndrome is an array of findings caused by toxoplasmosis, rubella, cytomegalic inclusion disease, syphilis, or herpes simplex virus; these are the classic agents associated with congenital eye infections. Discussion will be limited to these five agents, although it is well recognized now that ocular involvement may be seen in congenital herpes zoster virus, mumps virus, Epstein-Barr virus, and cryptococcal infections [1].

Toxoplasmosis

Janku [2] described the first human case of ocular toxoplasmosis in 1923 by finding parasite cysts in the eyes of a hydrocephalic infant. Until that time, the chorioretinal scar in the macula was thought to be a congenital coloboma, but this report opened the investigation of an infectious etiology. It is now felt that chorioretinal involvement with *Toxoplasma gondii* is the result of congenital infection only [1,3].

Congenital toxoplasmosis classically presents as a tetrad of retino-choroiditis, hydrocephaly, neurologic abnormalities, and random intra-cranial calcification, [4], but may be inactive and clinically inapparent at birth. In the inactive form, diagnosis may be delayed until neurologic abnormalities are noted or until the chorioretinitis causes visual disturbance. It appears that over 80 percent of children with subclinical congenital toxoplasmosis have ocular involvement [5]. In neonates with known infections, ocular involvement is seen in approximately 70 percent of cases [6].

The incidence of congenital toxoplasmosis shows regional differences with the probability variation of 1 in 10,000 in the United States to 1 in 500 in Norway [7]. A woman who is freshly infected with *Toxoplasma* during pregnancy has about a 40 percent chance of having an affected child. The clinical expression of the disease is more severe in infections acquired early in pregnancy [8].

Figure 25–1
Quiescent macular scar with dense pigmentation.

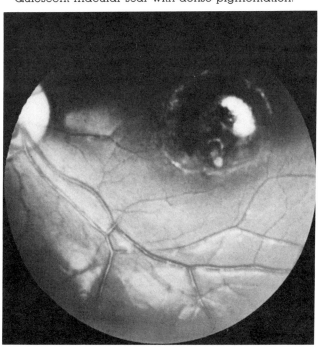

Microphthalmia is seen in over 20 percent of infants with ocular abnormalities and toxoplasmosis [4]. Leukocoria may be seen when intraocular inflammation causes cataracts or a severe central retinochoroiditis. In addition, an anterior uveitis may be present when associated with a retinochoroiditis [1].

The characteristic lesion on ophthalmoscopic examination in the neonate is a retinal lesion [6,8]. Acutely it appears as one or more yellowish-white, ill-defined lesions with a predilection for the posterior pole. They often show an overlying vitreous haze secondary to retinal involvement [9].

Indeed, the outer layers of the retina may also be secondarily involved with the inflammatory process, resulting in a focal panophthalmitis. The acute lesions subside with or without treatment over 6 to 10 weeks and undergo cicatricial change.

Quiescent retinal lesions of congenital toxoplasmosis are white chorioretinal scars with various degrees of pigmentation, particularly at its periphery (Figures 25–1 and 25–2). The lesions are, however, quite peomorphic and may be manifest as only small, nonpigmented lesions (Figures 25–3 and 25–4) or large, deeply pigmented scars. Visual morbidity is based on lesion size and location.

Figure 25–2
Large cystic lesion with atrophic, non-pigmented satellite lesions.

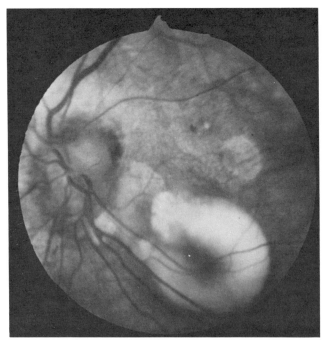

Figure 25–3

Small retinal lesion with densely pigmented center and atrophic edge showing pleomorphism of toxoplasmosis lesions.

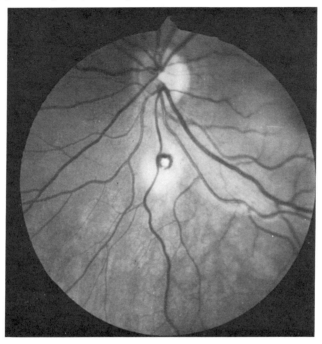

Reactivation of old lesions or late onset of subclinical lesions may occur from weeks to years after birth [5]. Recurrent lesions are usually small, yellow-white lesions at the border of a retinochoroidal scar (Figure 25–5). These lesions are often associated with mild iritis and visual disturbance (especially blurring secondary to vitritis), and it is this symptomatology that brings the patient to the ophthalmologist [4].

Optic atrophy, papillitis (Figure 25–6), nystagmus, and strabismus are also seen in congenital toxoplasmosis [4], and may be secondary to severe ocular involvement or intracranial disease.

The *Toxoplasma gondii* organism causes focal necrosis of the retina, with an associated inflammation of the other coats of the eye. It is probable that the natural cycle is initiated by the ingestion of infective oocysts from excreta of the cat family. In addition, a respiratory route of infection has been proposed [10].

Treatment of acute ocular toxoplasmosis is generally reserved for posterior pole uveitis where the macular region might be threatened. Combined use of systemic pyrimethamine, sulfadiazine, and folinic acid may be used in this situation, and systemic corticosteroids may also have

Figure 25–4
Retinal lesion with overlying vitreous veil.

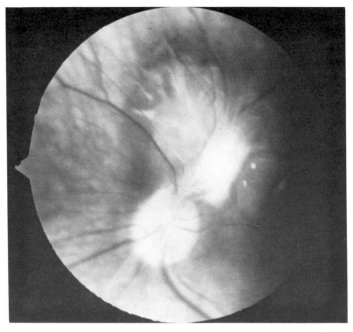

Figure 25–5
Small, yellow-white area of reactivation at edge of old scar in teenage girl.

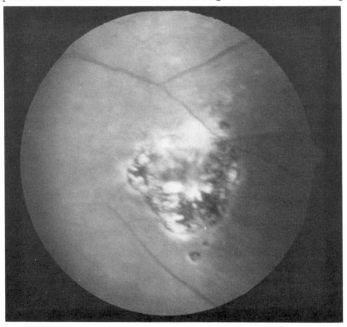

Figure 25–6
Optic papillitis seen in acute toxoplasmosis.

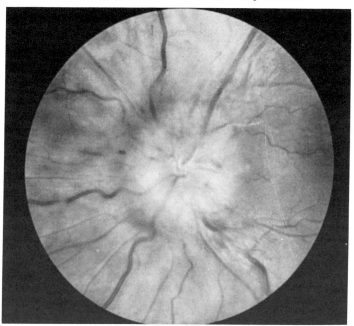

a place. Anterior uveitis is treated with cycloplegics and local steroids [11]. Clindamycin has been reported effective for recurrent disease [9].

Rubella

The effect of prenatal infection with rubella virus was first recognized by Sir Norman Gregg in 1941 [12]. He reported 78 infants who had ocular disorders born to mothers who had had rubella infections the first trimester of pregnancy. Classically a triad of findings are associated with congenital rubella: eye, ear and heart defects.

During the brief rubella viremia in a pregnant woman the virus crosses the placenta to the fetus. In 1968, Rawls et al. [13] demonstrated a widely uneven distribution of infected fetal cells that may lead to the wide variation in clinical manifestations of the syndrome. Adding to the variation, the incidence of embryopathy related to viral infection in the first month of the pregnancy is around 50 percent [14].

The systemic findings of congenital rubella syndrome include low birth weight, deafness, heart defects (especially patent ductus arteriosus), mental

319

Figure 25–7

Morgagnian cataract with nucleus displaced inferiorly in liquid cortical material.

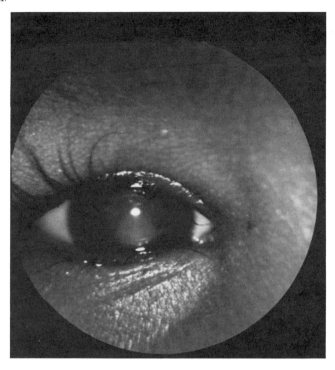

Figure 25–8
Nuclear cataract with poor iris dilation after atropine instillation.

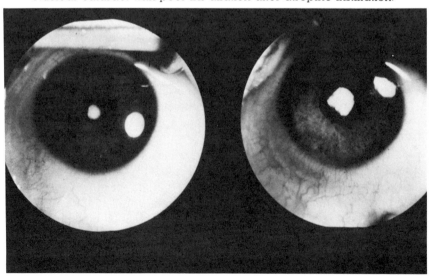

retardation, hepatosplenomegaly, thrombocytopenia and purpura, dental deformities, and osteomyelitis [15].

Every part of the eye may be involved with the organ odysgenesis seen in early gestational rubella, and ocular manifestations are reported in 30 to 70 percent of involved children [16]. Microphthalmia, cataracts, cloudy cornea, and pigmentary retinopathy were all reported by Gregg [12]. Microphthalmia may be unilateral or bilateral and is seen in about 20 percent of involved infants [17].

Cataracts occur in over half of affected children, and three-quarters of these are bilateral (Figure 25–7). Retention of cell nuclei in the lens fibers is characteristic of the rubella cataract [18], and the lens is most

Figure 25–9
Surgical iridectomy and aphakia in rubella syndrome.

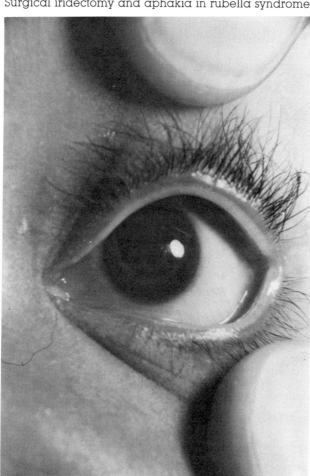

commonly affected when the maternal infection is between the second and eleventh weeks of gestation.

The technique and timing of surgical cataract removal have remained controversial (Figures 25–8 and 25–9). Wolf [15] recommended sector iridectomy as the initial procedure and then generally a two-step discission and aspiration. In children operated on before one year of age, significant postoperative complications were seen in 55.2 percent (29 eyes), and 21 percent of those children operated on after 18 months of age had complications. It was speculated that, since positive viral cultures of lens material were seen up to 22 months of age, liberating active viral particles in the eye with resultant inflammation was the etiology of the significant postoperative complications [18].

Cordes and Hertzberg established the efficacy of a one-step cataract procedure that was associated with fewer complications [19,20].

Corneal clouding may be a transient phenomenon in the affected neonate and may reflect viral involvement of the developing corneal endothelium [15]. Corneal clouding may also be seen in the eye with increased intraocular pressure. Such glaucoma (Figure 25–10) is seen in around 10 percent of rubella infants although the diagnosis may be quite difficult in the microphthalmic or cataractous eye. Late-onset glaucoma has been

Figure 25–10
Rubella cataract and corneal haze secondary to glaucoma.

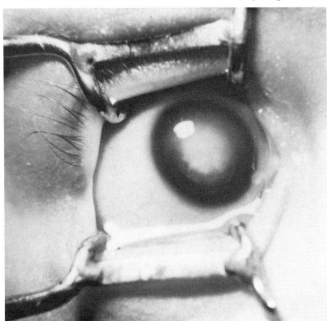

Figure 25–11
Fine, diffuse pigmentary retinopathy throughout retina.

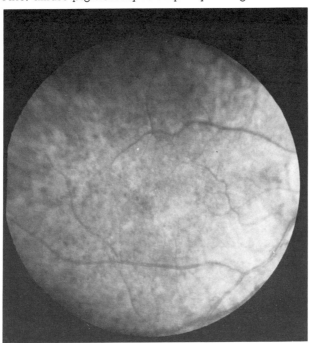

recognized as late as 22 years of age and is quite difficult to treat either medically or surgically [21].

Rubella retinopathy or "salt and pepper" pigmentary retinopathy (Figure 25–11) is seen in up to 70 percent of rubella cases [22]. Mild and moderate involvement is felt to be stable, nonprogressive, and not associated with visual acuity defects [15]. However, Krill [23] reported electroretinographic abnormalities in children with pigmentary retinopathy. Clinically the retinopathy of rubella syndrome is pleomorphic with patches of retinal pigment epithelium atrophy and hypertrophy (Figure 25–12) [24].

Other ophthalmological abnormalities of children with congenital rubella syndrome are dacryostenosis, chronic keratic precipitites [21], strabismus, amblyopia, optic atrophy, nystagmus, and high refractive errors [17].

Cytomegalic Inclusion Disease

Cytomegalovirus is one of the four known infectious herpesviruses in humans [25] and is the most common viral infective of the neonate, occurring

Figure 25–12
Atrophic areas of retinal pigment epithelium in diffuse "salt and pepper" retinopathy.

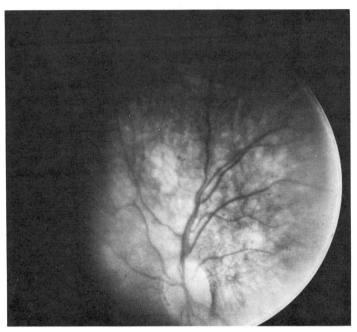

in 0.5 to 2.4 percent of live births in the United States [26]. The majority of affected infants are asymptomatic at birth, and few patients will have the full expression of the disease: hepatomegaly, microcephaly, periventricular calcification, mental retardation, motor disability, jaundice, petechiae, and chorioretinitis.

Ocular involvement in a patient with congenital cytomegaloviral infection was demonstrated [27] with inclusion bodies in the anterior corneal tract. The first isolation of cytomegalovirus from aqueous was in 1959 [28]. Since these reports, chorioretinitis, retinal hemorrhages, corneal clouding, conjunctivitis, cataract, optic atrophy, optic nerve hypoplasia and/or colomboma, and microphthalmia have been reported [1,29].

The most frequent site of involvement is the retina, and the lesions are seen at birth or shortly afterward. Characteristic acute retinal changes are small, yellow-white granular lesions with surrounding hemorrhagic patches in the posterior pole or midperiphery. In time, these lesions coalesce and form pale scars with little pigmentation (Figures 25–13 and 25–14). Pigmentary clumping may on occasion be so severe as to mimic toxoplasmosis. The hemorrhagic component of the acute process may also

Figure 25-13

Chorioretinal scar with little pigmentary reaction *(From Schaffer, D.B. Eye findings in intrauterine infections.* Clin. Perinatol. *8:434, 1981).*

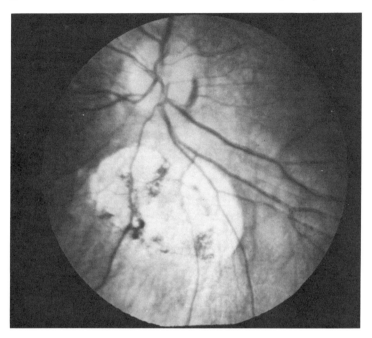

be so extensive as to resemble a branch vein occlusion [30]. The vitreous reaction in the region of an active lesion is minimal.

Of prognostic importance is that chorioretinitis in a child with cytomegaloviral infection is very likely to be associated with microcephaly, whereas in the child with toxoplasmosis it frequently occurs without major central nervous system abnormalities [25]. A similar observation might be made about the intracranial calcifications seen in the two diseases. The child with calcifications from toxoplasmosis may not have severe brain damage, but calcifications seen in cytomegaloviral disease almost always herald severe central nervous system damage.

Optic nerve abnormalities are the next most common ocular manifestations of cytomegalovirus infection and range from optic atrophy [31] to severe coloboma with microphthalmia [29].

Optic atrophy has been reported in 25 percent of congenitally affected children [31].

Frenkel et al. [32] reported a series of unusual eye findings in congenital cytomegalovirus infection. His series included two children with clinical anophthalmia (one unilateral, one bilateral) and one child with

Figure 25–14
Small atrophic retinal lesion from congenital cytomegalovirus infection.

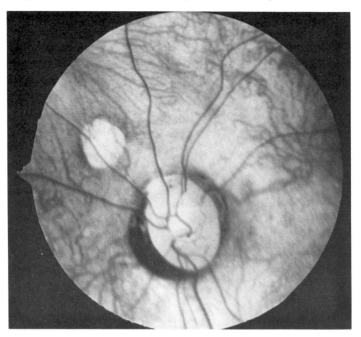

Peter's anomaly. Peter's anomaly is a congenital central corneal opacity with adherence of the lens. It is interesting that an infectious etiology was originally speculated, but the causal relationship of cytomegalovirus remains to be proven.

No specific therapy for congenital cytomegaloviral infections is available, and systemic adenine arabinoside and other antiviral agents have yet to be proven effective. Stagno et al. [31] reported that infants with congenital infections are most likely born to mothers with primary, not recurrent, infections.

Herpes Simplex Virus

Herpes simplex virus infections in the neonate may be acquired in three ways, and this probably accounts for the wide variability of ocular manifestations. Most herpes infections are acquired late in pregnancy, frequently in association with premature rupture of membranes in an affected mother and by direct contact with an active genital infection in the infant's passage through the vagina. Least common is fetal acquisition of the virus [33]. As most infections are acquired around the time of birth, one would expect, and indeed observes, that most neonatal ocular effects are inflammatory and not teratogenic [11]. In addition, the route of infection may explain the preponderance of herpes simplex virus type 2 as the etiologic agent in over 80 percent of neonatal herpes infections [34].

The ocular manifestations of neonatal herpes infection are conjunctivitis, keratitis, chorioretinitis, uveitis, cataracts (Figure 25–15), optic atrophy, and microphthalmia and vary widely as to manifestation over time. Ocular findings are present in about 17 percent of neonatal herpes simplex virus infections and may be unilateral or bilateral [35].

Conjunctivitis due to herpes simplex virus may mimic other causes of ophthalmia neonatorium. Onset is usually between days 3 and 14 of life with moderate injection and serous exudate. Of interest is the absence of conjunctival lymphoid follicle reaction common to newborns [17]. In the absence of central nervous system disturbance or skin lesions, confusion about diagnosis is likely.

Keratitis is uncommon at birth and occurs after the onset of conjunctivitis. It appears usually between the second and eighth week of life and presents as a diffusely opaque cornea with superficial epithelial defects

Figure 25–15
Intense anterior uveitis with cataract seen in congenital herpes simplex infection.

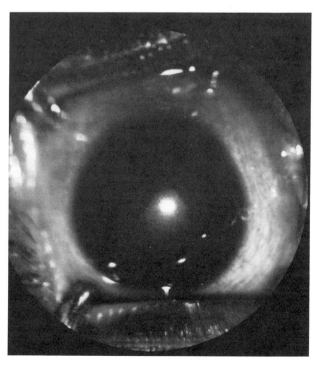

Figure 25–16

Small, non-pigmented retinal lesion of herpes simplex showing similarity to other congenital chorioretinal infections.

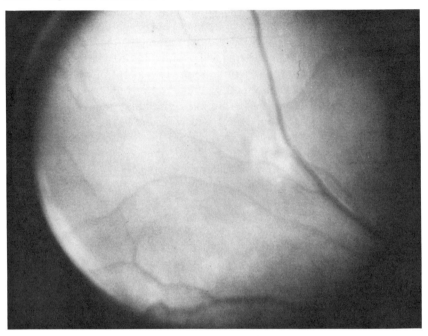

[36]. Epithelial dendrites and even geographic ulcers may occur, and deep disciform keratitis has been documented [33]. The long-term effects of ocular occlusion secondary to keratitis are yet to be determined.

Nahmias et al. [35] described chorioretinitis in 13 of 297 cases of neonatal herpes simplex virus infections and found a high correlation with central nervous system disease. When typing was done, herpes simplex virus type 2 was found in all cases of chorioretinitis. The retinal lesion seen varies greatly and, in the acute phase, is indistinguishable from other acute retinitis. It is yellowish-white with marked vitritis, may be extensive or small, and may be located in the periphery or posterior pole. As activity subsides, the intensity of pigmentation varies, and old scars may mimic toxoplasmosis or cytomegalovirus infections (Figures 25–16 and 25–17). In severe retinal involvement, cataracts, optic atrophy and severe global disruption may ensue [37].

Ocular involvement by herpes simplex virus of the neonate may be progressive, recurrent, and visually debilitating, so the diagnosis must be suspected early on in the clinical picture. Careful scraping of corneal or conjunctival epithelium may reveal a typical picture of multinucleated giant cells or intranuclear inclusions [33]. As herpes simplex virus type 2 is the

Figure 25–17

Small atrophic, punched-out chorioretinal lesions seen in an infant with herpes simplex infection.

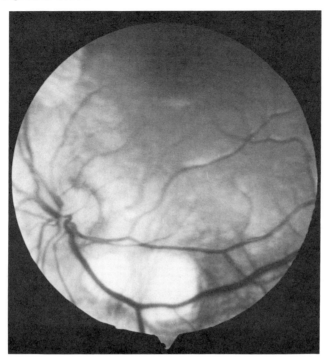

more common infective agent in this age group, initial medical treatment should be cytosine or adenine arabinoside rather than idoxuridine, which is less effective against herpes simplex virus type 2 [1]. The question of when to initiate systemic treatment in the absence of clinical or laboratory signs of disseminated herpetic involvement is still quite controversial [35].

Syphilis

Congenital syphilis is generally acquired by transplacental transmission of *Treponema pallidum* after the fourth gestational month; chorioretinitis, "salt and pepper" fundus, glaucoma, secondary cataract, uveitis, and eyelid chancres have been observed in the affected infant [38]. Approximately 5 percent of the children with congenital syphilis (and there were 300 in 1974) will have chorioretinitis as their earliest ocular finding [1].

Acute anterior or posterior uveitis may be present at birth and may lead to secondary cataracts and glaucoma from the chronic inflammation.

Figure 25–18

Pseudoretinitis pigmentosa seen in congenital syphilis. *(From Schaffer, D.B. Eye findings in intrauterine infections.* Clin. Perinatol. *8:417, 1981).*

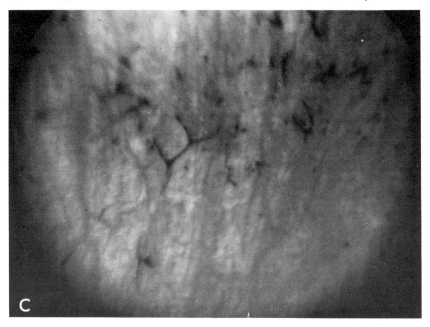

The posterior chorioretinal lesions vary in size, distribution, and location. Irregularity of the retinal pigment epithelium ("salt and pepper" appearance) is characteristic of the healed stage of inflammation where fibrosis, depigmentation, pigment clumping, and patches of chorioretinal atrophy are seen. Observed earlier, focal scattered deep retinal layers would predominate. In addition, a perivascular "bony spicule" picture may be seen that closely resembles primary retinitis pigmetosa (Figure 25–18) [39].

The most suggestive ocular finding in congenital syphilis is interstitial keratitis. It is rarely seen at birth, but occurs generally in the first decade of life in late congenital syphilis. An acute unilateral keratitis generally becomes bilateral in weeks to months and is manifest by severe photophobia, lacrimation, and blurring of vision. On examination these patients have conjunctival injection, miosis, corneal edema, and vascularization [38]. The vascularization proceeds so rapidly that the cornea becomes pink ("salmon-patch" appearance) and, untreated, will last 18 to 24 months. An intense anterior uveitis occurs at the same time. The corneal infiltrate clears from the periphery, and empty blood vessels ("ghost vessels") are identifiable under slit lamp examination [1]. The central haze may persist and cause visual difficulties. Approximately one-third of untreated cases have significant enough scarring to have vision below the 20/50 level [40]. Regardless of treatment, recurrences are common.

Interstitial keratitis appears due to a late hypersensitivity reaction rather than direct spirochete invation [38]. Indeed the organism is difficult to demonstrate in the acute process, whereas at birth, the cornea may have had abundant spirochetes with no evidence of keratitis [40].

Treatment of congenital syphilis requires systemic penicillin and local cyclopegics and systemic or local steroids as indicated. It appears that the late interstitial keratitis can be prevented by treatment of congenital syphilis before three months of age [41].

Acknowledgments

I thank my colleague, David B. Schaffer, M.D., who graciously permitted me to use photographs from his collection. He provided all prints for the figures.

References

1. Chandler, S.H. Ocular abnormalities associated with intrauterine infections. *Perspect. Ophthalmol.* 3:249–268, 1979.
2. Janku, J. Pathogenesis and pathologic anatomy of coloboma of the macula lutea in a microphthalmic eye with parasites in the retina. *Casop. Lek. Gesk.* 62:1021–1138, 1923.
3. Akstein, R.B., Wilson, L.A., Teutsch, S. Acquired toxoplasmosis (abstr.) *Ophthalmology* 58:49–67, 1981.
4. Remington, J.S., Desmonts, G. Toxoplasmosis. In Remington, J.S., Klein, J.O. (eds.), *Infectious Diseases of the Fetus and Newborn Infant*. Philadelphia: The W.B. Saunders Co., 1976, pp. 191–351.
5. Wilson, C.B., Remington, J.S., Stagno, S., Reynolds, D.W. Development of adverse sequelae in children born with subclinical congenital toxoplasma infections. *Pediatrics* 66:767–774, 1980.
6. Couvruer, J., Desmonts, G. Congenital and maternal toxoplasmosis: review of 300 congenital cases. *Dev. Med. Child Neurol.* 4:519–512, 1962.
7. Schlaegel, T.F. Toxoplasmosis. In Duane, T.D. (ed.), *Clinical Ophthalmology*, vol. 21. Philadelphia: Harper & Row, Publishers, 1981, pp. 2–17.
8. Desmonts, G., Couvreur, J. Pregnancy and the fetus. *Bull. N.Y. Acad. of Med.* 50:839–851, 1966.
9. Schlaegel, T.F. *Ocular Toxoplasmosis and Pars Planitis*. New York: Grune and Stratton, 1978, p. 251.
10. Editorial. Transmission of toxoplasmosis. *Br. Med. J.* 1:126–127, 1970.
11. Schaffer, D.B. Eye findings in intrauterine infections. *Clin. Perinatol.* 8:415–443, 1981.

12. Gregg, N.M. Congenital cataract following german measles in the mother. *Trans. Ophthalmol. Soc. Aust.* 3:35, 1941.

13. Rawls, W.E., Desmyter, J., Melnick, J.L. Serologic diagnosis and fetal involvement in maternal rubella. criteria for abortion. *J. Am. Med. Assoc.* 203:627–631, 1968.

14. Hardy, J.B., Monif, G.R.G., Sever, J.L. Studies in congenital rubella, Baltimore 1967–1965. *Bull. Johns Hopkins Hosp.* 118:97–108, 1966.

15. Wolf, S.M. The ocular manifestations of congenital rubella. *J. Pediatr. Ophthalmol.* 10:101–141, 1973.

16. Rudolph, A.J., Desmond, M.M. Clinical manifestations of the congenital rubella syndrome. *Int. Ophthalmol. Clinics.* 12:3–19, 1972.

17. Schaffer, D.B. Ophthalmia neonatorum. In Scheie, H.G., Albert, D.M. (eds.), *Textbook of Ophthalmology,* 9th ed. Philadelphia: The W.B. Saunders Co., 1977, pp. 321–323.

18. Yanoff, M., Schaffer, D.B., Scheie, H.G. Rubella ocular syndrome: clinical significance of viral and pathologic studies. *Trans. Am. Acad. Ophthalmol. Otolaryngol.* 72:896–902, 1968.

19. Cordes, F.D. Surgery of congenital cataracts. *Am. J. Ophthalmol.* 31:1073–1084, 1948.

20. Hertzberg, R. Twenty-five year follow-up of ocular defects in congenital rubella. *Am. J. Ophthalmol.* 66:269–271, 1968.

21. Boger, W.P. Late ocular complications in congenital rubella syndrome. *Ophthalmology* 87:1244–1252, 1980.

22. Schaffer, D.B. Congenital infections. In Scheie, H.G., Albert, D.M. (eds.), *Textbook of Ophthalmology,* 9th ed. Philadelphia: The W.B. Saunders Co., 1977, pp. 311–320.

23. Krill, A.E. The retinal disease of rubella. *Arch. Ophthalmol.* 77:445–449, 1967.

24. Yanoff, M. The retina in rubella. In Tasman, W. (ed.), *Retinal Diseases in Children.* New York: Harper & Row, Publishers, 1971, pp. 223–232.

25. Hanshaw, J.B. Cytomegalovirus. In Remington, J.S., Klein, J.C. (eds.), *Infectious Diseases of the Fetus and newborn Infant.* Philadelphia: The W. B. Saunders Co., 1976, pp. 107–164.

26. Pass, R.F., Stagno, S., Myers, G.J., Alford, C.A. Outcome of symptomatic congenital cytomegalovirus infection: results of long-term longitudinal follow-up. *Pediatrics* 66:758–762, 1980.

27. Kalfayan, B. Inclusion disease of infancy. *Arch. Pathol.* 44:467–476, 1947.

28. Burns, R.P. Cytomegalic inclusion disease uveitis: report of a case with isolation from aqueous humor of virus in tissue culture. *Arch. Ophthalmol.* 61:376–387, 1959.

29. Hittner, H.M., Desmond, M.M., Montgomery, J.A. Optic nerve manifestations of human congenital cytomegalovirus infection. *Am. J. Ophthalmol.* 81:661–664, 1976.

30. Boniuk, I. The cytomegalovirus and the eye. *Int. Ophthalmol. Clin.* 12:169–190, 1972.

31. Stagno, S., Reynolds, D.W., Amos, C.S., et al. Auditory and visual defects resulting from symptomatic and subclinical congenital cytomegaloviral and toxoplasma infections. *Pediatrics* 49:669–678, 1977.

32. Frenkel, L.D., Keys, M.P., Hefferen, S.J., et al. Unusual eye abnormalities associated with congenital cytomegalovirus infections. *Pediatrics* 66:763–766, 1980.

33. Nahmaias, A.J., Hagler, W.S. Ocular manifestations of herpes simplex in the newborn. *Int. Ophthalmol. Clin.* 12:191–213, 1972.

34. Florman, A.L., Gershon, A.A., Blackett, P.R., Nahmias, A.J. Intrauterine infection with herpes simplex virus: resultant congenital malformations. *J. Am. Med. Assoc.* 225:129–132, 1973.

35. Nahmias, A.J., Visintine, A.M., Caldwell, D.R., Wilson, L.A. Eye infections with herpes simplex virus in neonates. *Surv. Ophthalmol.* 21:100–105, 1976.

36. Hutchinson, D.S., Smith, R.E., Haughton, P.B. Congenital herpetic keratitis. *Arch. Ophthalmol.* 93:70–73, 1975.

37. Cogan, D.G., Kuwabara, T., Young, G.F., Knox, D.L. Herpes simplex retinopathy in an infant. *Arch. Ophthalmol.* 72:641–645, 1964.

38. Ingall, D., Norins, L. Syphilis. In Remington, J.S., Klein, J.O. (eds.), *Infectious Diseases of the Fetus and Newborn Infant*. Philadelphia: The W.B. Saunders Co., 1976, pp. 414–458.

39. Bernardino, V.B., Naidoff, M.A. Retinal inflammatory diseases. In Duane, T. (ed.), *Clinical Ophthalmology,* vol. 3. Philadelphia: Harper & Row, Publishers, pp. 1–11.

40. Smith, J.L. Congenital syphilis. In Smith, J.L. (ed.), *Spirochetes in Late Seronegative Syphilis, Penicillin Notwithstanding*. Springfield, Ill.: Charles C. Thomas, Publisher, 1969, pp. 252–260.

41. Tavs, L.E. Syphilis. *Maj. Probl. Clin. Pediatr.* 19:222–256, 1978.

26

Stimulation Programs in the Neonatal Intensive Care Nursery

Gail Liberg, M.P.A., O.T.R., Cheryl Ehrhart, R.N., M.S., and Manohar Rathi, M.D.

Current information indicates that low-birth-weight premature infants are at a high risk both in terms of actual survival and in terms of future neurologic development or intellectual, social, and emotional impairments. A large percentage of these survivors have problems that include retardation in growth, cerebral palsy, visual disturbances, behavioral problems, and mental retardation. Sonstegard et al. [1] Stewart and Reynolds [2] Grassey et al. [3] and Teberg et al. [4] have reported a decrease in mortality and morbidity rates for high-risk newborns because of changes in management that include regionalization of care, better coordinated maternal and neonatal programs, technological advances, and early identification of developmental defects. Despite this progress, the high-risk infant remains at risk for developmental delays, neuropsychiatric disabilities, and future learning disorders. Many workers in this field feel that more attention should be directed at assessing the infants' strengths and vulnerabilities so that ways can be found to help surviving infants lead full and more productive lives [5–11].

Under normal circumstances, the human infant receives a variety of stimulating, growth-facilitating experiences throughout the course of his or her intrauterine development. The intrauterine environment provides a continual and progressive bombardment of activity from the moment of conception to the moment of birth. This includes the stimulation and protection of the amniotic fluid; the tactile, kinesthetic, vestibular, and auditory stimulation provided by the mother's cardiovascular system and her physical movements; the tactile stimulation provided by the infant's body growth [12]; the effects on the infant's sleep-wake cycles provided by the maternal sleep cycles and neurohumoral secretions [13]; and the actual physical stimulation of the labor itself.

It has been demonstrated that there is a critical period during perinatal life when maximal brain growth occurs, and adequate conditions of stimulation are needed to facilitate genetically defined patterns of behavior. Autopsies show that a lack of stimulation may lead to a decrease in brain weight, lack of dendritic connections between nerve cells, and axons shrinking in diameter. Deprivation of stimuli also alters the rates of synthesis of protein and ribonucleic acid in brain cells. The growth and maintenance of neural structures are facilitated by any type of intermittent, patterned afferent stimulation in the tactile, auditory, visual, vestubular, and kinesthetic areas [14]. Early and systematic stimulation of the nerve cells can accelerate growth and development in the premature infant [15].

Normal development is believed to be contingent upon the impact of varied stimuli upon the human organism. Sensory input helps the infant to establish the first level of learning and cognitive growth by teaching him to distinguish himself from the external environment. Infants have tactile and kinesthetic needs that are separate from, but of equal importance to, the sensory needs of other stages. This tactile-kinesthetic phase in utero predates the oral phase, and motility may be a specific mode of expression [16].

The premature infant lacks control of this motility and thus may not have the ability the full-term baby has to discharge tension to reestablish homeostasis. Since the premature infant is deprived of his or her final weeks in utero, he or she not only is robbed of intrauterine stimulation, but also does not receive the type and amount of stimulation which the more routine hospital environment offers. Instead, he or she is placed in an isolette, which differs dramatically from the intrauterine or extrauterine environment of the healthy full-term infant [17,18]. Since the neonatal intensive care unit is basically an unhealthy environment, the stimulation the premature infant does receive is often noxious, intrusive, and irritating. This includes ventilator noises, the constant hum of isolettes, the noise from medical rounds, monitors, alarms, charting on isolettes, and loud music, as well as the irritation of injections, intravenous treatments, gavage feedings, and blood tests. Because of the babies' physical problems, parental visitation is limited and the babies receive limited handling. All of these factors combine to jeopardize the premature infant's chance for optimal neurologic and cognitive development. Some of the more recent research studies of infant stimulation in the neonatal intensive care nursery and their implications are discussed in this Chapter. We will also present an innovative approach for implementing a stimulation program in a neonatal intensive care unit which requires no specialized equipment but does require appropriately trained personnel.

Review of Literature

The major types of stimulation that researchers have studied when attempting to alter the early environment of the full-term, high-risk, and premature infant include vestibular, proprioceptive, tactile, auditory, and visual input. Two basic theoretical rationales for stimulation programs have been utilized, including 1) attempts to duplicate the womb environment and 2) attempts to modify the stimulation program depending on the infant's condition. The former assumes that the premature infant is an extrauterine fetus who continues to grow in the same pattern as the infant who will attain full-term gestation; whereas the latter assumes that the competencies of the premature infant differ from those of the fetus who will reach full term, because the sensory system, like the cardiovascular, respiratory, and digestive systems, undergoes a dramatic change at birth. We agree with the latter philosophy and feel that a careful assessment of the infant should be done to determine what stimulation is appropriate for a particular baby.

When reviewing the literature previously written on infant stimulation, we found some discrepancies in results; however, a general feeling was evident that careful stimulation causes positive changes in the full-term, preterm, or high-risk infant. A table of more current research projects is provided in Table 26-1. Some of the more pertinent effects of stimulation observed include increased weight gain, decreased incidence of central apnea, higher scores on mental and motor tests, less irritability, altered arousal levels, sleep states, and cardiac responses, and a more efficient utilization of calories. These results could all be considered reflections of greater maturation of the central nervous system.

Additional responses relate to the parent-infant attachment process, which is felt to be affected by the infant's response to his or her environment. We presume that it is easier for a parent to attach to an infant who appears more responsive and pleasant than to a scrawny, irritable, or lethargic infant. Thus, the initial bonding process is also affected by the stimulation program and can be thought to influence later psychosocial development [19].

Early stimulation can actually prevent parental attachment problems such as those evidenced by failure to thrive, neglect, and abuse. Every effort should be made to include parents in the stimulation program and to help parents feel that they can contribute to their child's well-being [20].

Table 26–1
Stimulation

Type of Stimulus	Results	Author(s)	Reference
Vestibular-Kinesthetic Stimulation			
Common maternal soothing techniques	On the shoulder position was more effective than touch alone in soothing and comforting infants	Korner and Thomas	[45]
Stroking, handling, rocking	No difference in weight gain; premature group was more quiescent	Hasselmeyer	[17]
Rocking	Temporary weight gain	Freedman et al.	[46]
Rocking in motorized hammock	Greater weight gain, better scores on Graham-Rosenblith for general maturation, visual & auditory responsiveness, pull to sit and displacement of limbs	Neal	[47]
Vertical vestibular stimulation	Rocking effect was a positive function of amplitude; higher frequency rocking was greater than low frequency rocking; effectiveness of rocking was positive function of frequency	Pederson and Ter Vrugt	[48]
Oscillating waterbeds	No significant effects on vital signs, weight gain, or emesis frequency; experimental group had less apnea	Korner et al.	[24]
Spinning clockwise and counterclockwise	Decreased incidence of central apnea	Korner et al.	[22]
	Decrease in postrotary nystagmus in both groups	Kantner et al.	[21]
Tactile Stimulation			
Rubbing of backs, arms, and necks	Temporary weight gain, less crying, more activity, higher Bayley scores, more optimal growth and home environment	Solkoff et al.	[28]
Stroking head, arms, legs, and back	Decreased incidence of respiratory problems in experimental group 2; more weight gain in handled infants who were exposed to a temperature change	Freeman	[29]

Intervention	Author	Findings	Ref.
Stroking and flexing of arms and legs	Solkoff and Matuszak	Did not affect weight gain positively; more positive changes on Brazelton	[32]
Extra handling	Powell	Increased development on Bayley scores through 6 months of age; mothers' handling did not affect maternal behavior	[30]
Nonnutritive sucking	Kattwinkel et al.	Decreased incidence of central apnea	[49]
	Kramer et al.	Improved social development	[31]
	Neeley	Experimental infants were less irritable, spent more time in alert wakeful states, and required less burping	[50]
Finger sucking	Anderson and Vidyasagar	Sucking opportunities seemed to facilitate neuromuscular coordination, alert activity, alert inactivity, and deep sleep	[51]
Auditory Stimulation			
Adult heartbeat	Palmquist	Failed to replicate Salk's findings; no significant weight gain difference between two groups	[34]
Recorded mother's voice	Katz	No differences in irritability; better scores on Graham-Rosenblith test in motor, tactile, auditory, and visual function	[35]
	Segall	Greater heart rate accelerations and habituation to white noise; greater heart rate deceleration to unfamiliar female and mother's voices (greater attentiveness)	[36]
Maternal voices and Brahm's Lullaby recordings	Salk	Increased weight gain; no significant increases in mental and motor development at 9 months of age	[33]
	Chapman	Gross motor activity not decreased; females showed less activity than males; maternal speech group developed laterality more often	[52]
Noise and stimuli	Bench and Mentz	Heart rate habituation reflects progressive state changes	[53]

338

Stimulus	Description	Author	Ref
Familiar and discrepant auditory stimulation	A habituation memory relationship for an infant's cardiac response to auditory stimulation	Horowitz	[54]
Continuous white noise	Continuous auditory stimulation was directly related to lowering arousal levels in unstressed newborns	Brackbill	[37]
Low-intensity (continuous) auditory stimulation for 20 seconds	Experimental group responded by change in heart rate followed by a normal heart rate	Neal	[15]
Visual Stimulation			
Novel visual stimuli	Showed a greater awareness of and hesitancy to approach novel stimulation in familiar environment than in unfamiliar environment	Parry	[38]
	On the shoulder position significantly increased quality of visual behavior	Frederickson and Brown	[23]
Hands in field of vision	When in asymmetrical tonic neck reflex position hands were more likely to be visualized, which would affect later eye-hand coordination	Coryell and Henderson	[43]
Blue and green mobiles	Responsive to blue and green mobiles, but visual attention less sensitive than motor movements such as foot kicking for assessing perceptual response capacities	Fagan	[42]
Multimodal Stimulation			
Extra handling and stroking	Increased appetite and weight gain	White	[55]
Stroking and flexing of arms and legs	Greater weight gain, greater formula intake, fewer feedings required	White and Labarba	[56]
Tactile and vestibular stimulation	Intervention altered preterm; sensory function during active sleep, not quiet sleep	Rose et al.	[57]

Stimulation	Author	Findings	Ref
Rocking motion and heart beat sound	Barnard	Quieter sleep and longer duration of quiet sleep; less active awake stages; no differences in active or quiet sleep; greater maturation scores on Dubowitz; greater weight gain	[58]
	Kang and Barnard	Temporal stimulation patterning, started early in neonatal life, helped infant organize and integrate behavior and sleep patterns	[59]
Rocking water bed, simulated heartbeat, tape of mother's voice played during rocking	Kramer and Pierpont	Greater weight gain, greater growth in head circumference and biparietal diameter of head; no difference on Dubowitz or Brazelton	[60]
Auditory buzzer and rattle; tactile plastic filament	Field et al.	Preterm infants did not show a cardiac decrement to repeated stimulation, but did show an integration of autonomic and motor responsivity patterns in second experiment	[61]
Auditory, kinesthetic, and vestibular stimulation	Neal	Premature infants who were exposed to auditory, kinesthetic, and vestibular stimulation showed higher level of maturation	[62]
Group 1: visual decorating Group 2: body rubbing and passive limb movements Group 3: both Group 4: control	Groom	No significant differences in: habituation to auditory stimulation prior to discovery, conditioned head-turning at 42 weeks, weight gain at 42 weeks, head circumference at 42 weeks, irritability at 42 weeks	[63]
	McNichol	No effect on weight gain; groups receiving tactile stimulation had more visual tracking and less visual attention to bullseye; visual group less attention to bullseye	[64]

At Home Program

Intervention	Result	Author	Ref
Specific cephalocaudal massage treatment and rocking administered by mothers	Better Brazelton at 4 weeks; greater weight gain at 4 weeks; better Cattell scores at 1 year	Rice	[65]
Visual, auditory, tactile, and kinesthetic in hospital home visits after discharge	Greater weight gain at 4 months; better Bayley scores; greater maturational development as indicated by assessments of reflexes at 4 months	Scarr-Salapatek and Williams	[66]
Proprioceptive stimulation	Increased parents' visiting from experimental group	Rosenfield et al.	[67]
Mothering and contingent stimulation for eye opening, handling during feeding	Better performance at 4 months on visual reinforcement control of sucking behavior and auditory reinforcement task	Siqueland	[68]
Group 1: handling by nurses Group 2: handling by mothers	Group 1 regained birth weight faster, had no differences in weight or height at 2, 4, or 6 months and had better Bayley mental scores at 4 months and Bayley behavioral scores at 6 months	Powell	[30]
Tactile, visual, kinesthetic, and auditory stimulation	Experimental group scored significantly higher on Bayley scales at 6 months; improved capacity to relate to care giver	Leib et al.	[44]

341

Another effect of early stimulation is that it may influence the brain's growth in ways that will actually prevent or lessen later learning disabilities. Currently there is a controversial category of school age children with normal IQs who show problems that result in behavior disorders or in difficulty processing information. Twenty percent of the high-risk population now shows this problem [1]. Occupational therapists testing learning-disabled children have found that numerous neurologic soft signs are present, motor control is poor, and processing of sensory stimulation is inadequate. Hence the terms sensory integration and sensorimotor integration developed, implying that there is a functional interrelationship among the various sensory and motor areas in the brain. Therapists working with these problems have found that providing sensorimotor experiences can help these children progress in learning areas and help "integrate" the nervous system by increasing the child's ability to organize and process information at lower levels of the brain. Early stimulation in the nursery may encourage integration of the nervous system.

The first major area of infant stimulation research is that of vestibular and proprioceptive input. One major deficit area found in some learning-disabled children is in the ability to adequately process vestibular input. This is evidenced by abnormal amounts of postrotary nystagmus after a specific spinning test as well as by poorly controlled eye movements after vestibular or proprioceptive input. Some of these children improve after being treated with exercises that utilize vestibular and proprioceptive input and that are aimed at eliciting specific adaptive responses. It is felt that these children need or were lacking this kind of sensation. One 1976 study by Kantner et al. [21] showed that a specific spinning program of both Down's syndrome and normal children 6 to 24 months of age produced improved motor performance in both groups as well as a decreased postrotary nystagmus response, reflecting greater central inhibition. This study would seem to support the sensorimotor integrative theory.

Earlier infant studies in the nursery demonstrated that visual alerting is related to vestibular and proprioceptive input. The 1966 Korner and Grobstein [22] study, which was later duplicated by Frederickson and Brown in 1975 [23], demonstrated that infants stimulated in an upright position on the shoulder became more alert and visually scanned the environment. This kind of stimulation can easily be incorporated into a nursery program. A 1975 study by Korner et al. [24] used an oscillating water bed to provide vestibular stimulation. They found that their infants experienced fewer episodes of apnea, although there were no significant effects on weight gain or frequency of emesis. In 1976, Gregg et al. [25] found that infants exposed to either horizontal or semivertical vestibular-proprioceptive stimulation showed more efficient visual pursuits than did those who remained in a stationary position. Both of these studies would seem to imply that movement has an impact on the nervous system in ways that increase autonomic function, which in turn may affect cortical responses.

A second area of stimulation that has been studied in the nursery and is recognized as an area of deficit in some learning-disabled children is related to tactile input. Ayres [26] notes that children who show a deficit in tactile perception often exhibit tactile defensiveness, which is a hypersensitive response to touch and is therefore perceived as noxious. Frequently, this response is also associated with hyperactivity, anxiety, and distractability—all behaviors that inhibit higher levels of learning.

Several studies in the nursery attempted to provide tactile stimulation and have shown some positive results. Ourth and Brown [27] reported significantly less crying in their sample of handled babies, whereas Solkoff et al. [28] reported that their handled infants, who were also stimulated by colored mobiles, scored higher on the Brazelton test upon discharge. It is interesting to note that Freeman [29] found no significant differences in weight gain or length of hospitalization in groups of infants who received handling before and after feedings; however, those infants who experienced a temperature change during the handling did gain weight faster. Some of these findings may possibly reflect an interrelationship between the different modalities of sensory stimulation and their affects on different areas of development. Later studies continued to support the value of stimulation in the nursery. In 1974, Powell [30] found that extra tactile stimulation increased low-birth-weight infants' development and performance through the six-month adjusted age period. In 1975, Kramer et al. [31] found that premature infants who were regularly handled had a faster rate of social development, whereas Solkoff and Matuszak [32] found that infants who received a stroking program performed better on the Brazelton test. Their handled infants were more alert, had better head control, were more consolable, habituated more rapidly to light and sound, showed improved body tonus, changed states more rapidly, had greater hand-to-mouth consolability, and showed more avoidance of noxious stimuli. Weight gain was not significantly affected. These findings would again seem to imply that early stimulation in the nursery will affect a variety of functions, not only through an increase in the amount of brain growth, but also in improved integration of the infant's neuromotor systems. This in turn may affect later learning by giving the child a better foundation for processing future experiences.

In the area of auditory stimulation, several infant researchers have measured babies' responses to tapes of mothers' voices and heart beats. Since the child has experienced the mother's constant heart beat while in utero, it is postulated that such stimulation helps the infant to organize his or her internal rhythms and establish a diurnal cycle. Perhaps infant-parent attachment can be facilitated through the imprinting phenomena experienced by both parent and child. This may be facilitated in the premature infant by providing the comforting and soothing sounds to which the child is accustomed. The fact that the child's cardiovascular system is influenced by auditory stimulation again implies that there is an inter-relationship among the various sensory and motor systems and that a primitive memory association may be involved.

In 1960, Salk [33] found that maternal heartbeat sounds led to infant quieting and increased weight gain over time. Palmquist, however, was unable to duplicate these findings in a replication study done in 1975 [34]. In 1971, Katz found that a tape of the mother's voice improved the pre-mature infant's motor and tactile adaptive scores and increased auditory and visual functions. [35]. In 1972, Segall [36] exposed premature infants to tapes of their mothers' voices and to white (meaningless) noise. Cardiac accelerations were considered a defensive reflex. Those infants who re-ceived exposure to white noise and their mother's voice showed greater heart beat accelerations initially, but then habituated to the auditory stim-uli. The control group, which did not receive a planned auditory stimulation program, showed no initial heart rate acceleration. This was interpreted to mean that the experimental group was able to react initially with greater "protective" reaction to novel stimuli. In 1975, Brackbill [37] found that continuous auditory stimulation lowered the levels of arousal of unstressed newborn infants. We presume that this demonstrated the habituation phe-nomenon. In 1979, Neal [15] demonstrated that infants responded to au-ditory input by a change of heart rate followed by a normal heart rate. This, again, would appear to imply habituation or adaption. This basic level of learning would appear to be necessary for future performance by allowing one to adapt by tuning out excessive stimulation.

When studying the areas of visual stimulation, researchers disproved prior notions that infants could not see. Their studies have centered on three main areas: 1) infants' responses to novel stimuli, 2) the types of visual stimulation that infants prefer, and 3) the effects of posturing on visual perception and eye-hand coordination.

Relating to novel stimuli, Parry in 1972 [38] found that infants show a greater awareness of and hesitancy to approach a novel stimulus in a familiar environment than in an unfamiliar environment, whereas Friedman [39] found that infants are receptive and respond to changes in their im-mediate visual environment.

When looking at specific types of stimulation that infants prefer, Fantz and Nevis [40] determined that infants older than three months prefer circular to noncircular visual patterns. In 1975, Bornstein [41] found that older infants prefer the colors red, yellow, blue, and orange. These colors and patterned objects have since been used in the development of infant toys and mobiles. In a more recent study in 1980, Kagan [42] found that infants respond to blue mobiles more than to green mobiles, but visual attention behavior was determined to be a less sensitive indicator for assessing the infant's perceptual response capacities than was motor behavior such as foot kicking or other negative cues.

Regarding the effects of posture on visual perception, Fredrickson and Brown [23] noted that the "on the shoulder" position significantly affects the quality of the infant's visual behavior by increasing the newborn's ability to follow. This was noted earlier in comments about vestibular and proprioceptive stimulation. In 1979, Coryell and Henderson [43] postulated that the asymmetrical tonic neck reflex posture places the hands in a position that can be easily visualized and that should help facilitate later eye-hand coordination.

Some of the more recent studies have focused on combining sensory modalities such as tactile and kinesthetic input or auditory with kinesthetic input. Attempts have been made to follow long-term effects and to determine how the programs have affected mother-infant bonding or behavioral outcomes. Some of the studies have been able to show a long-term effect. For instance, in 1980, Leib et al. [44] reported that their experimental group of premature infants exposed to a four-point enrichment program of tactile, visual, kinesthetic, and auditory stimulation scored significantly higher on the Bayley scales at six months of adjusted gestational age. They felt that a program designed to provide appropriate stimulation may increase the infant's capability to respond to the environment and, subsequently, positively effect the interaction with care giver in a way that may foster attachment and improve the care giver's sensitivity to the child's needs.

We feel that the trend of future research will be to implement specific stimulation programs based on past studies of infant responses and that longer-term follow-up studies to determine the long-range effects will be increasingly important. As yet little has been done to correlate problems such as learning disabilities, behavioral disorders, or parental attachment disorders with treatment received in the high-risk nursery. These problems should be explored from the perspective of prevention.

A Stimulation Program For The Neonatal Intensive Care Unit

The following program is one designed for three general levels of developing infants. Although we believe that it is best to individualize a stimulation program for a particular infant, it is possible to provide some general guidelines based on the infant's functional and medical level. This generalized program should not preclude the specialized therapy programs needed by infants with neurologic, orthopedic, or motor dysfunctions.

Some basic things that the staff can do to help most infants and their parents include the following. 1) Provide the infant with the same caretaker every day per shift. 2) Make the infant as attractive as possible by dressing him or her up with colored ribbons, blankets, clothes, and so on. 3) Place attractive pictures or mobiles in the infant's line of vision, but do not use too many objects as this may be too stimulating. 4) Help the infant establish a day-night cycle by covering the eyes at night or by turning lights out or down. 5) Encourage the infant to follow your head movements with his or her eyes (i.e., when the infant's eyes are open, place your head about nine inches from the eyes, talk to the infant, and slowly move your head up and down and back and forth to elicit visual tracking). 6) Talk to the infant and hold his or her hands. 7) Encourage parents to provide clothes, toys, and so on to reinforce their ability to care for their child. 8) Move slowly when you pick up a baby to avoid startling or overstimulation.

BABIES ON THE VENTILATOR FOR PROLONGED PERIODS OR WHO ARE ACUTELY ILL

Most infants on the ventilator are unable to perform comforting self-stimulation by moving their own bodies to provide tactile, kinesthetic, or proprioceptive input. We found no studies regarding stimulation for these infants; however, we feel that careful controlled stimulation could be provided for short periods to help stabilize the infant and further enhance his or her long-term developmental prognosis. Any exercises should be performed only by trained personnel who are familiar with the responses of very small infants. We hope that future studies will be done in this area.

The following activities provide gentle stimulation. a) Use a water bed or three-quarter-filled 1,000-L intravenous bags to provide a softer and more mobile surface. b) Periodically change the infant's position, using blanket rolls to hold the extremities in a variety of patterns. The rolls can also be used as a surface for the child to snuggle against to provide tactile stimulation as well as a more emotionally secure position. Using rolls along the outside of the legs in sidelying position will also prevent the typical "frogged" position we see in legs of premature infants. c) Slowly and gently stroke the infant's head, arms, legs, trunk, fingers, and toes. This should be done with a mild pressure; your pressure is too light if the baby shows a noxious response. You should spend only two to three minutes initially and watch the monitors and the child for his or her response. Wait for several seconds between maneuvers to give the baby time to adjust. d) Quietly talk to the infant, especially when the eyes are opened. e) Place a colorful picture or toy in the infant's visual range. This may be taped to the side rail of the open bed or suspended from overhead. f) Allow the baby to suck on a pacifier if he or she has a nasotracheal tube or is on nasal continuous positive airway pressure.

346

RECOVERING INFANTS RECEIVING INTERMEDIATE CARE IN THE ISOLETTE

The recovering infant should be observed to determine whether he or she is either hyperactive or lethargic. Your stimulation should be adjusted depending on his or her reactions. The hyperactive or irritable baby needs more soothing stimulation, whereas the lethargic baby needs gentle alerting. a) When possible, encourage parents to hold their infant outside of the bed. Encourage touching and massaging within the isolette or on the lap. b) Occasionally hold the infant upright in a sitting position to allow the body to adjust to postural changes and to encourage visual alerting. Allow the baby to hold his or her own head up as much as possible. Use a doll-sized infant seat within the isolette as an alternate positioning technique. c) Surround the active infant with rolled blankets to cuddle. d) If the infant appears hyperactive or irritable, muffle the noise level by partially lining the isolette with blankets. Swaddling may also be used during irritable periods. e) Slow rocking and slow, repetitive patting have a relaxing affect. Use these to comfort the hyper or irritable infant. They may also slow the heart rate of a tachycardic baby (watch the monitor!). With the baby's head turned to one side, slowly and rhythmically log roll the infant from his or her back to side. Reverse and rock to opposite side. Pause between repetitions. f) Rub the baby's hands over his or her own hair, face, arms, body and legs. g) Visually alert the child with gentle bouncing and by using an upright position. Place the infant in an enface position. Try to get him or her to focus on your eyes. Slowly move your face to the side to get visual tracking. Slowly move back to the opposite side. If infant cannot track, work first on focusing and then move only a couple inches to allow refocusing. Talk to the baby in a rhythmic pattern to encourage auditory orienting while focusing. Bright-colored baby toys or colored design cards may also be used for visual responses. h) Consider taping the mother's voice, especially for transport babies whose parents cannot visit frequently. Play this tape at a quiet level. i) Gently flex and extend the infant's arms and legs. Tickle the feet of the inactive or lethargic baby to get a motor response. j) Stimulate a sucking reflex using your finger or a nipple designed for premature infants and sealed with tape over the back. While gavage feeding, allow the infant to suck on the pacifier. k) Attempt to regulate lights and routines to foster time perception. Darken the room or cover the infant's eyes at night. Turn down radios and speak more softly during "quiet time."

INFANTS IN OPEN BEDS

Babies preparing to go home should be able to tolerate the stimulation noted above as well as additional routines that will help them adjust to

347

home. More time should be spent in the waking state. Quiet alert is the best state for utilizing visual and auditory routines. a) Use a mobile over the crib and occasionally play a music box or soft music. Avoid "hard rock" or loud music. b) Rub the baby's hands over toys of different textures and colors. Gently shake the arm for extra stimulation and wave it in front of the baby's eyes. Flex and extend arms. c) When bathing the baby, rub him or her gently with the wash cloth. Talk or sing during the bath. If time allows, play with the infant in a tub, massaging extremities, talking, making faces at the baby. Rub the baby with lotion for additional stimulation. d) Sit the infant in an upright position on your lap. Let the baby hold his or her own head up, keeping your hands around the shoulders to provide support. Use toys and facial expressions to stimulate vision. e) Sit in a rocker while feeding the baby. Talk to the baby and elicit visual responses while feeding. f) Walk around with the baby, holding him or her either supine or over the shoulder. The over-the-shoulder position stimulates more visual alerting. g) Hold the baby on his or her stomach over your forearm. Sway gently from side to side. h) Talk to the baby while changing the diaper or clothes. Massage can easily be done at this time. Flex and straighten the legs when changing the diaper. Gently flex and extend the feet and massage the toes and soles. i) On the tummy, prop the baby on his or her forearms. Try to get him or her to look up at you or at a toy. j) Promote self-quieting hand-to-mouth activity by placing your finger in the hand on the side to which baby is facing. This stimulates a reflexive hand-to-mouth movement.

Illustration: A Case Study

K.K. was a 32-week-gestation white male infant, twin number two born to a 27-year-old gravida 3, para 1, blood group A positive, woman by spontaneous breech vaginal delivery. There was no history of prolonged rupture of membranes. The Apgar score was 7 and 6 at 1 and 5 minutes, respectively. The birth weight was 1685 g (appropriate for gestional age). Because of signs of respiratory distress, he was put on mechanical ventilator therapy, and an imbilical arterial line was introduced to monitor blood gases. Blood and peripheral cultures were drawn, and antibiotic therapy was given for 10 days. A chest x ray showed moderate to severe respiratory distress syndrome. He required ventilatory assistance for three days. A modified exchange transfusion was done because of hyperviscosity syndrome on the first day of life. During this time the baby was placed on a water bed in the Ohio open bed. A position change and a three-minute tactile, vestibular, and auditory stimulation program were carried out every two to three hours. He was quite alert at times, sucked vigorously on a pacifier during those times, and watched a yellow toy elephant his parents had brought in for him.

On the third day of life he was weaned from the ventilator and placed in oxygen therapy by hood. He developed hyperbilirubinemia, which was treated by phototherapy for three days. The above stimulation program was continued. The tactile, vestibular, and auditory program was increased to five minutes every three to four hours.

On the seventh day of life, the baby no longer required oxygen or phototherapy. He was started on oral feedings, remained on intravenous therapy and was transferred to an isolette. Intravenous therapy was discontinued on the ninth day of life. He remained in the isolette for an extended period of time until weight gain and thermoregulation controls matured. During this time the parents were encouraged to visit daily with their child. They were taught a tactile massage program and encouraged to hold and rock their child outside of the isolette for at lease 15 minutes a day. When in the isolette, the baby was placed in a premature infant seat at least four times a day, and a mobile of nipples designed for premature infants was suspended in the isolette for him to look at. During sleeping periods, the isolette was lined with blankets, and blankets were draped over the isolette to darken the environment. The baby also received a 15-minute daily stimulation program that consisted of human interaction, a music box and human voice, massage, gentle flexion and extension of the extremities, rocking, prerolling, and head control exercises. During gavage feedings, he was encouraged to suck on a nipple. When he progressed to nipple feedings, the nurses and parents were encouraged to feed him outside of the isolette in a rocking chair.

Six days before discharge, he was transferred into an open crib. A mobile was attached to the side of the crib. The parents came in daily, participated in his bath, continued the tactile massage programs, and progressed to using toys. His yellow toy elephant traveled with him from open bed to isolette to open crib, and a few rattles and teething rings were added. He was held, fed, and rocked with each feeding. When not asleep, he spent much time sitting up in an infant seat or was carried by his nurse when she was not in direct contact with other babies.

Neurodevelopmental assessment of the baby revealed that the postural tone, head control, and activity level were within normal limits for infants at 36 weeks of gestational age. He could track visually, although some nystagmus was present after prolonged stimulation. Reflex activity was age appropriate. Before his discharge the parents were given guidelines for generalized stimulation and handling of the baby at home.

On his medical follow-up visit at term age, his postural tone and head control were good. He was alert and active and could focus and track well, and the nystagmus was no longer present. He responded appropriately to noise, and reflex activity was age appropriate.

Discussion and Conclusion

It has been our experience that critically ill infants, as well as full-term newborns, do benefit, often dramatically, both physically and psychologically from special stimulation. The above case study is a child who was at risk for a developmental delay or neuropsychiatric disorder by virtue of his birth history and medical complications; however, after receiving a consistent stimulation program, he is performing at an appropriate neurodevelopmental level for term age. The program allows and encourages the parents to form an emotional attachment and become well acquainted with their child before discharge. We feel that a specialized program can achieve the following goals. 1) It teaches the child body awareness. 2) It promotes motor control and development. 3) It utilizes positioning to prevent reflexive posturing. 4) It facilitates sucking and more controlled swallowing for feeding and often prevents feeding problems so common in the premature infant. 5) It establishes a wealth of perceptual and motor experiences upon which later learning will depend. 6) It familiarizes the child with the environment to promote future successful interactions with other individuals and the inanimate environment. 7) It facilitates parent-infant attachment by promoting positive social interactions.

Summary

There has been a dramatic improvement in the outcome of high-risk premature infants during the past 10 to 15 years, due to the advances in neonatal medicine and to new technology allowing closer monitoring. It appears that there is a growing awareness of the need for psychosocial care of the newborn and their families, although these advances have not been as rapid as the technological changes.

Providing appropriate sensory stimulation is an important aspect in supplying quality care for the high risk newborn. Some research studies have indicated that sensory stimulation programs using a variety of modalities lead to increases in weight gain, psychomotor maturation, reduction of central apnea, and increased responsiveness of the infant to his or her care giver. These effects have led to the facilitation of parental attachment, which may in the future promote a more holistic approach to health care in the neonatal intensive care unit.

References

1. Sonstegard, L., Scanlon, J., Knuppel, R.A., Plumer, M.H. (eds.) *Perinatal Press*, vol. 3. Perinatal Press, Inc., 1979, pp. 21–22.

2. Stewart, A., Reynolds, E. Improved prognosis for infants of very low birthweight. *Pediatrics* 54:724–735, 1974.
3. Grassy, R.G., Hubbard, C., Graven, S., Zachman, R. The growth and development of low birth weight infants receiving intensive neonatal care. *Clin. Pediatr.* 15:529–533, 1976.
4. Teberg, A., Hodgman, J., Wu, P., Spears, R. Recent improvement in outcome for the small premature infant: a follow-up of infants with a birthweight of less than 1,500 grams. *Clin. Pediatr.* 16:307–313, 1977.
5. Brazelton, T.B. Neonatal behavioral assessment. National Spastics Society monographs. *Clin. Developmental Med.* 50:1–3, 1973.
6. Avery, G.B. *Neonatology: Pathophysiology and Management of the Newborn.* Philadelphia: J.B. Lippincott Co., 1975, p. 12.
7. Schaffer, A.T., Avery, M.E. *Diseases of the Newborn.* Philadelphia: The W.B. Saunders Co., 1977.
8. Klaus, M.R., Fanaroff, A.A. *Care of the High Risk Neonate.* Philadelphia: The W.B. Saunders Co., 1977.
9. Kearsley, R.B., Sigel, Z.E. (eds.), *Infants at Risk: Assessment of Cognitive Functioning.* New York: John Wiley & Sons, Inc., 1979, pp. 582-590.
10. Babson, S.G., Pernoll, M.S., Benda, G.I., Simpson, K. *Diagnosis and Management of the Fetus and Neonate at Risk: A Guide for Team Care.* St. Louis, Mo.: The C.V. Mosby Co., 1980, p. 7.
11. Desmond, M., Wilson, G., Alt, E., Fisher, E. The very low birth weight infant after discharge from intensive care: Anticipatory health care and developmental course. *Curr. Probl. Pediatr.* 10:1–59, 1985.
12. Sweet, A. Classification of the low-birth-weight infant. In: Klaus, M., Fanaroff, A. (eds.) *Care of the High Risk Neonate.* Philadelphia, The W.B. Saunders Co., 1979, pp. 66–93.
13. Dreyfus-Brisae, C. Ontogenesis of sleep in human prematures after 32 weeks of conceptual age. *Dev. Psychobiol.* 3:91–121, 1970.
14. Purpura, D.P. Neuronal migration and dendritic differentiation: normal and aberrant development of human cerebral cortex. In *Biologic and Clinical Aspects of Brain Development.* Evansville, Ind.: Mead-Johnson Co., 1975, pp. 13–27.
15. Neal, M. Organizational behavior of the premature infant. In *Newborn Behavioral Organization: Nursing Research and Implication,* vol. 15. New York: Alan R. Lise, Inc., 1979, p.43–60.
16. Kula, A., Fry, C., Goldstein, F. Kinesthetic needs in infancy. *Am. J. Orthopsych.* 30:562–571, 1960.
17. Hasselmeyer, E.G. The premature neonates response to handling. *Am. Nurs. Assoc.* 1:15–24, 1964.
18. Rothchold, B.T. Incubator isolation as a possible contributing factor to the high incidence of emotional disturbances among prematurely born persons. *J. Gen. Psychol.* 110:287–304, 1967.
19. Bakeman, R., Brown, J. Early interaction: Consequences for social and mental development at three years. *Child Dev.* 51:437–447, 1980.
20. Metze, M. Teaching parents a strategy for enhancing infant development. *Child Dev.* 51:583–586, 1980.

21. Kantner, R., Clark, D., Allen, L., Chase, M. Effects of vestibular stimulation in nystagmus response and motor performance in the developmentally delayed infant. *Phy. Ther.* 56:414–421, 1976.

22. Korner, A.F., Grobstein, R. Visual alertness as related to soothing neonates; implications for maternal stimulation and early deprivation. *Child Dev.* 37:867–876, 1966.

23. Fredrickson, W., Brown, J. Posture as a determinant of visual behavior in newborns. *Child Dev.* 46:579–582, 1975.

24. Korner, A., Kraemer, H., Haffner, E., Casper, L. Effects of waterbed flotation on premature infants: a pilot study. *Pediatrics* 56:361–367, 1975.

25. Gregg, C., Haffner, M., Korner, A. The relative efficancy of vestibular-proprioceptive stimulation and the upright position in enhancing visual pursuit in neonates. *Child Dev.* 47:309–314, 1976.

26. Ayers, A. Tactile functions: their relation to hyperactive and perceptual motor behavior. In *The Development of the Sensory Integrative Theory and Practice.* Dubuque, Iowa: Kendall/Hunt Publishing Co., 1974, pp. 83–96.

27. Ourth, L., Brown, K. Inadequate mothering and disturbance in the neonatal period. *Child Dev.* 32:287–295, 1961.

28. Solkoff, N., Weintraub, D., Yaffe, S., Blase, B. Effects of handling on the subsequent development of premature infants. *Dev. Psychol.* 1:765–769, 1969.

29. Freeman, E. The Effects of Interpersonal Stimulation on Growth and Development of Premature Infants. Unpublished doctoral dissertation, The University of Florida, 1969.

30. Powell, L. The effect of extra stimulation and maternal involvement on the development of low birthweight infants and on maternal behavior. *Child Dev.* 45:106–113, 1974.

31. Kramer, M., Chamorro, I., Green, D., Knudtson, F. Extra tactile stimulation of the premature infant. *Nurs. Res.* 24:324–334, 1975.

32. Solkoff, N., Matuszak, D. Tactile stimulation and behavioral development among low birthweight infants. *Child Psych. Hum. Dev.* 6:33–37, 1975.

33. Salk, L. Effect of the normal heartbeat sound on the behavior of the newborn infant: implications for mental health. *World Mental Health* 12:168–175, 1960.

34. Palmquist, H. The effects of heartbeat sound stimulation on the weight development of newborn infants. *Child Dev.* 46:292–295, 1975.

35. Katz, V. Auditory stimulation and developmental behavior of the premature infant. *Nurs. Res.* 20:196–207, 1971.

36. Segall, M.E. Cardiac responsivity to auditory stimulation in premature infants. *Nurs. Res.* 21:369–378, 1972.

37. Brackbill, Y. Continuous stimulation and arousal level in infancy: effects of stimulus intensity and stress. *Child Dev.* 46:364–369, 1975.

38. Parry, M. Infants responses in familiar and unfamiliar settings. *Child Dev.* 43:233–237, 1972.

39. Friedman, S. Newborn visual attention to repeated exposure of redundant versus "novel" targets. *Percept. Psychophys.* 12:292–294, 1972.

40. Fantz, R., Nevis, S. Pattern preference and perceptual cognitive development in early infancy. *Merrill Palmer Q.* 13:77–108, 1967.

41. Bornstein, M. Qualities of color vision in infancy. *J. Child Psych.* 19:401–419, 1975.

42. Fagan, J. Stimulus preference, reinforcement effectiveness, and relationship responding in infants. *Child Dev.* 51:372–378, 1980.
43. Coryell, J., Henderson, A. Role of the asymmetrical tonic neck reflex in hand visualization in normal infants. *Am. J. Occup. Ther.* 33:255–260, 1979.
44. Leib, S., Benefield, G., Guidubaldi, J. Effects of early intervention and stimulation on the preterm infant. *Pediatrics* 66:83–90, 1980.
45. Korner, A., Thomas, E.B. The relative efficacy of contact and vestibular proprioceptive stimulation in soothing neonates. *Child Dev.* 43:443–453, 1972.
46. Freedman, D., Boverman, H., Freedman, N. Effects of kinesthetic stimulation on weight gain and on smiling in premature infants. Paper presented at the American Orthopsychiatric Association, San Francisco, Calif., April, 1966.
47. Neal, M. Vestibular stimulation and development of the small premature infant. *Nurs. Res. Rep.* 8, 1977, pp. 2–5.
48. Pederson, D., Ter Vrugt, D. The influences of amplitude and frequency of vestibular stimulation on the activity of two-month-old infants. *Child Dev.* 44:122–128, 1973.
49. Kattwinkel, J., Hearman, H., Fanaroff, A., et al. Apnea of prematurity. *J. Pediatr.* 86:588–592, 1975.
50. Neeley, C. Effects of non-nutritive sucking upon the behavioral arousal of the newborn. In *Newborn Behavioral Organization: Nursing Research and Implications*, vol. 15. New York: Alan R. Lise, Inc., 1979, pp. 173–196.
51. Anderson, G.C., Vidyasagar, D. Development of sucking in premature infants from 1 to 7 days postbirth. In *Newborn Behavioral Organization: Nursing Research and Implications*, vol. 15. New York: Alan R. Lise Inc., 1979, pp. 145–166.
52. Chapman, J.S. Influence of varied stimuli on development of motor patterns in the premature infant. *Newborn Behavioral Organization: Nursing Research and Implications*, vol. 15. New York: Alan R. Lise, Inc., 1979, pp. 61–80.
53. Bench, J., Mentz, L. Neonatal auditory habituation and state change. *Q. J. Exp. Psychol.* 30:355–362, 1978.
54. Horowitz, A. Habituation and memory: infant cardiac response to families and discrepant auditory stimulation. *Child Dev.* 43:43–53, 1972.
55. White, J.L. The effects of tactile and kinesthetic stimulation on neonatal development in the premature infant. *Disabil. Abstr. Int.* 30:3607–3612, 1975.
56. White, J., Labarba, R. The effects of tactile and kinesthetic stimulation on neonatal development in the premature infant. *Dev. Psychobiol.* 9:569–577, 1976.
57. Rose, S.A., Schmidt, K., Riese, M., Bridger, W. Effects of prematurity and early intervention on responsivity to tactile stimuli: a comparison of pre-term and full-term infants. *Child Dev.* 51:416–425, 1980.
58. Barnard, K. The effect of stimulation on the sleep behavior of the premature infant. *Commun. Nurs. Res.* 6:12–33, 1973.
59. Kang, R., Barnard, K. Using the neonatal behavioral assessment scale to evaluate premature infants. In *Newborn Behavioral Organization: Nursing Research and Implications*, vol. 15. New York: Alan R. Lise Inc., 1979, pp. 119–133.
60. Kramer, L., Pierpont, M. Rocking waterbeds and auditory stimulation to enhance growth of preterm infants. *J. Pediatr.* 8:279–299, 1976.

61. Field, T., Dempsey, J., Hatch, L., et al. Cardiac and behavioral responses to repeated tactile and auditory stimulation by pre-term and term neonates. *Dev. Psychol.* 15:406–416, 1979.
62. Neal, M.V. Organizational behavior of the premature infant. In *Newborn Behavioral Organization: Nursing Research and Implications*, vol 15. New York: Alan R. Lise, Inc., 1979, pp. 49–60.
63. Groom, G. Effects of Perinatal Factors and Supplemental Stimulation of Premature Infants upon Measures of Cognitive Behavior. Unpublished doctoral dissertation, Purdue University, 1973.
64. McNichol, T. Some Effects of Different Programs of Enrichment on the Development of Premature Infants in the Hospital Nursery. Unpublished doctoral dissertation, Purdue University, 1975.
65. Rice, R. Neurophysiological development in premature infants following stimulation. *Dev. Psychol.* 13:69–76, 1977.
66. Scarr-Salapatek, S., Williams, M. The effects of early stimulation on low birth weight infants. *Child Dev.* 44:94–104, 1973.
67. Rosenfield, A.B., Vohr, B.R., Cowett, R.W., Oh, W. The effects of an intervention program on parental visiting in a special care nursery. Paper presented at the meeting of the Society for Research in Child Development, New Orleans, 1977.
68. Siqueland, E.R. Biological and experiential determinants of exploration in infancy. In Stone, L., Smith, H., Murphy, C. (eds.), *The Competent Infant*. New York: Basic Books, Inc., 1963, pp. 822–823.

27

Drugs and Breast-Feeding

Jacob V. Aranda, M.D., Ph.D., and Judith Gibbs, M.D.

The growing consumer advocacy, coupled with increasing interest on breast-feeding, has heightened public awareness on the possible problems associated with the transfer of drugs from the mother to her infant via the breast milk. It is well known that many drugs, environmental pollutants, and recreational or "social" chemicals find their way into the human milk. Several reviews on this area have been published recently [1–5], and the present report, in addition to providing another overview on the subject, focuses on some of the evidence underlying the recommendations that certain drugs (Table 27-1) are contraindicated during lactation.

Factors Governing Passage of Exogenous Compounds from Maternal Blood to Milk

The presence and concentration of compounds in human milk depend on molecular weight, degree of ionization, protein binding in blood, lipid solubility, and specific uptake by mammary tissue. Drugs that are not absorbed after oral ingestion will obviously not appear in milk.

Small compounds of less than 200 molecular weight appear freely in milk and are presumed to have passed through pores in the mammary

Table 27–1
Drugs Contraindicated During Lactation

Drugs Not to be Given to Nursing Mothers
Antimetabolites
Some cathartics (e.g., phenolphtalein)
Radioactive drugs (therapeutic use)
Some anticoagulants (pheninacione ethyl biscoumacetate)
Iodides
Ergot alkaloids
Metronidazole
Dihidrotachysterol
Thiouracil
Diazepam
Chlorpromazine
Lithium carbonate
Chloromycetin
Tetracycline

Adapted from Giacoia, G.P., Catz, C.S. Drugs and pollutants in breast milk. *Clin. Perinatol.* 6:181–196. 1979.

alveolar cells. Large compounds such as insulin or heparin do not pass into milk. Intermediate-size compounds must penetrate the lipoprotein cell membrane by diffusion or active transport.

In general, drugs that are not ionized at blood pH will traverse the alveolar cell membrane with greater ease than will highly ionized compounds. Since milk pH is about 7 or slightly less, milk will act as a "trap" for weak bases.

Drugs pass the cell membrane only in their free form; thus, highly protein bound drugs are less available for passage. Drugs or other chemicals that are very lipid soluble readily cross the alveolar cell, and since milk contains a considerable amount of lipid, these compounds are also "trapped" in milk.

Finally, certain compounds are actively taken up by mammary tissue and are found in milk in concentrations substantially higher than in blood.

Modifications of Passage of Compounds into Milk

Drugs may be metabolized by the maternal body to active or inactive metabolites. These derivatives may then be secreted into milk more or less readily than is the parent compound. The timing of maternal ingestion of a drug in relation to the time of milk synthesis may influence the concentration of drug in a particular milk feeding.

In animals, changes in mammary gland blood flow control the amount of drug presented to the sites of uptake. Mammary tissue itself can metabolize certain compounds. Drugs already secreted into milk may be back secreted into the alveolar cell and thence into blood. Lastly, the stage of lactation plays a role; drugs may be secreted more easily in the colostral phase.

Delivery of Compounds to and Disposition by the Infant

The total volume of milk consumed in a known period of time determines the dosage to the infant. Since the daily volume intake of breast milk is exceedingly variable and impractical to rountinely measure, one could assume a high average daily milk consumption to be about one liter.

To produce an effect, the drug in the milk must either act locally in the gut or be absorbed. It is possible that the proteins of milk will bind certain drugs and thereby impede absorption; it is also possible that the bowel of a very young infant may permit absorption of normally excluded large molecules.

The infant's disposition of the drug in milk will change with postnatal age, as discussed elsewhere in this book: in addition, one must always be aware of the drug's potential for displacement of bilirubin from serum albumin.

Compounds in Human Milk

DRUGS

Anticoagulants   As mentioned above, heparin does not enter breast milk. Oral anticoagulants of the indandione group as well as bishydroxycoumarin and ethyl biscoumacetate are found in milk and have been associated with infant coagulopathies (see below). Warfarin must be considered the drug of choice, since by virtue of its acidity as well as its high degree of protein binding, it is undetectable in human milk [6,7].

Antiinflammatory and Analgesic Drugs   Acetylsalicylic acid appears to be without danger when used occasionally. It should be avoided in the neonatal period because of its displacement of bilirubin from albumin. Older infants have been found to receive 0.2 to 0.3 percent of a single dose of acetylsalicylic acid administered to the mother [8,9]. Although detailed studies do not exist, acetaminophen seems to be safe. Indomethacin taken by a nursing woman (200 mg daily) has been anecdotally associated with a convulsion by the infant; no milk or infant blood levels were reported [9]. Indomethacin is presently given directly to premature infants to close the patent ductus arteriosus. Propoxyphene, which

357

achieves milk levels half those of plasma, was implicated in one case of infant hypotonia [10]. Pentazocine has not been reported to be harmful.

Drugs Affecting the Cardiovascular System The amount of digoxin present in milk depends on the maternal dose; infants whose mothers received 0.25 mg per day did not ingest enough digoxin in milk to have detectable blood levels [11–13]. At a maternal dose of 0.75 mg per day, one infant's serum digoxin level was 0.2 n/ml, and the infant was asymptomatic [14]. Diuretics in general seem to be harmless, although were a nursing woman to become dehydrated because of diuretic use, lactation would be greatly depressed. The effects of diuretics on milk composition are unclear. Spironolactone and its less active metabolite are secreted in milk, and an estimated 0.2 percent of the mother's daily dose is received by the infant [15,16]. Chlorthalidone appears in small amounts in milk, but could potentially accumulate in the young infant [17]. Propranolol seems to be safe. Quinidine is secreted in milk to a concentration about 60 percent that of maternal blood; no ill effects have been observed [18].

Drugs Affecting the Central Nervous System Diazepam is converted in the body to an active metabolite, desmethyldiazepam, and both are excreted in milk. Both of these compounds have a prolonged half-life in infants, and chronic use of diazepam by nursing women has been associated with lethargy and weight loss in their babies [10,19]. Oxazepam, which is also a metabolite of diazepam, has a simpler disposition in the body, being converted to the inactive glucuronide; this drug might be considered an alternative to diazepam during lactation. The barbiturates appear in milk in concentrations that depend on their different degrees of ionization and lipid solubility. In anticonvulsant doses, they seem to be safe. Chlordiazepoxide in breast milk has been linked to depression of the nursing infant. Meprobamate should probably be avoided, since the drug achieves milk concentrations several times the maternal plasma levels [10].

Lithium is definitely contraindicated during lactation since it has been found to cause significant cardiovascular and central nervous system signs in the infants (see below). The phenothiazines have a very long half-life in adults; one infant whose mother ingested chlopromazine developed lethargy and sleepiness. In this case, milk chlorpromazine level was 92n/ml [20]. The use of phenothiazines as galactogogues in induced lactation or relactation [2] needs to be carefully evaluated. Small amounts of the tricyclic antidepressants have been found in breast milk. No effects were noted when the mother was taking low dosages of imipramine, in one case [21]; in another, in which the mother received amitriptyline, none was found in the serum of the infant [22]. Amoxapine and its metabolites have been detected in milk, with unknown effects on the infant [23]. The amphetamines appear in milk and have caused jitteriness in some instances.

Anticonvulsant drug use during lactation requires close clinical supervision. As mentioned above, barbiturates in usual dosage appear to be safe. Phenytoin is found in milk concentrations about one-fifth that of the maternal blood level [10,24]. Primidone [10,24] and ethiosuximide [25] both achieve milk levels near that of maternal blood, but significant symptoms in the infants have not been noted. Carbamazepine and its epoxide metabolite in milk are not known to affect the infant, but they could potentially accumulate [26,27]. Valproic acid is present in very small amounts, 1 to 2 percent of maternal blood levels [28].

Drugs Affecting the Endocrine System. Drugs of the thiouracil family, methimazole, carbimazole, and iodides have been contraindicated during breast-feeding; they achieve a high milk concentration and can suppress the infant's thyroid (see below). On the other hand, thyroxin and other thyroid hormone preparations seem to be safe; endogenous thyroid hormone naturally secreted in breast milk may mask congenital cretinism during breast-feeding. The long-term effects of exogenous glucocorticoids and their derivatives in milk are not known. Women receiving prednisone and prednisolone excrete very samll amounts of these compounds in milk.

A common dilemma is the use of oral contraceptives during lactation. Little is known about the effects of long exposure to small doses of these compounds in milk [29,30]. Contraceptives with a high concentration of estrogen and progestin will depress lactation, especially if they are begun soon after parturition [2,31]. If their use is imperative, it would seem wise to start treatment about four weeks postpartum, ensuring that lactation is already well established, and to use the lowest dosage possible. The infants should be followed with some care; there have been reports of gynecomastia and changes in vaginal epithelium [3,4]. A study of late effects in exposed infants is urgently needed.

Other Drugs Cimetidine, a histamine-H-2-receptor antagonist, has been reported in breast milk in concentrations 3 to 12 times greater than in maternal blood; this drug may be actively transported into milk. Until there is more information concerning its effects in infants, cimetidine should not be used during lactation [32,33]. Theobromine from chocolate has been found in milk at a level of 80 percent of that in maternal serum [34]. Theophylline ingestion by the mother has been associated with infant irritability. Caffeine is discussed below. Extracts of ergot have been responsible for toxic reactions in nursing infants and should be avoided. Methyl ergonovine will suppress lactation in repeated doses; in a single dose, as used intrapartum, milk levels are low [31,35]. The use of isotopes for diagnosis or therapy should be avoided during lactation. An acceptable level of isotope in milk is not known. It has been suggested that women not nurse for 10 days after exposure to $_{131}$I, for three days after $_{99m}$Tc, and for two weeks after $_{67}$Ga [1].

Drugs Contraindicated During Lactation

Table 27-1 lists those drugs contraindicated in nursing mothers as recommended in several reviews, more recently that of Giacoia and Catz [1]. The rationale for these recommendations is briefly reviewed below for the more commonly used agents.

Radiopharmaceuticals Table 27-2 shows some of the more commonly used radioactive agents used mainly for diagnostic procedures. Because of the great hazard of radioactive compounds these agents should not be used when breast-feeding. Whenever administration to the mother is necessary, breast-feeding should be stopped temporarily.

Ergot The basis for the contraindication comes from Fomina's study in 1934 whereby he found that 11 of 21 milk samples from 16 lactating women who ingested liquid ergot had this drug in the milk as measured by bioassays with rabbit uterus and cock's comb. In 90 percent of babies who ingested milk containing ergot, symptoms of ergotism (vomiting, diarrhea, weak pulse, and so on) were noted. More recent studies quantitating ergot transfer to milk with the doses currently used need to be done. Methylergonovine 0.2 mg three times daily has no effect on prolactin or milk secretion; however, neonatal ergotism was not evaluated in these studies by del Pozo in 1975.

Chloramphenicol The milk/plasma ratio of chloramphenicol is about 0.5, with 50 percent of the drug as inactive metabolite. The maximum breast milk concentrations have been reported to be as high as 3.5 mg/L. These doses are not sufficient to produce gray baby syndrome; thus, chlorampenicol is probably not a contraindicated drug during lactation.

Table 27–2
Radiopharmaceutics and Breast Milk

Drug (dose)	Concentration in Milk	Comments
[^{67}Ga]gallium citrate	70 nCi/ml at 96 and 120 hours	Contraindicated breast-feeding for 2 weeks
[^{125}I]albumin (6 and 10 μCi)	0.7 and 0.3 nCi/ml	Avoid drug; stop breast-feeding for 10 days
^{131}I(100 μCi orally)	1,3 and 2 nCi/ml 24 hours after dose, peaked 39 nCi/ml at 6 hours	Contraindicated with large doses; D/C breastfeeding for 24 hours for small dx doses
[^{131}I]hippurate (12 to 20 μCi intravenously)	0.37 nCi/ml	D/C breast-feeding for 24 hours
^{99}m TcO$_4$(4 mCi intravenously XI)	3 and 5.2 × cp at 17 and 20 hours	Concentrate in milk; Stop breast-feeding for 32 to 72 hours

Tetracyclines Tetracycline is excreted in breast milk with concentrations as high as 4 mg/L. There is minimal absorption by infants, but tetracycline may produce pigmentation of permanent dentition if given between the ages of two months and two years. The threshold dose is not conclusively established, and tetracycline should remain as a contraindicated drug.

Metronidazole The contraindication of metronidazole is based on carcinogenecity in rodents. Evidence to the contrary has been provided in humans. This drug is now used for the treatment of anaerobic infections in the newborn with little or no adverse effects. It should no longer be contraindicated in breast-feeding mothers.

Diazepam The contraindication of diazepam is based on one case report of a baby with lethargy after the mother received diazepam (10 mg twice daily) [50]. Systematic study to evaluate this problem further is necessary to generate meaningful recommendations regarding its use in nursing mothers.

Lithium Carbonate Reports that neonatal serum lithium concentrations of about 50 percent of maternal plasma concentration have been provided [51,52]. Since the long-term effect of psychoactive drugs during critical central nervous system development is not known and since infants absorb this drug, it should remain contraindicated. Mothers should be advised to formula feed if lithium is truly required.

Thiouracil The contraindication for thiouracil is based on Williams' observation in 1944 that the thiouracil concentration in milk is 3 times greater than serum concentrations [53]. More recently, it was found that the amount of drug in the breast milk is negligible. In two lactating women given $[_{35}S]$propylthiouracil and $[_{35}S]$carbimazole, only 0.077 percent of propylthiouracil and 0.47 percent of carbimazole were recovered during 24 hours [54]. In another study involving lactating women, propylthiouracil (400 mg orally) produced propylthiouracil concentrations in serum of 7.7 mg/L and in milk of 0.7 mg/L. Propylthiouracil milk excretion is 0.025 percent of the maternal dose per four hours [55]. Once suckling infant remained euthyroid during five months of follow-up. Thus, lactating mothers on propylthiouracil should continue nursing, if they wish, with close supervision of the infant.

RECREATIONAL CHEMICALS IN HUMAN MILK

Caffeine One hour after the ingestion of an average cup of coffee, a peak milk caffeine level of about 1.5 mg/ml is obtained. Caffeine levels in milk are about one-half the corresponding maternal blood level [36]. Although the daily amount of caffeine consumed by a nursing infant might be small, the long half-life of caffeine could cause symptoms such as wakefulness or jitteriness. In 23 mother-infant pairs, 16 of whom were breast-feeding and minimal coffee drinkers, negligble (<1 mg/L) amounts of caffeine were found in the infants' plasma.

Ingredients of Cigarettes The nicotine content of breast milk from women smoking one pack per day has been found to be about 100 to 500 parts per billion. No symptoms have been ascribed to this degree of contamination. Thiocyanate, which is elevated in the blood of smoking women, does not appear in elevated amounts of their milk [37].

Ethanol Ethanol, a small molecule, diffused freely into milk and achieves levels equivalent to those in blood. The metabolite acetaldehyde does not appear in milk. There has been a case of Cushingoid syndrome in a four-month-old nursing child whose mother drank heavily; a random milk ethanol level was 100 mg/dl [38].

Narcotics Heroin, methadone, morphine, and other opiate derivatives have been found in milk and may be responsible for both addiction and withdrawal symptoms in the nursing infant [10,39]. Opiates used briefly appear to have little clinical effect. It has been suggested that women on methadone maintenance take their daily dose after the last breast-feeding in the evening, since milk methadone levels are found to peak about four hours after administration of the drug by mouth [10].

ENVIRONMENTAL POLLUTANTS IN HUMAN MILK

Lead Lead has been found in both bovine and human milk as well as in commercial infant formulas. The lead content of human milk has remained rather constant over the past four decades, in contrast to levels of some other pollutants. One study found the lead level in human milk in the US to be about 0.03 μg/ml [4]. There are no reports of signs and symptoms of lead toxicity from this source.

Mercury Metallic or inorganic mercury poisoning in adults has usually been in association with occupational exposure. There are no reports of metallic mercury poisoning from human milk. Organic mercury, more specifically methylmercury, has been used industrially in fungicides, in pulp and paper factories, and in chlor-alkali plants. In the late 1950s, Minamata Bay in Japan was contaminated with industrial wastes containing methylmercury; the compound found its way into humans through contaminated fish. There was a high incidence of neurologic abnormalities in children born in this area, probably related to in utero exposure to the chemical rather than to exposure during lactation [1]. Methylmercury was found in human milk in a concentration about 5 percent of that in blood; the half-life for disappearance of mercury from milk was estimated to be about 70 days [40].

Several epidemics in Iraq in the last 15 years were traceable to the contamination of grains with methylmercury fungicides. A number of nursing infants ingested enough methylmercury in milk to achieve blood levels above the toxic limit [1].

Pesticides   Organic pesticides are concentrated in body fat; milk production, with its export of large quantities of lipid, is a very efficient way for the female to rid her body of these poisons. The nursing human infant thus becomes the highest animal in the "food chain." Dichlorodiphenyltrichloroethane (DDT) was first identified in breast milk in 1951, and milk levels have been slowly falling since its use was restricted in North America in the early 1970s. Current levels of DDT in human milk vary geographically and are related to agricultural use of the compound [41–43]. In Canada in 1979, average milk DDT was 44 n/g of human milk [44]. A 5-kg infant ingesting 1 kg of breast milk each day would thus take in about 0.009 mg/kg of body weight per day. The FAO-World Health Organization recommendations for maximum allowable intake by an adult is about 0.005 mg/kg of body weight per day. Nonetheless, there are no known harmful effects to the infant from the ingestion of human milk contaminated to this degree.

Many other pesticides have been found in human milk and reflect the current commercial use in the region or country. Dieldrin, for instance, which was banned in the United States after 1974, is decreasing in concentration in breast milk [44].

Industrial Byproducts   The extremely toxic dioxin (2,3,7,8-tetrachlorodibenzo-P-dioxin TCDD) caused environmental contamination in Seveso, Italy, in 1976. Children who were directly exposed developed chloracne; further effects remain to be determined. This toxin has been found in human milk.

There has been great public interest in the polychlorinated biphenyls (PCBs). This class of compounds has had 50 years of industrial usage, primarily in the manufacture of electrical apparatus (transformers, capacitors), although such usage seems to be declining. Due to contamination of rivers and lakes by industrial effluent, PCBs are widely distributed in freshwater fish and those animals who eat them. Like organic pesticides, PCBs remain in body fat; stores are excreted with the fat of breast milk. An epidemic of poisoning by PCBs (Yusho disease) occurred in 1968 in Japan, when a commercial rice oil product was inadvertently contaminated with PCBs. Fetuses exposed in utero suffered growth retardation both antenatally and postnatally. Several infants whose only exposure was via human milk developed weakness and apathy [45,46]. It is of great concern that milk levels of PCBs in North America appear to be increasing; in Canada in 1979, the average PCB level in human milk was 12 ng/g [44], whereas women who are exposed occupationally to PCBs or who consume game fish from contaminated waters may have much higher levels in milk.

The polybrominated biphenyls (PBBs) were brought to attention by an incident in Michigan in 1973 and 1974, in which several hundred pounds of PBBs, normally used as fire retardants in the plastics industry, accidently contamined cattle feed; widespread intoxication of farm animals resulted. PBBs have the usual propensity to lodge in fat tissue and to persist in the body. To date, no ill effects have been noted in infants exposed to PBBs through their mother's milk. In Michigan, breast milk PBB surveillance has provided an accurate picture of the contamination of the general population [47]. This method of epidemiologic analysis for fat-soluble poisons has much to recommend it, since the collection of milk samples is far easier than the collection of adipose tissue specimens. Breast milk PBB levels in the contaminated areas of Michigan averaged 0.07 parts per million.

An interesting case reported in 1977 concerned a nursing infant who developed obstructive jaundice; the illness was attributed to the presence of tetrachloroethylene in breast milk. The child's mother had been repeatedly exposed to this common solvent while visiting her husband in a dry-cleaning plant [48].

The contamination of human breast milk in North America by chlorinated hydrocarbon insecticides and industrial pollutants has been extensively reviewed recently [49]. It has become increasingly clear that human breast milk is a significant source of exposure to these contaminants and that the human infant may imbibe amounts greater than the levels allowed by the Food and Drug Administration. The acute and long-term effects of such exposure are matters of concern and require evaluation.

Conclusion

Like the helpless fetus in utero, the nursing infant is exposed to nearly everything entering the body of its mother. The dangers, especially over the long term, are quite unclear. Environmental pollutants are almost impossible to avoid, and elimination of recreational compounds involves changing lifestyles. Drug administration is the easiest to control, yet often a difficult choice must be made between maternal therapy and potential infant harm. The following are some simple guides to be observed. 1) A lactating woman should not receive a drug that one would be reluctant to give directly to her infant at that particular postnatal or gestational age. 2) Drug secretion into milk is so variable that one should not attempts to treat an infant by administering the drug to the lactating mother. 3) Milk that is donated to milk banks must be free from contamination. 4) When maternal drug administration is necessary, one may attempt to minimize the dosage to the infant by withholding nursing at the time of maximum secretion of the drug into milk. 5) Signs and symptoms in a nursing child should be correlated with drug ingestion by the mother. In investigation, it is perhaps most useful to measure levels of the drug and its metabolites in the infant's body fluids. rather than at isolated times in maternal blood or milk.

With the advent of sensitive and precise technology for drug and chemical assays and with the increased understanding of pharmacologic and pharmacokinetic principles, systematic studies on drug breast milk transfer and quantitative measurements of infants' drug intake via this route are now highly feasible to provide meaningful applicable data on this important area of pediatric pharmacology and nutrition.

References

1. Giacoia, G.P., Catz, C.S. Drugs and pollutants in breast milk. *Clin. Perinatol.* 6:181, 1979.
2. Lawrence, R.A. *Breast Feeding: A Guide for the Medical Profession.* St. Louis: C.V. Mosby 1980.
3. Anderson, P.O. Drugs and breast feeding. *Semin. Perinatol.* 3:271, 1979.
4. Levin, R.H., and Pagliaro, L.A. Drugs excreted in breast milk. In Pagliaro, L.A., Levin, R.H. (eds.), *Problems in Pediatric Drug Therapy.* Hamilton, Ill.: Drug Intelligence Publications, 1979, p. 51.
5. Update. Drugs in breast milk. *Med. Lett. Drugs Ther.* 21:21, 1979.
6. deSwiet, M., Lewis, P.J. Excretion of anticoagulants in human milk. *N. Engl. J. Med.* 297:1471, 1977.
7. Orme, M.L., Lewis, P.J., et al. May mothers given warfarin breast-feed their infants? *Br. Med. J.* 1:1564, 1977.
8. Erickson, S.H., Oppenheim, G.L. Aspirin in breast milk. *J. Fam. Pract.* 8:189, 1979.
9. Eeg-Olofsson, O., Malmros, I., et al. Convulsions in a breast-fed infant after maternal indomethacin. *Lancet* 2:215, 1978.
10. Anath, J. Side effects in the neonates from phychotropic agents excreted through breast feeding. *Am. J. Psychiatry* 135:801, 1978.
11. Chan, V., Tse T.F., et al. Transfer of digoxin across the placenta and into breast milk. *Br. J. Obstet. Gynaecol.* 85:605, 1978.
12. Levy, M. Granit, L., et al. Excretion of drugs in human milk. *N. Engl. J.Med.* 297:789, 1977.
13. Loughnan, P.M. Digoxin excretion in human breast milk. *J. Pediatr.* 92:6:1019, 1978.
14. Finley, J.P., Waxman, M.B. et al. Digoxin excretion in human milk. *J. Pediatr.* 94:339, 1979.
15. Karum, A. Spironolactone: disposition, metabolism, pharmacodynamics and bioavailability. *Drug Metab. Rev.* 8:151, 1978.
16. Phelps, D.L., Karim, A. Spironolactone: relationship between concentrations of dethioacetylated metabolite in human serum and milk. *J. Pharm. Sci.* 66:1203, 1977.
17. Mulley, B.A., Parr, G.D., et al. Placental transfer of chlorthalidone and its elimination in maternal milk. *Eur. J. Clin. Pharmacol.* 13:129, 1978.

18. Hill, L.M., Malkasian, G.D. The use of quinidine sulfate throughout pregnancy. *Obstet. Gynecol.* 54:366, 1979.
19. Mandelli, M., Tognoni, G., et al. Clinical pharmacokinetics of diazepam. *Clin. Pharmacokin.* 3:72, 1978.
20. Wiles, D.H., Orr, M.W., et al. Chlorpromazine levels in plasma and milk of nursing mothers. *Br. J. Clin. Pharmacol.* 5:272, 1978.
21. Sovner, R., Orsulak, P.J. Excretion of imipramine and desipramine in human breast milk. *Am. J. Psychiatry* 136:451, 1979.
22. Erickson, S.H., Smith, G.H., et al. Tricyclics and breast feeding. *Am. J. Psychiatry* 136:1483, 1979.
23. Gelenberg, A.J. Amoxapine, a new antidepressant, appears in human milk. *J. Nerv. Ment. Dis.* 167:635, 1979.
24. Kaneko, S., Sato, T., et al. The levels of anticonvulsants in breast milk. *Br. J. Clin. Pharmacol.* 7:624, 1979.
25. Koup, J.R., Rose, J.Q., et al. Ethosuximide pharmacokinetics in a pregnant patient and her newborn. Epilepsia 19:535, 1978.
26. Niebyl, J.R., Blake, D.A., et al. Carbamazepine levels in pregnancy and lactation. *Obstet. Gynecol.* 53:139, 1979.
27. Phynnonen, S., Kanto, J., et al. Carbamazepine: placental transport, tissue concentrations in fetus and newborn and level in milk. *Acta Pharmacol. Toxicol.* 41:244, 1977.
28. Dickinson, R.G., Harland, R.C., et al. Transmission of valproic acid (Depakene) across the placenta:half-life of the drug in mother and baby. *J. Pediatr.* 94:832, 1979.
29. Nilsson, S., Nygren, K., et al. d-Norgestrel concentrations in maternal plasma, milk and child plasma during administration of oral contraceptives to nursing women. *Am. J. Obstet. Gynecol.* 129:178, 1977.
30. Nilsson, S., Nygren, K., et al. Transfer of estradiol to human milk. *Am. J. Obstet. Gynecol.* 132:653, 1978.
31. Dickey, R.P. Drugs affecting lactation. *Semin. Perinatol.* 3:279, 1979.
32. Karpow, S., Gotz, V., et al. Climetidine. *J. Am. Med. Assoc.* 239:402, 1978.
33. Somogyi, A., Gugler, R. Cimetidine excretion into breast milk. *Br. J. Clin. Pharmacol.* 7:627, 1979.
34. Resman, B.H., Blumenthal, H.P., et al. Breast milk distribution of theobromine from chocolate. *J. Pediatr.* 91:477, 1977.
35. Erkkola, R., Kanto, J., et al. Excretion of methylergometrine (methylergonovine) into the human breast milk. *Int. J. Clin. Pharmacol.* 16:579, 1978.
36. Tyrala, E.E., Dodson, W.E. Caffeine secretion into breast milk. *Arch. Dis. Child.* 54:787, 1979.
37. Meberg, A., Sande, H., et al. Smoking during pregnancy: effects on the fetus and on thiocyanate levels in mother and baby. *Acta. Paediatr. Scand.* 68:547, 1979.
38. Binkiewicz, A., Robinson, M.J., et al. Pseudo-Cushing syndrome caused by alcohol in breast milk. *J. Pediatr.* 93:965, 1978.
39. Ghodse, A.H., Reed, J.L., et al. The effect of maternal narcotic addiction on the newborn infant. *Psychol. Med.* 7:667, 1977.
40. Fujita, M., Takabatake, E. Mercury levels in human maternal and neonatal blood, hair and milk. *Bull. Environ. Contam. Toxicol.* 18:205, 1977.

41. Jonsson, V., Liu, G.J.K., et al. Chlorohydrocarbon pesticide residues in human milk in greater St. Louis, Missouri. *Am. J. Clin. Nutr.* 20:1106, 1977.
42. Olszyna-Marzys, A.E. Contaminants in human milk. *Acta. Paediatr. Scand.* 67:571, 1978.
43. Vuori, E., Tyllinen, H., et al. The occurrence and origin of DDT in human milk. *Acta. Paediatr. Scand.* 66:761, 1979.
44. Nes, J., Davies, D.J. Presence of polychlorinated biphenyl and organochlorine pesticide residues and the absence of polychlorinated terphenyls in Canadian human milk samples. *Bull. Environ. Contam. Toxicol.* 21:381, 1979.
45. Kuwabara, K., Yukushiji, et al. Levels of polychlorinated biphenyls in blood of breast-fed children whose mothers are non-occupationally exposed to PCB's *Bull. Environ. Contam. Toxicol.* 21:458, 1979.
46. Yoshida, S., Nakamura, A. Residual status after parturition of methylsulfone metabolites of polychlorinated biphenyls in the breast milk of a former employee in a capacitor factory. *Bull. Environ. Contam. Toxicol.* 21:111, 1979.
47. Billiant, L.B., Wilcox, K., et al. Breast-milk monitoring to measure Michigan's contamination with polybrominated biphenyls. *Lancet* 2:643, 1978.
48. Bagnell, P.C., Ellenberger, H.A. Obstructive jaundice due to a chlorinated hydrocarbon in breast milk. *Can. Med. Assoc. J.* 117:1047, 1977.
49. Calabrese, E.J. Human breast milk contamination in the United States and Canada by chlorinated hydrocarbon insecticides and industrial pollutants: current status. *J. Am. Coll. Toxicol.* 1:91, 1982.
50. Patrick, M.J., Tilston, W.J., Reavey, P. Diazepam and breast feeding. *Lancet* I:542, 1972.
51. Schou, M., Amdisen, A. Lithium and pregnancy. III. Lithium ingestion by children breastfed by women on lithium treatment. *Br. Med. J.* II:138, 1973.
52. Sykes, P.A., Quarrie, J. and Alexander, F.W. Lithium carbonate and breast feeding. *Br. Med. J.* II:1299, 1976.
53. Williams, R.H., Kay, G.A., Jandorf, B.J. Thiouracil: Its absorption, distribution and excretion. *J. Clin. Invest.* 23:613, 1944.
54. Low, L.C.K., Lang, J., Alexander, W.D. Excretion of carbimazole and propylthiouracil in breast milk. *Lancet* II:1011, 1979.
55. Kampmann, J.P., Johansen, K., Hansen, J.M., Helweg, J. Propylthiouracil in human milk. *Lancet* I:736, 1980.

Index

A

Abdominal wall defects, congenital, 269–280
  defined, 269–270
  embryology, 272–278
  evaluation and treatment of infants with, 278–280
  historical perspective, 272
  incidence, 270, 272
Abdominal wall folding, 273
Abdominal wall muscular deficiency syndrome, congenital, 270
Abortion, therapeutic, 114
Abruptio placentae, mild, 6
Abuse Prevention and Treatment Act, Federal Child, 175, 177
Acacia, intravenous, 97
Accomplishment as coping mechanism, 159–160
Acetaldehyde, 362
Acetaminophen, 357
Acetylsalicylic acid, 357
Actin-myosin interaction, 3–4
Adenine arabinoside, 329
Adenosine monophosphate, cyclic, 39
Adenyl cyclase, 39
Administrative education, 183
Age, gestational, 36
Air leaks, pulmonary, 227–228
Airway trauma, direct, 265
Alcohol, ethyl, 9–10, 362
Aldosterone, 40
Alpha-fetoprotein, 277–278
Alpha-tocopherol, see Vitamin E
Alveolar pressure, 229
Ambulation versus recumbency in labor, 53
Aminophylline, 85
Amitriptyline, 358
Amniocentesis, premature uterine activity and, 5–6
Amniotic fluid, 257
  meconium-stained, 252
Amniotic fluid aspiration, 254–258
Amoxapine, 358
Amphetamines, 358
Ampicillin, 113, 116

Analgesic drugs, 357–358
Anemia, 113
Anesthesia
  conduction, 88
  epidural, see Epidural anesthesia
  general, 112
Angiography, 84
Anophthalmia, 325
Antecubital hematocrit, 295–296
Antepartal hospitalization, see Psychosocial effects of long-term antepartal hospitalization
Anterior uveitis, 319
  intense, 327
Antiarrhythmic drugs, 124–125
Antibiotic therapy, prophylactic, 113
Anticoagulant drugs, 124, 357
Anticoagulation, 85–86
  indications for, 86
  oral, 117–118, 124
Anticonvulsant drugs, 359
Antidepressants, tricyclic, 358
Antidiuretic hormone, 40
Antiinflammatory drugs, 357–358
Antiplatelet antibody, 75
Antithrombin III, 87
Aorta, coarctation of, 119–120
Aortic rupture, 119
Aortic valve, bicuspid, 119
Aortic valve prostheses, 118
Apgar scores, 77
Arabinofuranosyladenosine (Ara-A) or arabinofuranosylcytosine (Ara-C), 139
Arrhythmias, cardiac, 116
Arterial blood pressure, 92–93
  mean, see Mean arterial blood pressure
Arterial oxygen monitoring, 193–207
Arterial oxygen tension, 193
Asphyxia, 249–250, 258
Aspiration
  amniotic fluid, 254–258
  meconium, see Meconium aspiration
  neonatal, of first feeding, 258–261
Aspiration syndromes, perinatal, 249–261

Atelectasis, 225
ATP, *see* Autoimmune thrombocytopenia
Atrial fibrillation, 116
Attachment process, parent-infant, 336
Auditory stimulation, 338–339, 343–344
Autoimmune thrombocytopenia (ATP), 74–80
  cesarean section and, 79
  clinical course of, 75
  management for, 80
  vaginal delivery and, 78
Autopsy of newborns, 169

B

Bacterial endocarditis, 110–111, 116
Baptism, 167
Barbiturates, 358, 359
Barotrauma, 210, 235
Bed rest, 7
Beds, stimulation in, 347–348
Benzathine penicillin, 116
Beta-adrenergic agonists, 39–42
Beta-methasone, 80
Beta-receptors, 12, 39
Beta-sympathomimetics, 1–2
  administration of, 19
  clinical use of, 17–19
  tocolysis with, 12–19
Bicuspid aortic valve, 119
Biphenyls
  polybrominated (PBBs), 363–364
  polychlorinated (PCBs), 363
Birth, premature, *see* Prematurity
Birth weight, 36
Bishop score, 29–30
Bleeding, *see* Hemorrhage/bleeding
Blood
  maternal, passage to milk from, 355–356
  whole, 291
Blood flow
  mammary gland, 356–357
  uteroplacental, 102–103

Blood gas analyzer, 199–200
Blood pressure, 111
  arterial, *see* Arterial blood pressure
  clinical measurement of, 92–94
  diastolic, 93
  placental perfusion and, 101–104
Blood viscosity, *see* Viscosity, blood
Blood volume
  increment in, during gestation, 111
  pulmonary, 116
Body organs, transplantation of dead infant's, 179–180
BPD, *see* Bronchopulmonary dysplasia
Bradycardia, 112
Bradyzoites, 132
Brain growth, 335
Breast-feeding, drugs and, 355–365
Breast milk, *see* Milk
Breathing, fetal, 258
Breech presentation
  cesarean section and, 70–71
  preterm, 44
Bronchopleural fistulas, 227–228
Bronchopulmonary dysplasia (BPD), 211, 233, 264–267
Burial, neonates and, 169–170

C

C_3, platelet-associated, 74–75
Caffeine, 361–362
Calcium channel blockers, 20
Carbamazepine, 359
Carbimazole, 359, 361
Carbogen, 239
Cardiac arrhythmias, 116
Cardiac glycosides, 125–126
Cardiac hypertrophy, 215
Cardiac output, 111
Cardiac patient, pregnant, 112–113
Cardiomyopathy, peripartum, 111, 122
Cardiopulmonary resuscitation, 178
Cardiovascular disease, congenital, 118–122
Cardiovascular drugs and fetus, 124–126

Cardiovascular lesions during
    pregnancy, 110–127
  most common dangerous, 115–122
  recommendations regarding
    pregnancy, 127
Cardiovascular physiology
  hypertension and, 94–99
  in pregnancy, 111–112
Cardiovascular surgery during
    pregnancy, 114–115
Cardiovascular system, drugs
    affecting, 358
Carotid artery ligation, 241
Cataract removal, 322–323
Cataracts
  morgagnian, 320
  rubella, 320–321
Catheter-tip electrodes, 194
  Searle, see Searle umbilical artery
    catheter-tip electrode
Caudal fold defect, omphalocele, 274
Centipoise (unit), 290
Central nervous system, drugs
    affecting, 358–359
Cephalic fold defect, omphalocele,
    275
Cephalic version, external, 70–71
Cervical dilatation, 55–56
  early, 4
Cervical priming with prostaglandins,
    33
Cervix, unfavorable or unripe, 29
Cesarean section, 67–72
  ATP cases and, 79
  breech presentation and, 70–71
  fetal distress and, 71–72
  prostaglandin and, 33
  repeated, 70
  rising rate of, 67
  safety of, 68
Chemicals, recreational, in human
    milk, 361–362
Child Abuse Prevention and
    Treatment Act, Federal, 175, 177
Chloramphenicol, 360
Chlordiazepoxide, 358
Chlorinated hydrocarbon insecticides,
    364

Chlorpromazine, 358
Chlorthalidone, 358
Chorioretinal lesions, 329
Chorioretinal scar, 325
Chorioretinitis, 133, 134, 325
  in herpes simplex virus infections,
    328
Cicatricial ROP, 303, 307
Cigarettes, 362
Cimetidine, 359
Circulation
  extracorporeal (ECC), 232
  persistent fetal (PFC), 210
Civil liability, 177
Clark cell, 193
Clindamycin, 319
Clouding, corneal, 322
CMV, see Cytomegalovirus infections
Coarctation of aorta, 119–120
Coffee, 361–362
Comfort, maternal, position in labor
    and, 59, 61–62
Compromise, fetal, hypertension and,
    99–100
Conduction anesthesia, 88
Conjunctivitis, 327
Contraceptives, oral, 359
Contractions, see Uterine
    contractions
Control as coping mechanism, 159
Coping mechanisms in long-term
    hospitalization, 158–162
Cord, see also Umbilical entries
  nuchal, 61
Cord blood hemoglobin concentration,
    283–284
Cornea, "salmon-patch" appearance,
    330
Corneal clouding, 322
Corticosteroids, 76
  systemic, 317, 319
Cortisol, 9, 216
Coumarin agents, 86–87
CPAP, 253
Cyclic adenosine monophosphate,
    39
Cytomegalic inclusion disease, 323–
    326

Cytomegalovirus infections, 137–139
  diagnosis, 139
  fetal, 137–138
  management, 139
  maternal, 137
  neonatal, 137–138
Cytosine arabinoside, 329

D

D⁵W administration, 12
D⁵W aspiration, 260
Dane particle, 140
Dating information, pregnancy, 43
DDT
  (dichlorodiphenyltrichloroethane),
  363
Death of newborn, 167–170
Decision to resuscitate or not
  resuscitate, 178–179
Deep vein thrombosis (DVT), 83–88
Defective newborns, 172–178
Delalutin (17-hydroxyprogesterone
  caproate), 9
Denial as coping mechanism, 158
Deprivation, sleep, 154
Desmethyldiazepam, 358
Desoxycorticosterone, 96
Dexamethasone, 80, 277
Dextran, 97
Diabetic mother, infant of, see Infant
  of diabetic mother
Diaphragmatic hernia, 210, 234–235
Diastolic blood pressure, 93
Diazepam, 358, 361
Diazoxide, 104
Dichlorodiphenyltrichloroethane
  (DDT), 363
Dieldrin, 363
Diffuse lung disease, HFV in, 225–227
Digitalis, 116, 125–126
Digoxin, 358
Dilatation, cervical, see Cervical
  dilatation
Dioxin (TCDD), 363
Disciform keratitis, 328
Disopyramide, 125

Distress, fetal, cesarean section and,
  71–72
Diuretics, 358
  thiazide, 126
DNR (decision not to resuscitate),
  178–179
Dopamine, 85
Down's syndrome, 176
Drugs
  affecting cardiovascular system, 358
  affecting central nervous system,
    358–359
  affecting endocrine system, 359
  antiarrhythmic, 124–125
  anticoagulant, 124, 357
  anticonvulsant, 359
  antiinflammatory and analgesic,
    357–358
  breast-feeding and, 355–365
  cardiovascular, fetus and, 124–126
  contraindicated during lactation,
    356, 360–361
  initiation of parturition with, 28–34
  in milk, 357–359
DVT (deep vein thrombosis), 83–88
Dystocia, 69–70
  oxytocin and, 69–70

E

ECC (extracorporeal circulation), 232
ECMO, see Extracorporeal membrane
  oxygenation
Edema, pulmonary, see Pulmonary
  edema
Education
  administrative, 183
  medical staff, 184
  nursing, 183–184
  paramedical staff, 183–184
  of parents, 184–185
Eisenmenger's syndrome, 121–122
Electroshock therapy, 125
Embolus, pulmonary (PE), 83–88
Emotional issues in failed pregnancy,
  164–170

Emphysema, pulmonary interstitial, 227–228
Endocarditis, bacterial, 110–111, 116
Endocrine system, drugs affecting, 359
Endotheliosis, glomerular, 91–92
Environment, intrauterine, 334–335
Environmental pollutants in human milk, 362–364
Epidural anesthesia, 45–46, 112
  segmental, 116–117
Epinephrine, 13
Equal protection principle, 176–177
Ergot, 359, 360
Ergotism, 360
Erythrocyte, *see also* Red cell *entries*
Erythrocyte aggregation, 291
Erythrocyte deformability, 291
Erythropoiesis, fetal, 286
Erythropoietin, 287–288
Estrogen, 125–126, 359
Estrogen surge, 28
Ethanol, 9–10, 362
Ethics committee, 177
Ethiosurimide, 359
Exaggerated lithotomy position in labor, 49
Exchange transfusion, partial, 296–299
External cephalic version, 70–71
Extracorporeal circulation (ECC), 232
Extracorporeal membrane oxygenation (ECMO), 209–211
  circuit diagram for venoarterial, 236
  coagulation problems with, 239–241
  complications, 244–245
  development of, 233–234
  diagnoses in patients treated with, 244
  indications for, 234–236
  management of patient on, 236–242
  for newborn respiratory failure, 232–246
  results of, 243–245
  venoarterial (VA), 243–245
    circuit diagram for, 236
  venovenous (VV), 241–245
Eye infections, congenital, 314–331

F

Factor X, activated, 87
Family law priniciples, 172–175
Family relationships, stressors related to, 155–156
Federal Child Abuse Prevention and Treatment Act, 175, 177
Feeding, neonatal aspiration of first, 258–261
Fetal breathing, 258
Fetal circulation, persistent (PFC), 210
Fetal compromise, hypertension and, 99–100
Fetal cytomegalovirus, 137–138
Fetal distress, cesarean section and, 71–72
Fetal erythropoiesis, 286
Fetal hypoxemia, 287
Fetal monitoring in preterm labor, 45
Fetal scalp pH evaluation, 71
Fetal toxoplasmosis, 133
Fetus
  cardiovascular drugs and, 124–126
  heart disease and, 123–124
Fibrillation, atrial, 116
Fibroplasia, retrolental, *see* Retinopathy of prematurity
Finger sucking, 338
Fistulas, bronchopleural, 227–228
Folinic acid, 317
Furosemide, 15

G

Gap junctions between myometrial cells, 2–3
Gastroschisis, 269–270, 271, 272
  embryogenesis, 276–277
  management, 280
General anesthesia, 112
Gentamicin, 113, 116
Gestation, preterm, *see* Preterm labor
Gestational age, 36
Gestational hypertension, *see* Hypertension, pregnancy-induced
Glaucoma, 322–323

Glomerular endotheliosis, 91–92
Glucocorticoids, 359
Glucose, 215
Glucose solutions, 259–260
Glutamic-pyruvic transaminase, 141
Glycosides, cardiac, 125–126
Guardians for defective infants, 173–174

H

Halothane, 196
Hartmann's solution, 12
HBIg (hepatitis B immune globulin), 143
HBV (hepatitis B virus), 139–142
Health care professionals, relationships with, 156–158
Heart disease
  congenital, 110
  fetus and, 123–124
  during pregnancy, 110–111
  rheumatic, 110, 115
Heart rate, 111
Heartbeat sounds, maternal, 344
Heel stick hematocrit, 295
Hematocrit, 283–285
  antecubital, 295–296
  heel stick, 295
  maternal, 123–124
  viscosity and, 291
Hemodilution, isovolemic, 296–297
Hemodynamics, maternal, see
  Maternal hemodynamics
Hemoglobin, 112, 113
  cord blood concentration, 283–284
Hemorrhage/bleeding
  intracranial, 210–211
  postpartum, 76
  vaginal, 6–7
  vitreous, 305
Heparin, 85–88, 124, 210, 233
  complications of, 86
  low-dose, 87
  not entering breast milk, 356, 357
  in sampling fluid infusion, 203

Hepatitis B immune globulin (HBIg), 143
Hepatitis B infections, 139–143
  epidemiology, 140–141
  maternal, 141–143
  neonatal, 143
Hepatitis B vaccine, 143
Hepatitis B virus (HBV), 139–142
Hepatosplenomegaly, 138
Hernia
  diaphragmatic, 210, 234–235
  ruptured cord, see Gastroschisis
  umbilical cord, 269, 270, 271, 275–276
Heroin, 362
Herpes simplex virus, 326–329
Herpes simplex virus (HSV)
  infections, 143–146
  diagnosis, 145–146
  epidemiology, 144–145
Hexoprenaline, 8, 16, 40
HFJV (high-frequency jet ventilation), 222–224
HFOV (high-frequency oscillatory ventilation), 224–229
HFPPV (high-frequency positive-pressure ventilation), 222
HFV, see High-frequency ventilation
High-frequency jet ventilation (HFJV), 222–224
High-frequency oscillatory ventilation (HFOV), 224–229
High-frequency positive-pressure ventilation (HFPPV), 222
High-frequency ventilation (HFV)
  complications, 228–229
  delivery methods, 222–224
  neonatal, 221–230
  uses in pathologic conditions, 224–228
High-risk pregnancy, 149–150
Homan's sign, 83–84
Hospitalization
  antepartal, see Psychosocial effects of long-term antepartal hospitalization
  perinatal, stressors related to, 154

HSV, *see* Herpes simplex virus infections
Human milk, *see* Milk
Humidification, HFV, 229
Hyaline membrane disease, 215, 264–267
HFV in, 224–225
Hydralazine, 104
parenteral, 105
Hydrocarbon insecticides, chlorinated, 364
Hydrocortisone, 218, 254
17-Hydroxyprogesterone caproate (Delalutin), 9
Hyperbilirubinemia, 138
Hyperglycemia, 12, 15, 216
Hyperoxia, 304
Hyperoxygenation, 206
Hyperproteinemic states, 292
Hypertension
pregnancy-induced (PIH), 90–105
blood pressure measurement and, 92–94
cardiovascular physiology and, 94–99
clinical management of, 99–101
defined, 91
diagnosis, 91
renal pathology in, 91
therapeutic agents for, 104–105
pulmonary, 121–122, 234, 254
Hypertonus, uterine, 30–31
Hyperviscosity, 283
incidence, 286
neonatal polycythemia/*see* Polycythemia/hyperviscosity, neonatal
Hypervolemia, 95
Hypoglycemia, transient, of newborn, 261
Hypokalemia, 12
Hypovolemia, 95
Hypoxemia
fetal, 287
neonatal, 206
Hysterosalpingogram, 4

I

^{125}I scanning, 84
IDM, *see* Infant of diabetic mother
Idoxuridin, 329
IFA (indirect fluorescent antibody assay), 135
IgG antibodies, 74, 134, 136
platelet-associated, 74–75
IgM, 134–135
Imipramine, 358
Immunoglobular (IgG) antibody, *see* IgG antibodies
Immunoglobulin M (IgM), 134–135
IMV (intermittent mandatory ventilation), 266
Indirect fluorescent antibody assay (IFA), 135
Indomethacin, 19, 357
Industrial byproducts, 363
Infant of diabetic mother (IDM)
experimental studies of, 216
polycythemia and, 287
respiratory distress in, 215–218
Infants, *see* Neonates
Infections
cytomegalovirus, 137–139
eye, congenital, 314–331
hepatitis B, 139–143
herpes simplex virus, 143–146
perinatal, 131–146
toxoplasmosis, 131–136
Infraumbilical omphalocele, 274
Insecticides, chlorinated hydrocarbon, 364
Insulin, 215, 356
effects of, 216–217
Insurance coverage, 191
Intensive care nursery, stimulation programs in, *see* Stimulation programs in neonatal intensive care nursery
Intermittent mandatory ventilation (IMV), 266
Interstitial emphysema, pulmonary, 227–228
Interstitial keratitis, 330–331

Intracranial hemorrhage, 210–211
Intrauterine environment, 334–335
Intrauterine pressure, 55
Iodides, 359
IQs, 342
Iridectomy, 321, 322
Iron, 112
  supplemental, 113
Isolettes, 335
  stimulation in, 347
Isoproterenol, 85
Isotopes, radioactive, 359, 360
Isovolemia, 95
Isovolemic hemodilution, 296–297
Isoxsuprine, 16

J

Jet ventilation, high-frequency
  (HFJV), 222–224

K

Keratitis, 327–328
  disciform, 328
  interstitial, 330–331
Ketoacidosis, 12
Kinase, MLC, 3–4
Kinesthetic needs, 335
Korotkoff phases, 93

L

Labor, 4–5
  induction of
    with oxytocin, 29–31
    with prostaglandins, 31–34
  onset of, 2–4
  position in, see Position in labor
  premature, see Prematurity
  preterm, see Preterm labor
  spontaneous, 28–29
Labor patterns in preterm gestation,
  43–44

Labor progress and positions, 57, 58
Lactation, 112
  drugs contraindicated during, 356,
    360–361
  drugs during, 355–365
Lateral recumbent position in labor,
  52, 60
Lavage, tracheobronchial, 253
Lead toxicity, 362
Lecithin, 217
Lecithin/sphingomyelin ratio, 43
Legal aspects of perinatal care, 171–
  180
Leukocoria, 316
Leukotrienes, 103
Liability, civil, 177
Lithium, 358, 361
Lithotomy position in labor, 51
Low-birth-weight premature infants,
  334
Lumen, sampling, see Sampling
  lumen entries
Lung deflation curves, 259
Lung diseases
  chronic, 264
  diffuse, HFV in, 225–227
  parenchymal, 235
Lung injuries, oleic acid, 225–226
Lung rest, 211

M

Macular scar, 315
Madrid units, 56
Magnesium sulfate ($MgSO_4$), 42–43
  as antihypertensive, 105
  clinical use of, 18
  dosage, 42–43
  tocolysis with, 10–12
Mammary gland blood flow, 356–357
Mannitol, 97
MAP, see Mean arterial pressure
Marfan's syndrome, 120–121
MAS, see Meconium aspiration
  syndrome
Maternal blood to milk, passage from,
  355–356

Maternal comfort, position in labor and, 59, 61–62
Maternal cytomegalovirus, 137
Maternal heartbeat sounds, 344
Maternal hematocrit, 123–124
Maternal hemodynamics, 50–51
  parturition and, 112
Maternal hepatitis B infections, 141–143
Maternal mortality, 110
Maternal position in labor, *see* Position in labor
Maternal smoking, 286, 362
Maternal toxoplasmosis, 133
Mean arterial pressure (MAP), 94
  reductions in, 102–104
Meconium, prevention of passage of, 250
Meconium aspiration, 249–254
  etiology, 249–250
  management, 253–254
  pathophysiology, 250
  prevention, 251–252
Meconium aspiration syndrome (MAS), 210
  HFV in, 225
Meconium-stained amniotic fluid, 252
Medical staff education, 184
Megakaryocytes, 75
Meprobamate, 358
Mercury poisoning, 362–363
Methadone, 362
Methimazole, 359
Methyldopa, 97–98
  oral, 105
Methylergonovine, 359, 360
Methylmercury, 362–363
Metronidazole, 361
MgSO₄, *see* Magnesium sulfate
Microphthalmia, 316, 321
Milk
  compounds in, 357–364
  drugs in, 357–359
  environmental pollutants in, 362–364
  modifications of passage into, 356–357

passage from maternal blood to, 355–356
  recreational chemicals in, 361–362
Mitral stenosis, 115–117
Mitral valve prosthesis, 117–118
Mitral valvotomy, 117
MLC (myosin light chain), 3–4
MLC kinase, 3–4
MLC phosphatase, 3
Monitoring, fetal, in preterm labor, 45
Montevideo units, 56
Morbidity, ocular, 307–309
Morgagnian cataract, 320–321
Morphine, 362
Morphine sulfate, 7
Mortality, maternal, 110
  perinatal, 1
Mucociliary transport, 229
Mucus, respiratory, 229
Multimodal stimulation, 339–340
Myocarditis
  acute, 245–246
  viral, 111
Myometrial cells, gap junctions between, 2–3
Myosin light chain, *see* MLC *entries*

N

Narcotics, 362
Nasopharyngeal suctioning, 252
Necrotizing tracheitis, 229
Neonatal aspiration of first feeding, 258–261
Neonatal cytomegalovirus, 137–138
Neonatal hepatitis B infections, 143
Neonatal herpes infections, 326–329
Neonatal high-frequency ventilation, 221–230
Neonatal intensive care nursery, stimulation programs in, *see* Stimulation programs in neonatal intensive care nursery
Neonatal polycythemia/hyperviscosity, *see* Polycythemia/hyperviscosity, neonatal

Neonatal pulmonary air leaks, 227–228
Neonatal pulmonary insufficiency index, 235
Neonatal respiratory distress syndrome, 20–21
Neonatal respiratory failure, ECMO for, 232–246
Neonatal stimulation, *see* Stimulation
Neonatal toxoplasmosis, 136
Neonates/infants/newborn
  acute respiratory failure in, 209–213
  autopsy of, 169
  baptism of, 167
  burial of, 169–170
  catheter-tip electrode in, *see* Searle umbilical artery catheter-tip electrode
  death of, 167–170
  defective, 172–178
  terminally ill, 178–179
  transient hypoglycemia of, 261
  transplantation of body organs of dead, 179–180
  transportation of, 204–206
Neonatology practice, 182–192
  education in, 183–185
  organization of, 190–191
  problems in, 191–192
  special care nursery in, 185–189; *see also* Special care nursery
Nephroscoliosis, 92
Nervous system, central, drugs affecting, 358–359
Neural structures, growth of, 335
Newborn, *see* Neonates
Nicardipine, 20
Nicotine, 362
Nifedipine, 20
Nuchal cord, 61
Nursery
  ophthalmologists in, 310–311
  special care, *see* Special care nursery
  stimulation programs in, *see* Stimulation programs in neonatal intensive care nursery

Nurses, 183
Nursing education, 183–184

O

Occlusion, sampling lumen, 202–203
Ocular infections, congenital, 314–331
Ocular morbidity, 307–309
Ocular toxoplasmosis, 314–319
Oleic acid lung injuries, 225–226
Omphalocele, 269–270, 274, 275
  caudal fold defect, 274
  cause of, 272–275
  cephalic fold defect, 275
  infraumbilical, 274
  supraumbilical, 275
  treatment, 278–279
"On the shoulder" position, 345
Oocysts, 132
Ophthalmologists, 310–311
Opiates, 362
Optic atrophy, 325
Optic nerve abnormalities, 325
Optic papillitis, 317, 319
Oral contraceptives, 359
Ordinary/extraordinary treatment approach, 175
Organs, transplantation of dead infant's, 179–180
Oropharyngeal suctioning, 252
Oscillatory ventilation, high-frequency (HFOV), 224–229
Oxazepam, 358
Oxygen, arterial, *see* Arterial oxygen *entries*
Oxygen electrodes, transcutaneous, 206–207
Oxygen therapy, 85
Oxygen treatment and ROP, 302–303
Oxygenators, 232, 233
Oxygenation, extracorporeal membrane, *see* Extracorporeal membrane oxygenation
Oxyprenolol, 97
Oxytocin
  contraindications to, 30–31

dystocia and, 69–70
induction of labor with, 29–31
Oxytocin theory, 28

P

PA-IgG (platelet-associated IgG), 74–75
Packed red cell volume, 284–285
Papillitis, optic, 317, 319
Paramedical staff, 183
Paramedical staff education, 183–184
Parenchymal lung diseases, 235
Parens patriae doctrine, 172
Parent-infant attachment process, 336
Parents, education of, 184–185
Partial exchange transfusion, 296–299
Parturition
    initiation of, with drugs, 28–34
    maternal hemodynamics and, 112
    onset of, 2–4
PBBs (polybrominated biphenyls), 363–364
PCBs (polychlorinated biphenyls), 363
PE (pulmonary embolus), 83–88
Penicillin
    benzathine, 116
    systemic, 331
Pentazocine, 358
Perfusion, uterine, *see* Uterine perfusion
Perinatal aspiration syndromes, 249–261
Perinatal care, 182
    legal aspects of, 171–180
Perinatal infections, 131–146
Perinatal mortality, 1
Peripartum cardiomyopathy, 111, 122
Persistent fetal circulation (PFC), 210
Pesticides, 363
Peter's anomaly, 326
PFC (persistent fetal circulation), 210
PGE and PGF, *see* Prostaglandins
pH evaluation, fetal scalp, 71
Phenothiazines, 358
Phenytoin, 359

Phosphatase, MLC, 3
Photocoagulation, xenon-arc, 310
Physical stimulation, 335
PIH, *see* Hypertension, pregnancy-induced
Pitocin, *see* Oxytocin
Placenta, abruption of, *see* Abruptio placentae
Placental perfusion, blood pressure and, 101–104
Plasma protein substrate, stable (SPPS), 97, 98
Plasma volume, 94–96, 111
Platelet-associated C_3, 74–75
Platelet-associated IgG (PA-IgG), 74–75
Poise (unit), 290
Poiseuille's law, 288
Polarizing voltage, 194–195
Polarogram, 195
Pollutants, environmental, in human milk, 362–364
Polybrominated biphenyls (PBBs), 363–364
Polychlorinated biphenyls (PCBs), 363
Polycythemia, 283
Polycythemia/hyperviscosity, neonatal, 283–299
    blood viscosity and, 288–293
    clinical signs, 294
    diagnosis and treatment, 295–299
    etiology, 286–288
    fetal hypoxemia and, 287
    incidence, 283–286
    infants of diabetic mothers and, 287
    laboratory abnormalities in, 294
    outcome, 298–299
    signs of, 293–294
Position in labor, 48–62
    ambulation versus recumbency, 53
    changing, 49
    clinical phenomena related to, 50
    clinical studies of, 52–54
    comparisons of specific, 54–59
    exaggerated lithotomy, 49
    labor progress and, 57, 58
    lateral recumbent, 52, 60

Position in labor (*continued*)
  lithotomy, 51
  maternal comfort and, 59, 61–62
  recumbent, 49
  rocking, 62
  squatting, 48–49
  standing, 60
  subject as own control of, 54
  Trendelenburg, 51
  upright, 48–50
  uterine contractions and, 52, 56–58
  uterine efficiency and, 58, 59
  Walcher's, 48
Positive-pressure ventilation, high-
  frequency (HFPPV), 222
Postnatal surfactant replacement
  therapy, 211–213
Postpartum hemorrhage, 76
Potassium, 12
Potassium supplementation, 126
Practice, neonatology, *see*
  Neonatology practice
Prednisolone, 77, 359
Prednisone, 76, 77, 359
Preeclampsia, 90
  etioloty of, 91
  proteinuric, 92
  treatment of, 100–101
Pregnancy
  ATP and, 74–80; *see also*
    Autoimmune thrombocytopenia
  cardiovascular lesions during,
    110–127
  cardiovascular physiology and, 111–
    112
  cardiovascular surgery during, 114–
    115
  heart disease during, 110–111
  high-risk, 149–150
  recommendations regarding
    cardiovascular lesions in, 127
  spiritual and emotional issues in
    failure of, 164–170
  toxemia of, *see* Hypertension,
    pregnancy-induced
Pregnancy dating information, 43
Pregnancy-induced hypertension, *see*
  Hypertension, pregnancy-induced

Pregnant cardiac patient, 112–113
Prematurity, 1
  low-birth-weight infants and, 334
  retinopathy of, *see* Retinopathy of
    prematurity
Presentation
  breech, *see* Breech presentation
  vertex, preterm, 44–45
Pressure
  alveolar, 229
  blood, *see* Blood pressure
  intrauterine, 55
Preterm breech presentation, 44
Preterm labor
  conduct of, 45–46
  defined, 36
  fetal monitoring in, 45
  labor patterns in, 43–44
  management of, 36–46
  prenatal assessment for, 36–37
  risk factors for, 37, 38
Preterm vertex presentation, 44–45
Primidone, 359
Privacy, lack of, 154
Professionals, health care,
  relationships with, 156–158
Progesterone, 8–9
Progestin, 359
Prophylactic antibiotic therapy, 113
Propoxyphene, 357–358
Propranolol, 120, 125, 358
Proprioceptive input, 342
Propylthiouracil, 361
Prostacyclin, 103
Prostaglandin inhibitors, 19
Prostaglandin theory, 28
Prostaglandins, 19
  E$_2$
    cervical priming with, 33
    oral, systemic side effects with,
      32
    induction of labor with, 31–34
Prosthesis
  aortic valve, 118
  mitral valve, 117–118
Proteinuric preeclampsia, 92
Prune belly syndrome, 270
Pseudoretinitis pigmentosa, 330

Psychosocial effects of long-term
    antepartal hospitalization, 149–
    162
    conceptual framework of study,
        150–151
    coping mechanisms in, 158–162
    data analysis in, 152
    methodology in, 151–152
    stressors in, 152–158
Pulmonary air leaks, 227–228
Pulmonary blood volume, 116
Pulmonary edema
    beta-mimetics and, 13–15, 40
    HFV in, 225–227
Pulmonary embolus (PE), 83–88
Pulmonary hypertension, 121–122,
    234, 254
Pulmonary insufficiency index,
    neonatal, 235
Pulmonary interstitial emphysema,
    227–228
Pyrimethamine, 135, 317

Q

Quadrant summary score, 307–308
Quality of life approach, 174–175
Quinidine, 124, 358

R

Radioactive isotopes, 359, 360
"Random zero" sphygmomanometer,
    93
Rationalization and coping
    mechanism, 159
RDS (respiratory distress syndrome),
    adult, 210–213
Recreational chemicals in human
    milk, 361–362
Recumbency versus ambulation in
    labor, 53
Recumbent position in labor, 49
Red cell, see also Erythrocyte entries
Red cell volume, packed, 284–285
Referral centers, 191

Relationships
    family, stressors related to, 155–156
    with health care professionals, 156–
        158
Renal pathology in hypertension, 91
Respiratory distress in infant of
    diabetic mother, 215–218
Respiratory distress syndrome (RDS)
    adult, 210–213
    neonatal, 20–21
Respiratory failure
    acute, in neonates, 209–213
    newborn, 232–246
Respiratory mucus production, 229
Rest
    bed, 7
    lung, 211
Resuscitate, decision not to (DNR),
    178–179
Resuscitation, cardiopulmonary, 178
Reticuloendothelial system, 75
Retinal lesions, 316–318
Retinal vascularization, 304
    abnormal, 304–305
Retinitis pigmentosa, primary, 330
Retinopathy, rubella, 323
Retinopathy of prematurity (ROP),
    302–311
    active, 305–307
    cicatricial, 303, 307
    grading of, 306
    historical perspective, 302–304
    quadrant grading of, 307–308
    surgical treatment of, 310
    vitamin E and, 309–310
Retrolental fibroplasia, see
    Retinopathy of prematurity
Rheumatic fever, 111
Rheumatic heart disease, 110, 115
Rheumatic valvular disease, 115
Ritodrine (Yutopar), 8, 13–16, 40
    clinical use of, 18
    dosage, 41
    side effects, 153
RLF, see Retinopathy of prematurity
Rocking, 337
Rocking position in labor, 62
ROP, see Rentinopathy of prematurity

Rubbing, 337
Rubella cataract, 320–321
Rubella retinopathy, 323
Rubella syndrome, congenital, 319–323
Ruptured cord hernia, *see* Gastroschisis

S

Sabin Feldman dye test, 135
"Salmon-patch" cornea appearance, 330
"Salt and pepper" pigmentary retinopathy, 323, 324
Sampling lumen management, 201–203
Sampling lumen occlusion, 202–203
Scalp pH evaluation, fetal, 71
Searle umbilical artery catheter-tip electrode, 193–207
  comparative characteristics of, 206–207
  complications, 204
  construction, 197
  description, 196
  failure rates, 202
  functional lifetime, 203–204
  initial calibration, 198
  insertion, 196–197
  positioning, 200–201
  principles of operation, 194–196
  recalibration, 198–199
  relationship between monitor and blood gas analyzer readings, 199–200
  sampling lumen management, 201–203
  use during transportation of neonates, 204–206
Segmental epidural anesthesia, 116–117
Self, sense of loss of, 153–154
Sensorimotor integration, 342
Sensory input, 335
Sensory stimulation, 343

Shear rate
  defined, 290
  viscosity and, 290
Sleep deprivation, 154
Smoking, maternal, 286, 362
Social support systems as coping mechanism, 161–162
Sodium
  requirements, 113
  restriction, 116
Soothing techniques, 337
Sounds, maternal heartbeat, 344
Special care nursery, 185–189
  incidence of high-risk infants against live births, 186
  mortality rate, 189
  organization of, 185
  results in, 185–189
  statistics on admissions from 1975 through 1981, 188 in 1978, 187
Sphygmomanometer, 93
Spiramycin, 135
Spiritual issues, 164–170
Spiritual needs, 167
Spironolactone, 358
Spleen, 75
Splenectomy, 76
Spontaneous labor, 28–29
SPPS (stable plasma protein substrate), 97, 98
Squatting position in labor, 48–49
Stable plasma protein substrate (SPPS), 97, 98
Standing position in labor, 60
Stenosis, mitral, 115–117
Sterile water, aspiration of, 260
Sterilization, 114
Steroids, 254
Stimulation
  in beds, 347–348
  in isolettes, 347
  lack of, 335
  major types of, 336
  multimodal, 339–340
  in ventilators, 346
Stimulation programs in neonatal intensive care nursery, 334–350
  case study, 348–349

generalized, 345–348
review of literature, 336–341
Stressors, categories of, 152–158
Stroke volume, 111
Stroking, 337–338, 343
Succinylcholine, 42
Sucking, nonnutritive, 338
Suctioning, tracheal, 252
Sulfadiazine, 135, 317
Supraumbilical omphalocele, 275
Surfactant replacement therapy,
    postnatal, 211–213
Swann-Ganz catheter, 238
Syphilis, congenital, 329–331

Tachycardia, relative, 115
Tachypnea, transient, 256
Tactile defensiveness, 343
Tactile stimulation, 335, 337–338, 343
TCDD (dioxin), 363
TED, see Thromboembolic disease
Terbutaline, 8, 16–19, 40
clinical use of, 18
Terminally ill infants, 178–179
Tetrachloroethylene, 364
Tetracycline, 361
Theobromine, 359
Theophylline, 359
Therapeutic abortion, 114
Thiazide diuretics, 126
Thiocyanate, 362
Thiouracil, 361
Thiouracil family of drugs, 359
Thrombocytopenia, autoimmune, see
    Autoimmune thrombocytopenia
Thromboembolic disease (TED), 83–
    88
diagnosis, 83–84
predisposition to, 83
treatment, 85–88
Thrombosis, deep vein (DVT), 83–88
Thyroxin, 359
Tidal volume, 221
Tocolysis, 1–2
beta-sympathomimetic, 12–19

candidates for, 37–39
contraindications to, 6
evaluation of, 20–21
long-term, 17
magnesium sulfate, 10–12
Tocopherol, see Vitamin E
Tolazoline, 234
TORCH syndrome, 314
Toxemia, 91
of pregnancy, see Hypertension,
    pregnancy-induced
Toxoplasma gondii, 131–132, 317
Toxoplasmosis, 131–136
diagnosis, 134–135
fetal, 133
incidence, 131–132
management, 135–136
manifestations, 133–134
maternal, 133
methods of transmission, 132
neonatal, 136
ocular, 314–319
prevention, 136
Tracheal obstructions, 229
Tracheal suctioning, 252
Tracheitis, necrotizing, 229
Tracheobronchial lavage, 253
Trajectory, defined, 150–151
Trajectory definition as coping
    mechanism, 160–161
Transcutaneous oxygen electrodes,
    206–207
Transient hypoglycemia of newborn,
    261
Transient tachypnea, 256
Transplantation of dead infant's body
    organs, 179–180
Transportation of neonates, 204–206
Trendelenburg position in labor, 51
Treponema pallidum, 329
Tricyclic antidepressants, 358
Trophozoites, 132

U

UACs (umbilical artery catheters),
    194

Umbilical, *see also* Cord *entries*

Umbilical artery catheter-tip electrode, *see* Searle umbilical artery catheter-tip electrode

Umbilical artery catheters (UACs), 194

Umbilical cord hernia, 269, 270, 271, 275–276

Unfavorable or unripe cervix, 29

Uniform Anatomical Gift Act, 179–180

Upright position in labor, 48–50

Uterine activity
  control of, 1–21
  premature, 4–5

Uterine contractions
  measurements of, 56
  normal, intensity of, 30
  position in labor and, 52, 56–58

Uterine efficiency, 58, 59

Uterine hypertonus, 30–31

Uterine perfusion, 51

Uterine relaxation, 20

Uteroplacental blood flow, 102–103

Uveitis
  acute, 329
  anterior, 319
  intense anterior, 327

V

VA (venoarterial) ECMO, 243–245
  circuit diagram for, 236

Vaginal bleeding, 6–7

Valproic acid, 359

Valvotomy, mitral, 117

Valvular disease, rheumatic, 115

Vascular volume, 94–97

Vascularization, retinal, *see* Retinal vascularization

Vasoactive amine, 85

Vasospasm, 96

Vein thrombosis, deep (DVT), 83–88

Venoarterial (VA) ECMO, 243–245
  circuit diagram for, 236

Venography, 84

Venous return, 112, 113

Venovenous bypass, 241–243

Venovenous (VV) ECMO, 241–245

Ventilation
  high-frequency, *see* High-frequency ventilation
  high-frequency jet (HFJV), 222–224
  high-frequency oscillatory (HFOV), 224–229
  high-frequency positive-pressure (HFPPV), 222
  intermittent mandatory (IMV), 266

Ventilators, stimulation in, 346

Version, external cephalic, 70–71

Vertex presentation, preterm, 44–45

Vestibular input, 342

Vestibular-kinesthetic stimulation, 337

Viral myocarditis, 111

Viscometer, Wells-Brookfield, 289

Viscosity, blood, 288–293
  apparent, tube diameter and, 292
  defined, 290
  hematocrit and, 291
  shear rate and, 290

Visual stimulation, 339, 344

Vitamin E, retinopathy of prematurity and, 303, 309–310

Vitrectomy, 310

Vitreous hemorrhage, 305

Voltage, polarizing, 194–195

Volume
  blood, *see* Blood volume
  packed red cell, 284–285
  plasma, 94–96, 111
  stroke, 111
  tidal, 221
  vascular, 94–97

VV (venovenous) ECMO, 241–245

W

Walcher's position in labor, 48

Warfarin, 87, 357

Water, sterile, aspiration of, 60

Weight, birth, 36

Wells-Brookfield viscometer, 289

Whole blood, 291

X

Xenon-arc photocoagulation, 310

Y

Yusho disease, 363
Yutopar, *see* Ritodrine